ENERGY INTAKE AND ACTIVITY

CURRENT TOPICS IN NUTRITION AND DISEASE

Series Editors

Anthony A. Albanese
The Burke Rehabilitation Center
White Plains, New York

David Kritchevsky
The Wistar Institute
Philadelphia, Pennsylvania

ENERGY INTAKE AND ACTIVITY

Editors

Ernesto Pollitt, PhD
Professor, Nutrition and Behavioral Sciences
University of Texas School of Public Health
Houston, Texas

Peggy Amante, MPH
Coordinator of Public Nutrition Education
University of Texas School of Public Health
Houston, Texas

**Published by Alan R. Liss, Inc.
for the United Nations University**

W. SUSSEX INSTITUTE
OF
HIGHER EDUCATION
LIBRARY

Address all Inquiries to the Publisher
Alan R. Liss, Inc., 150 Fifth Avenue, New York, NY 10011

Copyright © 1984 Alan R. Liss, Inc.

Printed in the United States of America.

Library of Congress Cataloging in Publication Data
Main entry under title:

Energy intake and activity.
    (Current topics in nutrition and disease;11)

    Supported by the United Nations University and
organized by the committees of the International Union of
Nutritional Sciences.
    Includes bibliograhical references and index.
    1. Nutrition–Congresses.   2. Energy metabolism–Congresses.   3. Physical fitness–Congresses.   4. Malnutrition–Congresses.   I. Pollitt, Ernesto.   II. Amante,
Peggy.   III. United Nations University.   IV. International
Union of Nutritional Sciences.   V. Series.   [DNLM:
1. Exertion–congresses.   2. Energy Metabolism–congresses.   3. Nutrition–congresses.
W1   CU82R v.11/ QU 125 E556 1983]
QP141.E55   1984   612'.39   84-9738
ISBN 0-8451-1610-X

Contents

Contributors and Participants

Linda S. Adair, Department of Anthropology, Rice University, Houston, TX **[33]***

Peggy Amante, School of Public Health, University of Texas Health Science Center, Houston, TX *

George H. Beaton, Department of Nutritional Sciences, Faculty of Medicine, University of Toronto, Toronto, Canada **[395]***

Thierry Brun, Unité de Recherches sur la Nutrition et L'Alimentation (U.1.INSERM), Paris, France **[131]***

Adolfo Chávez, Instituto Nacional de Nutrición Mexico, Tlalpan D.F., Mexico **[303]***

J.V.G.A. Durnin, Institute of Physiology, University of Glasgow, Glasgow, Scotland **[101]***

Anna Ferro-Luzzi, National Institute of Nutrition, Rome, Italy **[79]***

Rafael Flores, Institute of Nutrition of Central America and Panama, Guatemala, Guatemala **[355]**

Charles F. Halverson, Jr., Department of Child and Family Development, University of Georgia, Athens, GA **[185]***

Edward S. Horton, Metabolic Unit, University of Vermont College of Medicine, Burlington, VT **[115]***

Maarten D.C. Immink, School of Public Health, The University of Texas Health Science Center, Houston, TX **[355]***

Insun Kim, School of Public Health, University of Texas Health Science Center, Houston, TX*

Robert M. Malina, Department of Anthropology, The University of Texas, Austin, TX **[285]***

Sheldon Margen, Public Health Nutrition Program, University of California at Berkeley, Berkeley, CA **[57]***

Celia Martinez, Instituto Nacional de Nutrición Mexico, Tlalpan D.F., Mexico **[303]**

Susan C. McDonough, Institute for the Study of Development Disabilities, University of Illinois, Chicago, IL **[331]**

Ernesto Pollitt, School of Public Health, University of Texas Health Science Center, Houston, TX **[ix]***

Joan C. Post-Gorden, Department of Psychology, University of Southern Colorado, Pueblo, CO **[185]**

Andrew M. Prentice, Dunn Nutrition Unit, Cambridge, United Kingdom; and Keneba, The Gambia **[3]***

Merrill S. Read, Clinical Nutrition and Early Development Branch, Na-

*Participant in conference
The number in brackets is the opening page number of the contributor's article.

tional Institute of Child Health and Development, Bethesda, MD*

J.C. Reina, Departamento de Pediatría, División de Salúd, Universidad del Valle, Cali, Colombia **[263]***

Shlomo Reutlinger, Agriculture and Rural Development Department, World Bank, Washington, DC **[377]***

Piero Salzarulo, Institut National de la Santé et de la Recherche Médicale (INSERM U3), Bd de l'Hôpital, Paris, France **[323]***

Arnold J. Sameroff, Institute for the Study of Development Disabilities, University of Illinois, Chicago, IL **[331]***

Nevin S. Scrimshaw, Food, Nutrition and Poverty Programme, United Nations University, Massachusetts Institute of Technology, Cambridge, MA **[ix]**

G.B. Spurr, Department of Physiology, Medical College of Wisconsin, Milwaukee, WI **[207,263]***

Kraisid Tontisirin, Ramathibodi Hospital, Bangkok, Thailand*

R. Brook Thomas, Department of Anthropology, University of Massachusetts, Amherst, MA*

Benjamin Torún, Institute of Nutrition of Central America and Panama, Guatemala, Guatemala **[159,355]***

Fernando E. Viteri, Pan American Health Organization, Washington, DC **[355]**

Theodore Wachs, Department of Psychological Sciences, Purdue University, West Lafayette, IN*

Preface

The contents of this volume are based on the latest of a series of related workshops supported by the United Nations University (UNU) and organized by committees of the International Union of Nutritional Sciences (IUNS). Its immediate predecessor was also organized by IUNS Committee 111/2 on Nutrition and Behavior, and the Proceedings were co-published in 1982 by Raven Press and the UNU as *Iron Deficiency: Brain Biochemistry and Behavior*. That volume reviewed evidence showing that important brain substrates are iron dependent, and that iron deficiency may affect thermoregulation, work productivity, and cognitive function.

It has long been recognized that malnourished children are apathetic and less active than well nourished children. A number of investigators (Chavez and Martinez 1982; Lester 1979; Pollitt 1969) in the last two decades have proposed that these behavioral effects may impose limitations on the cognitive development of children through reduction of exploratory behavior and of meaningful social interactions with peers and adults. Moreover, among populations whose subsistence depends on manual labor, malnutrition may reduce life time earnings by limiting the availability of energy for work. Despite the obvious social and economic importance of these functional effects of malnutrition, surprisingly few relevant studies have provided quantitative data.

A critical question raised in this volume is the validity of our views on energy balance. Current theoretical propositions on energy intake and expenditure cannot explain satisfactorily some of the data from field studies in populations whose diets are evidently low in calories and protein. This discrepancy between constructs and data encourages the search for new concepts and explanations that are theoretically sound and that would provide more reasonable guidelines to planners and economists concerned with health and nutrition policies.

The first section of this volume presents evidence suggestive of the adaptation and reproductive competence of populations with energy intakes that are inappropriate according to current views on dietary requirements. A proposition is presented on how energy balance is maintained across time under variable conditions of intake; however the data necessary to test this hypothesis are unavailable. In a refreshingly frank chapter, Beaton takes up the issues of low dietary intakes, adaptation, and energy balance, exposes some of the inconsistencies of the data, and states that "Either our concepts are wrong or the data are wrong!"

Our understanding of the dynamics of energy expenditure is limited partly because of the lack of substantive and systematic information on activity among adults and children. Reduction of activity level is a way of achieving energy balance; however, this adaptive mechanism may prove costly to the individual by imposing restrictions on the adjustment to the ecological and cultural context. Little is known about the behavioral nature of the activities that may be affected by such an adjustment, or to what extent other energy expenditure processes, such as growth, are protected by reductions in activity level. Specifically, does reduced activity in play or exploratory behavior protect the growth of children in populations with restricted food availability? Although some data suggest that this is the case (Ruthishauer and Whitehead 1972) more information is necessary before conclusive inferences can be drawn. Similarly, how are energy savings achieved among women with low calorie intakes who, nevertheless, maintain reproductive competence and perform heavy agricultural tasks? One reason for the scarce information in these areas has been that the methodologies for measuring activity have been poorly defined. These methodological issues for adults and children are addressed in the second and third sections of this volume respectively. Important differences in the conceptualization of activity, as well as in its measurement, occur as a function of the disciplines of the investigators. Physiological approaches to activity require precise measures of metabolic rate, oxygen utilization, and cardiac output, without necessarily defining the behavioral constructs involved with the activities in question. Psychologists and anthropologists, on the other hand, are concerned with measures of activity that will help explain the adaptive and developmental significance of specific behaviors. Thus, for some, activity represents an outcome variable; for others it is an intervening variable in a behavioral-sociological chain.

Section four includes reviews and new evidence of the effects of reduced energy intake on agricultural productivity, activity and metabolism, motor development, and sleep. The data on sleeping patterns of malnourished children are novel and point to a new direction for research in the area of nutrition and biobehavioral function. Sleep follows a developmental sequence that reflects brain maturation; at the same time disturbances in sleep may affect the wake cycle. An important question in this regard is whether such disturbances restrict the stimulation a child receives.

The final section deals with the consequences of reduced activity. From a behavioral perspective we are still at the level of hypothesis generation and testing. Some of the data currently available indicates that physical activity is a mediating variable in brain function and possibly in cognitive development. Research with animals suggests that motor activity may be a necessary condition for the development of specific sensory functions (Held and Heim 1963). Piaget's (1963) theoretical formulations concerning the infants' need to act on the environment also suggest that this is the case. Research on the characteristics of cognitive function among developmentally disabled children with motor restrictions is an approach which may prove valuable, but conclusive inferences are unwarranted thus far.

The economic consequences of reduced individual productivity among sugar cane cutters in Guatemala have been explored. Increase in labor productivity as a result of an increase in energy intake has face validity, particularly among populations whose energy balance is at risk because of low energy intake. It is generally difficult, however, to determine the factors underlying human behavior, and what would be logical on the basis of an econometric equation may not be observed under field conditions. This issue leads naturally to policy considerations. Can nutritionists provide specific guidelines to economists and social planners regarding the caloric or other nutrient needs of populations? If not, is it possible to provide guidelines for specific populations? Relevant information on these issues shows that there is little overlap among the guidelines provided by international organizations and experts; in fact, significant discrepancies exist between some of these recommendations. Thus, it would appear that we can only aspire to temporary policies which are likely to be changed substantively in relatively short periods of time. While these gaps may not represent a significant problem in developed nations, they are less easily endured by developing countries.

The field covered by this volume is too young to permit a systematic and cohesive review, but the book defines the problems, discusses appropriate experimental designs, and presents important new data and concepts. It is hoped that it will be a guide and a stimulus to the further studies required to settle the issues raised and that it will provide a firmer basis for national policies with which to address the nutritional, educational, and economic problems posed.

REFERENCES

Chavez A and Martinez C (1982). "Growing up in a Developing Community." Mexico: Instituto Nacional de la Nutricion.

Held R and Heim A (1963). Movement-produced stimulation in the development of visually guided behavior. J Comp and Phys Psych 56:872–876.

Lester BMA (1979). A synergistic process approach to the study of prenatal malnutrition. Int J Behav Dev 2:377–393.

Piaget J (1963). "The Origins of Intelligence in Children." (Translated by M. Cook.) New York: W.W. Norton.

Pollitt E (1969). Ecology, malnutrition and mental development. Psychosomatic Med 31:193–200.

Rutishauser IHE and Whitehead RG (1972). Energy intakes and expenditure in 1–3 year old Ugandan children living in a rural environment. Brit J Nutr 28:145–157.

Nevin S. Scrimshaw, MD, PhD
Ernesto Pollitt, PhD

Acknowledgments

This volume is based on the invited papers presented at the meeting on Energy Intake and Activity convened in May 1983, at Villa Serbelloni, the Rockefeller Foundation Study and Conference Center in Bellagio, Italy. The meeting was organized as one of the activities of Committee 111/2 on Nutrition and Behavior of the International Union of Nutritional Sciences (IUNS) and was sponsored by the Food, Nutrition and Poverty Programme of the United Nations University. The Gerber Products Company also contributed toward Conference expenses. The editorial work for the publication of the Proceedings was funded by the National Institute of Child Health and Human Development, United States Public Health Service. This support allowed us to organize the Conference and we gratefully acknowledge the generosity of the contributors.

We are particularly indebted to Gay Robertson and the Word Processing Staff at the University of Texas School of Public Health in Houston for their dedication, competence and good humor in the preparation of the final manuscript.

ENERGY BALANCE IN
POPULATIONS

Energy Intake and Activity, pages 3–31
© *1984 Alan R. Liss, Inc., 150 Fifth Avenue, New York, NY 10011*

ADAPTATIONS TO LONG-TERM LOW ENERGY INTAKE

Andrew M. Prentice

Dunn Nutrition Unit
Cambridge, CB4 1XJ, U.K.
and Keneba, The Gambia

INTRODUCTION

Food intake measurements in developing countries generally reveal that the study communities are existing on far lower levels of dietary energy than would be recommended, and that these populations maintain energy balance in spite of apparently high levels of physical activity (Durnin 1979; Prentice 1980). There are several possible explanations for the disparity between our predictions, based generally on physiological measurements of well-nourished subjects, and observations in the field. The first possibility is that all such studies of food intake have systematically underestimated the true energy intake of their subjects (James and Shetty 1982). The second possibility is that long-term physiological adaptations can occur which increase the efficiency of energy utilization sufficiently to account for the differences in observed food intakes. Changes in activity patterns or changes in the energy cost of activity may be components of these adaptations. The possible existence of individuals with a high level of metabolic efficiency now forms the basis of one explanation for obesity (James and Trayhurn 1976; Jung and James 1980), but an extension of the same hypothesis to explain the apparent low energy requirements of many communities in the developing world seems to be less readily accepted (James and Shetty 1982).

This review will present comparative data relating to energy balance during pregnancy and lactation in affluent women from Cambridge, UK and in poor rural women in Keneba, The Gambia. The measurements of food intake were made for both groups by the same research unit and it will be argued that neither estimate is subject to significant bias, and that the gestational and lactational performance of the women in Keneba is comparable to that of the women in Cambridge in spite of a substantial difference in energy intake. Finally, it will be concluded on the basis of a literature review that there is ample experimental evidence to support the hypothesis that people in certain communities are more metabolically efficient than others, and that mechanisms exist which could theoretically spare sufficient energy to account for the observed differences in energy intake.

COMPARATIVE STUDIES IN KENEBA, THE GAMBIA AND CAMBRIDGE, UK

The Dunn Nutrition Unit has been conducting nutritional research on pregnant and lactating women in the contrasting environments of Keneba and Cambridge over the past 7 years. Only a brief summary of the methodology is presented here since much of the data and detailed methodology has been published elsewhere (Paul and Muller 1980; Prentice 1980; Prentice et al. 1981; Roberts et al. 1982; Whitehead et al. 1981)

Methods

All pregnant and lactating women in Keneba, a rural subsistence farming community in sub-Sahelian Gambia, took part in the studies. There are marked seasonal variations in both energy intake and expenditure in Keneba. The "hungry period" coincides approximately with the wet season when agricultural tasks result in the greatest energy expenditure. During the dry season, following the harvest, food is relatively plentiful. Women in Cambridge were self-selected by volunteering to participate in the studies after being approached at an ante-natal clinic. They tended to be of high socio-economic status and highly motivated towards breast-feeding. None were consciously slimming at the time of the study. A comparison of the two groups is contained in Table 1.

Food energy intake was measured using techniques appropriate for each community. In Keneba this consisted of

Table 1   Comparison of subjects in Keneba and
               Cambridge.

	Keneba (N = 156)		Cambridge (n = 59)	
	mean	range	mean	range
Age (Y)	27.3	16-43	28.1	19-36
Parity	4.7	1-12	1.8	1-5
Weight (kg)[a]	52.7	37-78	56.1	44-69
Height (cm)	157.4	141-174	162.5	151-174

[a]Weights refer to non-pregnant state and dry season for Keneba.

24-hour weighed dietary intakes in conjunction with 3-4 hourly recall for the limited variety of snack foods. The measurements were made by carefully trained indigenous field-workers on one day in each week for all subjects. Energy intake was calculated from a food table based on bomb calorimetry of 10-100 samples of each food type to determine gross energy (GE). Metabolizable energy (ME) was calculated as:

$$ME = GE \times 0.977 - N \times 6.6 - UC \times 4$$

(Hudson et al. 1980)

where nitrogen (N) was determined by a semi-automated micro Kjeldahl procedure and unavailable carbohydrate (UC) according to Southgate (1969).

In Cambridge the women carried out their own weighed intake over 4 consecutive days at monthly intervals. The energy content of the diet was calculated using standard food tables (Paul and Southgate 1978). In both studies changes in subcutaneous fat deposits were assessed through-out pregnancy and lactation by regular measurements of weight and skinfold thicknesses at several sites. Birth weights were measured in Keneba, and were obtained from hospital records in Cambridge. Breast-milk output was estimated by test-weighing over 12 or 24 hours in Keneba (Whitehead et al. 1978), and over 72 hours in Cambridge where the mothers performed their own measurements. The particular test-weighing technique used has been validated in

Keneba using the D_2O dilution techniques (Coward et al. 1982; Coward et al. 1979).

Results

Energy intake. The average levels of dietary energy intake during pregnancy and lactation are shown in Tables 2 and 3, together with comparable data published from similar studies. The energy intakes in Keneba (dry season) and in Cambridge are fairly close to the median values for developing and industrialized nations respectively and, therefore, represent a meaningful comparison in a wider perspective. The percentage energy deficit of the Keneba women compared with the Cambridge women was 29% during pregnancy and 27% during lactation. This compares with an estimated deficit in the mean per capita energy supply for developing nations of 21% when compared with industrialized nations (United Nations University 1979).

The energy intakes were qualitatively similar in the two communities and during early lactation both showed an increase of 20% above the level during pregnancy. As lactation progressed the energy intake decreased slightly, and at the end of lactation averaged only 10% above the level during pregnancy in both groups.

The Cambridge data will not be considered in any further detail since the ability of these women to obtain adequate energy is not in question. However, several important points concerning the data from industrialized nations as a whole should be noted. First, in most of the studies the average intakes fall well below currently recommended daily allowances for energy during pregnancy and lactation (N.R.C. 1980). This is partly due to the fact that the womens' non-pregnant energy intakes are low and partly because they are not increasing their energy intake by the calculated additional requirements for pregnancy and lactation, 301 and 500 Kcal/day respectively. Second, the values quoted are averages about which there is a wide variation. This means, in practice, that there are women in Cambridge who go through pregnancy and lactation in apparent overall energy balance despite having a measured energy intake typical of a woman in Keneba. The possibility that such individuals were concealing their true energy intake is unlikely since they were highly motivated breast-feeders who

Table 2   Published estimates of energy intake during pregnancy and lactation in developing countries.

Country — Dietary energy intake	KCal/day
Pregnancy	
Gambia - wet season (Prentice et al. 1981)	1299
New Guinea (Oomen & Malcolm 1958)	1359
India (Gopalan 1962)	1400
India (Venkatachalam 1962)	1409
New Guinea - lowland (Norgan et al. 1974)	1414
Gambia - dry season (Prentice 1981)	1483
Guatemala (Lechtig et al. 1972)	1500
Ethiopia (Gebre-Medhin & Gobezie 1974)	1538
India (Rajalakshmi 1971)	1569
Columbia (Mora et al. 1978)	1619
India (Devadas 1978)	1624
Guatemala (Arroyave 1975)	1720
Tanzania (Maletnlema & Bavu 1974)	1849
Iraq (Demarchi 1966)	1880
India (Bagchi & Bose 1962)	1918
Thailand (Thanangkul & Amatyakul 1975)	1980
New Guinea - highland (Norgan et al. 1974)	1999
Guatemala (Mata et al. 1972)	2059
Lactation	
Gambia - wet season (Prentice 1981)	1299
India (Karmarkar et al. 1963)	1299
India (Devadas & Murthy 1977)	1400
India (Karmarkar et al. 1959)	1440
New Guinea - lowland (Norgan et al. 1974)	1459
Guatemala (Arroyave 1975)	1600
India (Rajalakshmi 1971)	1619
Gambia - dry season (Prentice 1981)	1681
Guatemala (Schutz et al. 1980)	1927
Mexico (Martinez & Chavez 1971)	1949
New Guinea - highland (Norgan et al. 1974)	2166

Table 3 Published estimates of energy intake during pregnancy and lactation in industrialized countries.

Country	Dietary energy intake	KCal/day
Pregnancy		
England (Smithells et al. 1977)		1956
England (Whitehead et al. 1981)		1980
Australia (English & Hitchcock 1968)		2090
England (Darke et al. 1980)		2152
Sweden (Lunell et al. 1969)		2152
Scotland (Thomson 1958)		2503
Lactation		
USA (Sims 1978)		2123
Sweden (Abrahmsson & Hofvander 1977)		2279
England (Whitehead et al. 1981)		2293
Australia (Rattigan et al. 1981)		2305
Australia (English & Hitchcock 1968)		2460
Scotland (Thomson et al. 1970)		2716
England (Whicelow 1976)		2728
England (Naismith & Ritchie 1975)		2928

were aware of the importance of satisfactory maternal nutrition during lactation. People such as these, with exceptionally low energy requirements, are not necessarily abnormal but merely represent the extreme end of the normal distribution.

The food intake data from Keneba requires detailed consideration if the mechanisms by which these women manage to achieve overall energy balance through repeated child-bearing cycles under such harsh dietary conditions are to be understood. The energy intake during pregnancy is summarized in Table 4. Intakes during the dry season, when food was relatively plentiful following the harvest, averaged 1483 Kcal/day. However, there was a decrease in energy intake during the wet season (July-October), with a minimum intake of 1302 Kcal/day in August. The energy intake during lactation (Table 5) showed a similar seasonal variation, decreasing from a dry season mean intake of 1684

Table 4 Energy intake of pregnant women in Keneba analysed according to trimester[a].

Tri-mester	May	June	July	Aug	Sep	Oct	Nov	Dec	Jan	Feb	Mar	Apr	Dry Season[b]
1	2138 ±289 12	1720 ±60 3	1467 ±148 15	1378 ±112 10	-	-	-	1681 ±189 12	1469 ±74 22	1564 ±112 9	1392 ±150 9	1478 ±150 12	1615 ±67 79
2	1383 ±62 54	1500 ±72 54	1557 ±64 81	1309 ±55 87	1521 ±76 31	1541 ±86 37	1502 ±98 30	1638 ±129 20	1354 ±107 27	1311 ±103 29	1490 ±129 30	1495 ±88 38	1452 ±330 282
3	1287 ±103 29	1419 ±91 43	1541 ±72 57	1280 ±60 80	1299 ±60 80	1438 ±64 81	1581 ±69 60	1560 ±103 40	1572 ±76 58	1354 ±79 40	1459 ±81 40	1450 ±98 28	1481 ±31 338
Total	1447 ±62 95	1471 ±55 100	1543 ±45 153	1302 ±38 177	1369 ±48 102	1469 ±53 118	1557 ±57 90	1603 ±74 72	1488 ±53 107	1361 ±57 78	1459 ±67 79	1476 ±62 78	1483 ±21 699

[a]Values (Kcal/day) are means of all dietary days ± SEM, and number of days.   [b]Dry season is defined as November to June inclusive.

Table 5 Energy intake of lactating women in Keneba[a]

Stage of lactation	May	June	July	Aug	Sep	Oct	Nov	Dec	Jan	Feb	Mar	Apr	Dry Season[b]
0-3 mos. post-partum	2066 76 23	1591 112 23	1591 93 42	1414 100 33	1314 96 28	1533 115 27	1588 91 61	1863 93 58	1911 62 97	1720 96 55	1677 76 47	1722 84 51	1772 31 415
4-18 mos. post-partum	1667 55 144	1693 43 223	1631 48 201	1187 31 249	1204 38 216	1469 45 244	1787 50 211	1703 50 176	1703 38 225	1595 45 197	1533 38 245	1619 41 229	1662 21 1648
Total	1722 48 167	1684 36 246	1593 38 243	1201 26 282	1242 33 244	1493 36 271	1741 43 272	1744 45 234	1765 36 322	1622 41 252	1555 31 292	1638 36 280	1684 14 2063

[a]Values (Kcal/day) are means of all dietary days ± SEM, and number of days.   [b]Dry season is defined as November to June inclusive.

Kcal/day to a minimum wet season intake of 1202 Kcal/day. The lactating women, therefore, suffered a much greater percentage and absolute restriction of energy intake during the wet season. Although measurement of energy intake is considerably easier than measurement of energy expenditure it is sometimes suggested that subjects may have a conscious or subconscious desire to conceal their true energy intake. This suggestion is usually made with reference to obese subjects for whom it may be valid. It is unlikely that such an artifact is present in the Keneba data; indeed the reverse is more likely to be true, since there is a degree of shame associated with an inability to meet the food requirements of a family. An analysis of possible sources of error and bias in the dietary data presented here leads us to conclude that although individual values, in the most extreme case, may have been in error by as much as 50%, these errors were not associated with a particular bias and will be largely eliminated in the overall mean values from such a large study group.

Maintenance of energy balance. Changes in body weight indicate that all adults in Keneba are in negative energy balance during the farming/hungry season and in positive energy balance during the dry season (Prentice et al. 1981; Thomson et al. 1966). Although in the short-term these individuals are rarely in true equilibrium they maintain constant body weights from year to year and can, therefore, be presumed to be in long-term energy balance. The seasonal pattern of weight change is illustrated for the pregnant and lactating women in Figure 1. During the dry season pregnant women gained an average of 1.35 kg per month in spite of an energy intake of only 1483 Kcal/day. Changes in skinfold thicknesses showed that this weight gain included substantial fat deposition in early pregnancy when the metabolic demands of the fetus were small (Prentice et al. 1981). The corresponding weight gain in the pregnant Cambridge women was only slightly greater at 1.48 kg per month. However, the pregnancy weight gain during the wet season in Keneba was severely reduced and averaged only 0.3 kg per month.

Lactating women in Keneba gained weight during the dry season at a rate which was significantly greater than the weight gain of non-pregnant, non-lactating women (+0.59 vs. +0.33 kg/month). This may indicate a raised capacity for fat mobilization and deposition in lactating women. During

Figure 1

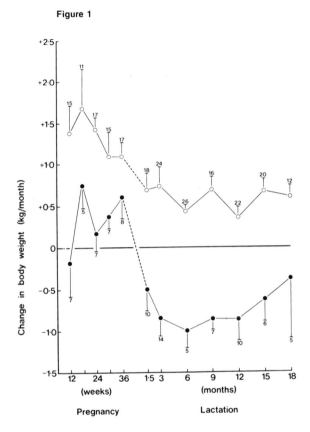

Weight changes in pregnant and lactating women in dry (○) and wet (●) seasons in Keneba. Values are means ±SEM, and number of subjects.

(Prentice et al. 1983 a)

the wet season lactating women in Keneba lost 0.74 kg per month; lactating women in Cambridge lost 0.57 kg per month.

The fact that lactating women in Keneba gained weight in the dry season was probably due to the fact that the impetus to regain weight lost during the wet season was more powerful than the normal physiological mechanism of gradual weight loss during lactation which was observed in the Cambridge women. Whatever the cause of the weight gain, the important fact is that such a rate of weight gain was possible on an energy intake on only 1684 Kcal/day.

An estimate of the residual energy available for resting metabolism (RMR) and activity has been made by correcting the energy intake data of the lactating women for changes in subcutaneous fat stores and for the energy cost of milk production. The resultant values, shown in Table 6, show a remarkable degree of internal consistency despite the wide variations in energy intake. Furthermore they demonstrate that the residual energy available in the wet season was actually higher than that available during the dry season since mobilization of adipose tissue more than compensated for the reduced energy intake. The average residual energy values of 1089 Kcal/day and 1125 Kcal/day are very low and approximate the predicted basal metabolic rate (BMR), of 1202 Kcal/day calculated according to Cunninghan (1980) on the basis of lean body mass and formulae derived from data on Western subjects. It should be noted that the assumed efficiency of conversion of dietary energy to milk energy

Table 6   Calculation of residual energy available to lactating women in Keneba

Trimester	Dietary energy	Change in adipose tissue	Energy to/ from fat stores[a]	Milk output	Energy to milk[b]	Residual energy
	Kcal/day	g/month	Kcal/day	g/day	Kcal/day	Kcal/day
Dry season						
0-3 months	1772	+700	-162	653	-499	1111
3-6 months	1658	+450	-105	614	-471	1082
6-9 months	1674	+700	-162	574	-439	1072
9-12 months	1648	+400	-93	583	-447	1108
12-15 months	1672	+700	-162	583	-447	1063
15-18 months	1653	+600	-141	536	-411	1101
					Mean	1089
Wet season						
0-3 months	1471	-700	+162	640	-490	1144
3-6 months	1314	-1000	+234	580	-444	1103
6-9 months	1392	-800	+186	611	-468	1111
9-12 months	1421	-900	+210	574	-439	1192
12-15 months	1390	-600	+141	564	-432	1099
15-18 months	1414	-350	+81	511	-392	1103
					Mean	1125

[a] One kilogram adipose tissue was assumed to represent (6998 Kcal) available energy

[b] An efficiency of conversion (dietary energy to milk energy) of 90% was assumed.

influences the residual energy value. If the efficiency of conversion were closer to 100%, which may be possible since energy lost as heat during milk production conceivably may be regained by a reduction in thermoregulatory thermogenesis, then the residual energy available would be increased by about 60 Kcal/day.

A similar calculation has been performed using the data from the pregnant women and published values for the energy cost of growth and maintenance of the products of conception, but excluding fat deposition since this is already accounted for in the calculation (Hytten and Leitch 1971). The results, given in (Table 7), show that in spite of the lower intakes of the pregnant women, their available residual energy for RMR and activity was 20-30% higher than that for the lactating women. These values are consistent with the increased tissue mass and higher energy cost of activity during pregnancy. Once again the residual energy during the wet season (1459 Kcal/day) was higher than during the dry season (1308 Kcal/day) in spite of the lower dietary energy intake in the wet season. This result is consistent with observations of activity patterns which would predict a

Table 7   Calculation of residual energy available to pregnant women in Keneba

Trimester	Dietary energy	Change in adipose tissue	Energy to/from fat stores[a]	Energy to fetus[b]	Residual energy
	Kcal/day	g/month	Kcal/day	Kcal/day	Kcal/day
Dry Season					
1	1615	+1000	-234	-43	1338
2	1452	+250	-57	-88	1306
3	1478	0	0	-201	1278
				Mean	1306
Wet season					
1	1438	-500	+117	-43	1512
2	1459	-500	+141	-88	1512
3	1381	-750	+174	-201	1354
				Mean	1459

[a]One Kilogram of adipose tissue was assumed to represent 6998 Kcal available energy.

[b]Calculated from Hytten and Leitch (Hytten & Leitch 1971).

slightly higher energy expenditure on farm work in the wet season as it is defined here (Mata et al. 1972). The residual energy available to the pregnant women also approximated the value for BMR (1439 Kcal/day) calculated in the same way as for the lactating women.

Adequacy of gestational and lactational performance.
There is no doubt that gestational and lactational performance during the wet season in Keneba were unsatisfactory. Mean birth weight was about 250 g lower than during the dry season and there was a high prevalence of low birth weight babies (< 2.5 kg) (Prentice et al. 1981). Milk output was also reduced in the wet season and milk quality was compromised (Prentice 1980). Dry season births in Keneba averaged 3.0 kg (sexes combined); the mean birth weight in the Cambridge study was 3.3 kg. However, the Keneba women were of smaller stature, suffered a higher incidence of infectious disease, particularly malaria with its known effect on birth weight, and had at least part of their pregnancy during the debilitating wet season. The prevalence of low birth weight babies was low during the dry season and their survival prospects were excellent (Prentice et al. 1981). The breast milk output of Keneba women during the dry season was very similar to that of the Cambridge women in early lactation and they sustained lactation for far longer (Whitehead et al. 1980). Milk quality was also virtually identical in the two communities with the exception of several water-soluble vitamins (Prentice 1980).

There was, therefore, very little indication during the dry season that either the gestational or lactational performance of women in Keneba was handicapped by inadequate maternal nutrition. This conclusion is further supported by the results of detailed maternal dietary supplementation studies (Prentice et al. 1980; Prentice et al. 1983b). Provision of a balanced dietary supplement to lactating women caused a net increase of 723 Kcal/day in maternal energy intake, after correction for a slight reduction in home food intake, but had no effect on breast milk output or milk energy content. When the same supplement was given to pregnant women, resulting in a net energy increment of 431 kcal/day, mean birth weights were substantially improved during the wet season, but there was no effect during the dry season. These supplement results show that the womens' customary energy intake was certainly lower than their preferred intake since they increased their energy consumption by a large amount. It is also noteworthy that the final voluntary intakes in supplemented Keneba women almost exactly matched the Cambridge womens' intakes (Pregnancy, K = 1895 Kcal/day, C = 1979 Kcal/day; lactation, K = 2289 Kcal/day, C = 2292 Kcal/day). It is clear, however, that although their pre-supplementation intakes were sub-optimal, women in Keneba managed somehow to make sufficient economies in the dry season to maintain energy balance and to preserve gestational and lactational performance close to the optimum. It appears that such findings are not unusual in developing countries. For instance, Adair and Pollitt (1982) have published preliminary information suggesting that a very similar pattern of energy balance existed in a group of 225 Taiwanese women whom they were studying.

The remainder of this review will explore possible explanations for the disparity between expectations, which are based upon extrapolation from limited physiological measurements made almost entirely on well-nourished subjects, and field observations of energy balance. Consideration will be given to the most likely areas in which metabolic economies could be made by undernourished subjects.

POTENTIAL ENERGY SPARING MECHANISMS

Reduced Physical Activity

Savings in energy expenditure are most likely to occur through reduction in physical activity. These reductions could take the form of gross changes in the number and duration of activities, or very subtle changes in the physical economy with which various movements and tasks are accomplished. In either case, detection of such changes would be difficult. Because we have only recently begun measurements of energy expenditure in Keneba it is not yet possible to make definitive statements regarding physical activity, but a number of observations are relevant. The women are certainly not inactive and they perform some physical tasks which would not be contemplated by most Western women. The question remains, however, as to whether they are able to be as active as they wish to be. In this respect it is instructive to consider their response to dietary supplementation. The lactating women will be considered here since their incremental energy intake was greater than that of the pregnant women, but the same conclusions could also be drawn from the latter. None of the 723 Kcal/day net increase in energy intake was transferred to the infant; both breast milk volume and milk energy content were entirely unaffected by supplementation. The supplement did cause a slight increase in mean maternal body weight in the first two months after its introduction, but thereafter the weight changes showed a pattern, including weight loss during the wet season, identical to the pre-supplementation group (Figure 2). Going on the assumption that all of the additional weight consisted of adipose tissue, the overall weight gain of 1.8 kg accounted for only 7% of the additional energy supplied by the supplement. The remaining 93% or 671 Kcal/day remained unaccounted for. The similarity of the seasonal changes in body weight,

Figure 2

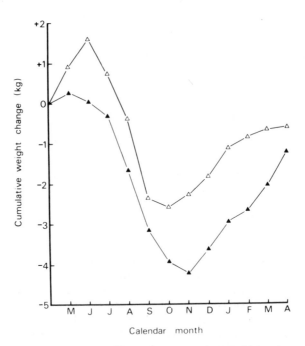

Cumulative weight changes in supplemented (△) and unsupplemented (▲) lactating women in Keneba. Each point represents data from approximately 85 subjects.

(Prentice et al. 1981)

which were also similar in the supplemented and unsupplemented pregnant women, suggest that increased physical activity could account for some of the 'missing' energy. It appears that there may be a maximum rate of weight loss which the women will tolerate and that, following supplementation, they may have adjusted their activity until this limit was again reached. The women certainly reported reduced fatigue and an increased feeling of well-being, but such subjective comments must be treated with scepticism. Even if changes in activity could account for some of the difference in energy intake between unsupplemented Keneba women and supplemented Keneba or Cambridge women it is most unlikely that this could account for the extra 723 Kcal/day since this would indicate that they had more than doubled their amount of physical activity. Furthermore, the supplemented women showed evidence of some profound changes in their handling of energy metabolites and in their hormonal profiles (Prentice et al. 1983). This suggests that changes in their overall metabolic efficiency may have occurred and these will be discussed below.

Reduction in Active Tissue Mass

People from developing countries are often shorter and lighter than people from industrialized nations. Much of this difference probably results from inadequate nutrition during childhood and adolescence since, with a few exceptions, the genetic potential for growth does not vary markedly between races. Smaller stature is often cited as an example of and adaptation to low food intakes. For certain nutrients this may be so, but it does not appear to confer an advantage in terms of energy requirements since fat-free mass is seldom found to be reduced. Measurements of total body water in Keneba yielded group mean values ranging from 59.1 to 64.3% in lactating women depending upon the time of year. Although total body water has not been estimated in the Cambridge subjects, Hytten et al. (1966) have obtained a value of 52.5% for 94 British women in the early post-partum period. Applying these values together with an assumed water content of 72.5% for fat-free tissue (Garrow 1978) yields estimates of fat-free mass of 40.6 kg in Cambridge and 43.1 kg in Keneba even when the lowest total body water estimate is used for the Keneba data. The differences in body weight are therefore accounted for by differences in body fat. In Keneba this represents only 18.1% of body weight compared to 27.6% in Cambridge. James and Shetty (1982) reached the same conclusion when comparing data from New Guinean women of mean body weight 46.9 kg (Norgan 1974) and a different group of Cambridge women with a mean body weight of 55.1 kg. Thus, although a reduction in active tissue mass may be one mechanism whereby energy is conserved in individuals subjected to semi-starvation on an experimental basis (Grande et al. 1958; Keys et al. 1950), it does not appear to be an explanation for the energy conservation shown by women in Keneba.

Reduction in Basal Metabolic Rate

Since it has been demonstrated above that women in Keneba do not have a reduced active tissue mass compared to their Cambridge counterparts, any reduction in BMR must consist of a change per unit active tissue mass if it is to represent an economy. A number of studies in the literature indicate that underfeeding is accompanied by a decrease in metabolic rate greater than can be accounted for by loss of active tissue (Garrow 1974; Garrow and Warwick 1978; Keys et al. 1950); similarly, overfeeding appears to be associated with an increased metabolic rate (Garrow 1978). Thus, whether one considers people from developing countries as undernourished or those from industrialized countries as overnourished, there appears to be at least some ability to alter metabolic rate in order to achieve energy balance. The important question concerns the extent to which this single mechanism can compensate for low energy intakes. A recent review (James and Shetty 1982) of the work of Keys et al. (1950) suggests that the 16% fall in BMR per unit active tissue mass which they observed would not explain the apparent low food intakes in developing countries. Even a decrease of this magnitude, however, could account for at least one third of the 27-29% difference between energy intakes in Keneba and Cambridge.

Although the experimental evidence quoted above confirms that adaptations in RMR are possible, it should be emphasised that actual measurements of RMR in undernourished subjects in developing countries have yielded variable results. Some studies report metabolic rates lower than would be predicted (Edmundson 1979), while others suggest that RMRs are normal (Ashworth 1968; Norgan 1974).

Reduction in Thermoregulatory Non-shivering Thermogenesis

Evidence in both experimental animals and man suggests that non-shivering thermogenesis (NST) may have a vital role to play in the maintenance of energy balance (James and Trayhurn 1976; Jung & James 1980), and that an abnormal thermogenic response may contribute to obesity (Jung et al. 1979; Miller 1974; Shetty et al. 1981). The extent to which NST influences energy balance in man is still unclear, but it is theoretically possible that people on a restricted energy intake conserve energy by a reduction in NST. This may be particularly likely in the case of developing countries since most of them have considerably higher ambient temperatures than most temperate industrialized nations. James and Trayhurn (1976) have suggested that in societies where food supplies are very limited, children who are genetically more thermo-responsive, and therefore less efficient, will die and the more efficient storers of fat will survive. They quote supportive evidence in the form of studies showing that adult Kalahari bushmen (Wyndham 1958) and Aborigines (Scholander et al. 1958) have a reduced response to the cold, and that they allow their core temperatures to fall during a cool night, thus reducing the temperature gradient and hence the heat loss. On being acculturated in urban societies such individuals are prone to obesity. Subjective observation in Keneba also suggests that thermorespon-siveness may be reduced and that there is a marked tendency toward obesity among migrants to urban areas.

It has been suggested that there are two components to NST: futile cycles occurring mostly in muscle (Jansky 1973), and uncoupling or respiration of ATP synthesis in brown adipose tissue (Nicholls 1979). The relative impor-tance of these two mechanisms in different species and in young and old animals is still unclear, particularly as futile cycles now appear to be of little importance, at least in small mammals. However, it has been suggested that the fructose-6-phosphate/fructose-1, 6-diphosphate futile cycle in man is stimulated by T_3 through an increase in plasma free fatty acid levels. It is somewhat difficult to interpret the data on Keneba women in this respect since two appar-ently contradictory findings were observed. Supplementation of lactating women caused a significant reduction in T_3 levels (suggestive of an increased efficiency), but at the same time a significant increase in plasma free fatty acid levels

(Prentice et al. 1983a) which, according to the above hypothesis, should stimulate wastage of energy through heat production by the futile cycle. The paradoxical fall in T_3 levels might be explained by the fact that the supplement also resulted in a large improvement in the severe riboflavin deficiency exhibited by these women. Riboflavin deficiency has been associated with a diminished responsiveness to T_3 (Rivlin and Wolf 1969).

Recent work in mice (Trayhurn et al. 1982) suggests that energy can be conserved very efficiently during pregnancy and particularly during lactation by a reduction in the degree of uncoupling, and hence heat production, in brown adipose tissue. Both thermoregulatory and diet-induced thermogenesis are suppressed. It is suggested that either the increased metabolic heat production which results from fetal growth and milk production obviate the need for any specific thermoregulatory heat production, or that there is a distinct physiological adaptation for energy conservation, possibly mediated by prolactin. Although the relevance of these findings to adult humans is not clear, they may provide an explanation for the fact that women rarely increase their energy intakes during pregnancy and lactation by the theoretical additional requirements. The suggestion that prolactin, which rises to high levels during pregnancy and lactation, may mediate changes in NST is of particular interest since prolactin levels in women in Keneba are many times higher than in Cambridge, and are reduced (with a possible rise in NST) by dietary supplementation (Lunn et al. 1980). It should be stressed, however, that the possible involvement of prolactin is still unclear since reduced thermogenic drive in grossly obese women and in pre-obese ob/ob mice is associated with lowered prolactin levels (Jung et al. 1982; Kopelman et al.; Larson et al. 1976). Although this entire area of research is still in its infancy, it is already clear that changes in NST conceivably could constitute a substantial energy sparing mechanism.

Reduction in Diet-Induced Thermogenesis

Diet-induced thermogenesis (DIT), or luxusconsumption, has two components: a relatively long-term adjustment in metabolic rate and heat dissipation following overfeeding (Garrow 1978) and a short-term post-prandial increase in metabolic rate (specific dynamic action).

It is possible that people consuming Western levels of dietary energy continually waste some of this energy by the latter mechanism and that such wastage is eliminated when energy intake is restricted. However, in reviewing the evidence that overfeeding causes an increase in energy expenditure, Garrow (1978) has concluded that there is probably a threshold below which this adaptation is not elicited, and that this explains the failure to detect such an effect when small energy overloads are used (Glick et al. 1977). If this is the case then it is unlikely that long-term changes in DIT contribute to the different efficiency of women in Keneba and Cambridge.

Changes in post-prandial thermogenesis may be important for several reasons. First, the meal frequency is low in Keneba (usually 2 meals per day) and snacking is also less common than in Cambridge. The period over which post-prandial DIT can operate is therefore reduced. Second, women in Keneba have a lower protein intake than women in Cambridge, and protein is known to be particularly thermogenic (Blaxter 1976). Furthermore, there are genetic factors which determine the extent of post-prandial thermogenesis since an abnormally low response in obese subjects has been shown following both glucose (Pittet et al. 1976) and a mixed diet (Shetty et al. 1979). In addition there appears to be a complex interrelationship between exercise and post-prandial thermogenesis (Zahorska-Markiewicz 1980). Miller and Wise (1975) showed that the energy cost of a standard activity was dependent upon the previous day's energy intake when the activity was performed in the post-prandial period, but not if the activity was performed before the meal. Exercise training also influences both DIT and BMR in experimental animals (Gleeson et al. 1982). Such considerations, together with the technical difficulties of measuring post-prandial thermogenesis (Garrow 1978), make it difficult to assess the effect of changes in this component of energy expenditure on increased metabolic efficiency, beyond recognizing it as a likely area for economies. It should be noted that the failure to show impaired heat production following a standard meal in malnourished children (Ashworth 1969) does not preclude the possibility of a genetically selected tendency towards lowered post-prandial thermogenesis as has been suggested. Indeed, according to the hypothesis being developed here, the children may have been malnourished partly because they did not have the ability to modify the DIT component of their energy expenditure.

Increased Metabolic Efficiency Caused by 'Gorging' as Opposed to 'Nibling'

As indicated above, women in Keneba tend to follow a gorging pattern of feeding while those in Cambridge are likely to be nibblers. This pattern may be fairly characteristic of developing and industrialized nations respectively. It has often been suggested that feeding frequency has a role in energy balance in man, with gorging being associated with a higher efficiency of energy utilization. However, a carefully conducted whole-body calorimeter study, while demonstrating an altered pattern of energy expenditure, could detect no difference in the overall 24-hour expenditure on a nibbling or gorging regime (Dallosso et al. 1982), that conclusions reached on the basis of early work with experimental animals were erroneous, and that feeding frequency is not an important factor in determining metabolic efficiency (Adams and Morgan 1981). It appears unlikely, therefore, that the difference in eating habits between Keneba and Cambridge contributes to the difference in metabolic efficiency.

Reduction in the Energy Cost of Muscular Activity

In addition to possible differences in the absolute amount of activity performed in Keneba and Cambridge, there may also be differences in the energy cost of specific activities. The 6% lower body weight in Keneba should immediately result in a comparable reduction in the energy cost of many activities. It is also conceivable that energy deficient people find ways of doing set tasks very efficiently. Such an inverse relationship between dietary energy intake and work efficiency has been reported in a study of East Javanese peasant farmers (Edmundson 1977). However, since physical activity probably only accounts for up to one third of the daily energy expenditure, any savings in the energy cost of activity must be proportionately reduced before inclusion in the overall energy balance sheet.

Increased Efficiency of Absorption of Dietary Energy

In normal subjects the efficiency of absorption of dietary energy varies between 90% and close to 100%, but there appear to be fairly consistent differences between individuals within this range. Some reported ranges of daily fecal losses in normal adults are 8-146 Kcal/day (Heymsfield et al. 1981) and 74-199 Kcal/day (Dallosso et al. 1982), and a variability of 50-60 Kcal/day has been reported in children (Widdowson 1947). Thus, while certain individuals may easily absorb over 95 Kcal/day more than others on the same diet, it is unlikely that a difference of this magnitude exists between the group mean values for Keneba and Cambridge. If differences of absorption do exist they are unlikely to contribute very significantly to the enhanced metabolic efficiency of women in Keneba.

Evolution or Adaptation?

The increased metabolic efficiency of populations existing on the low energy intakes described above may occur by means of genotypic evolution, phenotypic adaptation or even a genetically determined ability to adapt. It is suggested that no single explanation will be found for enhanced efficiency, and that further research will reveal close similarities between successful survivors in developing countries and those prone to obesity in the west. It is probable that both groups merely represent one end of a normal distribution of metabolic efficiencies and that this trait has been heavily selected for in conditions of food shortage. The selection drive could be extremely powerful, particularly in the case of child-bearing women, since the ability to produce a viable baby and to sustain it through its largely breast-fed infancy may be largely dependent on a mother's metabolic efficiency. Successful child-bearing women exist in Keneba who have 10 live offspring from 10 live births, in contrast to others who have only 1 or 2 living children from the same number of births. Part of the success may be due to a high level of metabolic efficiency, and under such conditions it would take only a few generations for the successful woman's genes to predominate. In the case of obesity, it seems increasingly likely that there is an important genetic component (James and Trayhurn 1976), and it may be that such people are those who have failed to readapt to a raised level of energy intake.

Longterm adaptation to low intakes for many nutrients is well documented, and evidence that it can occur for low energy intakes has been summarized above. However, the frequently cited adaptation of maintaining a relatively small adult stature needs to be re-examined on the basis of differences which may or may not exist in active tissue mass. As with the genetic selection pressure, the selection of infants capable of metabolic adaptation would also be extremely rigorous in most developing countries. In Keneba, prior to the installation of research clinic facilities, only 50.2% of all children reached their 5th birthday. Although most of the deaths resulted from acute infections, malnutrition was considered a contributory cause in a large proportion of the cases. Present evidence suggests that a combination of both evolution and adaptation results in the maintenance of a population characterized by high metabolic efficiency.

CONCLUSIONS

The conclusions are that many populations exist in genuine energy balance on surprisingly low energy intakes and that this finding is not the result of incorrect estimates of their food intakes. The magnitude of the energy deficit is probably 20-30% when compared with well-nourished communities. There appear to be several possible mechanisms for saving energy which when summed could readily account for a difference of this magnitude, and in conditions of food shortage the selection pressures towards making such economies are probably very powerful. It seems plausible, therefore, that people in developing countries are more efficient than those in developed countries, particularly since differences in metabolic efficiency are now accepted as at least part of the explanation of obesity.

This controversy will be resolved only when energy expenditure can be measured under more realistic free-living conditions than is currently possible. The doubly-labelled water technique (Lipson and McClintock 1966; Schoeller and van Santen 1982) presently being developed in several laboratories, including The Dunn Nutrition Unit, should satisfy the above criteria and will probably be used in Keneba and Cambridge in the near future to test the hypotheses outlined above.

Finally, when considering the implications of such long-term adaptations to low energy intake, it must be remembered that although survival can be achieved on intakes much lower than hitherto considered possible, such dietary conditions are almost certainly incompatible with the optimum quality of life we wish to see achieved for such communities, and must be regarded only as minimum requirements.

Acknowledgements

Many people, whose names appear on the original publications, assisted in the collection and analysis of the data presented here. Their contributions, in particular those of Roger G. Whitehead, Alison A. Paul and Tim J. Cole, are gratefully acknowledged.

REFERENCES

1. Abrahamsson L and Hofvander Y (1977). Naringsintaget hos ammande modrar. Resultat fran 3-dagars Kostregistrering av 25 modrar i Uppsala. Naringsforskning 21:93-94.
2. Adair LS and Pollitt E (1982). Energy balance during pregnancy and lactation. Lancet 2:219.
3. Adams CE and Morgan KJ (1981). Periodicity of eating: Implications for human food consumption. Nutr Res 1:525-550.
4. Arroyave G (1975). Nutrition in pregnancy in Central America and Panama. Am J Dis Child 129:427-430.
5. Ashworth A (1968). An investigation of very low calorie intake reported in Jamaica. Br J Nutr 22: 342-355.
6. Ashworth A (1969). Metabolic rates during recovery from protein-calorie malnutrition: the need for a new concept of specific dynamic action. Nature 223:407-409.
7. Bagchi K and Bose AK (1962). Effect of low nutrient intake during pregnancy on obstetrical performance and offspring. Am J Clin Nutr 11:586-592.
8. Blaxter KL (1976). Energy utilization and obesity. In Bray G (ed): "Obesity in Perspective," Washington, DC: Fogarty International Centre, US Govt Printing Office, pp. 127-135.
9. Coward WA, Cole TJ, Sawyer MB, Prentice AM and Orr-Ewing AK (1982). Breast-milk intake measurement in mixed-fed infants by administration of deuterium oxide to their mothers. Human Nutr: Clin Nutr 36C: 141-148.

10. Coward WA, Whitehead RG, Sawyer MB, Prentice AM and Evans J (1979). New method for measuring milk intake in breast-fed babies. Lancet 2:13-14.
11. Cunningham JJ (1980). A re-analysis of the factors influencing basal metabolic rate in normal adults. Am J Clin Nutr 33:2372-2374.
12. Dallosso HM, Murgatroyd PR and James WTP (1982). Feeding frequency and energy balance in adult males. Human Nutr: Clin Nutr 36C:25-39.
13. Darke SJ, Disselduff MM and Try GP (1980). Frequency distribution of mean daily intakes of food energy and selected nutrients obtained during nutrition surveys of different groups of people in Great Britain between 1968 and 1971. Br J Nutr 44:243-252.
14. Demarchi M, Isa A, Al-Saidi S, Al-Azzawee M, Ali M and Elmilli N (1966). Food consumption and nutrition status of pregnant women attending a Maternal Child Health Centre in Baghdad. J Fac Med Baghdad 8:20-30.
15. Devadas RP and Murthy NK (1977). Nutrition of the pre-school child in India. World Rev Nutr Diet 27:1-33.
16. Devadas RP, Vijayalakshmi P and Vanitha R (1978). Impact of nutrition on pregnancy, lactation and growth performance of the extero-gestate foetus. Ind J Nutr Dietet 15:31-37.
17. Durnin JVGA (1979). Energy balance in man with particular reference to low intakes. Biblthca Nutr Dieta 27:1-10.
18. Edmundson W (1977). Individual variations in work output per unit energy intake in East Java. Ecol Food Nutr 6:147-151.
19. Edmundson W (1979). Individual variations in basal metabolic rate and mechanical work efficiency in East Java. Ecol Food Nutr 8:189-195.
20. English R and Hitchcock NE (1968). Nutrient intakes during pregnancy, lactation and after the cessation of lactation in a group of Australian women. Br J Nutr 22:615-624.
21. Galton DJ (1971). "The Human Adipose Cell: a Model for Errors in Metabolic Regulation." London: Butterworth & Co.
22. Garrow JS (1978). "Energy Balance and Obesity in Man, 2nd edition." Amsterdam: North-Holland Publishers.
23. Garrow JS and Warwick PM (1978). Diet and obesity. In Yudkin J (ed): "The Diet of Man: Needs and

Wants." Barking: Applied Science Publishers, pp 127-144.

24. Gebre-Medhin M and Gobezie A (1975). Dietary intake in the third trimester of pregnancy and birth weight of offspring among non-privileged and privileged women. Am J Clin Nutr 28:1322-1329.

25. Gleeson M, Brown JF, Waring JJ and Stock MJ (1982). The effects of physical exercise on metabolic rate and dietary induced thermogenesis. Br J Nutr 47:173-181.

26. Glick Z, Shvartz E, Magazanik A and Modan M (1977). Absence of increased thermogenesis during short-term overfeeding in normal and overweight women. Am J Clin Nutr 30:1026-1035.

27. Gopalan C (1962). Effect of nutrition on pregnancy and lactation. Bull WHO 26:203-211.

28. Grande F, Anderson JT and Keys A (1958). Changes of basal metabolic rate in man in semi-starvation and refeeding. J Appl Physiol 12:230-238.

29. Heymsfield SB, Smith J, Kasriel S, Barlow J, Lynn MJ, Nixon D and Lawson DH (1981). Energy malabsorption: measurement and nutritional consequences. Am J Clin Nutr 34:1954-1960.

30. Hudson GJ, John PMV and Paul AA (1980). Variation in the consumption of Gambian foods: The importance of water in relation to energy and protein content. Ecol Food Nutr 10:9-17.

31. Hytten FE and Leitch I (1971). "The Physiology of Human Pregnancy, 2nd edition." Oxford: Blackwell.

32. Hytten FE, Thomson AM and Taggart N (1966). Total body water in normal pregnancy. J Obstet Synaec Brit Cwlth 73:553-561.

33. James WPT and Shetty PS (1982). Metabolic adaptations and energy requirements in developing countries. Human Nutr: Clin Nutr 36C-331-336.

34. James WPT and Trayhurn P (1976). An integrated view of the metabolic and genetic basis for obesity. Lancet 2:770-773.

35. Jansky L (1973). Non-shivering thermogenesis and its thermoregulatory significance. Biol Rev 48:85-132.

36. Jung RT, Campbell RG, James WPT and Callingham BA (1982). Altered hypothalamic and sympathetic responses to hypoglycaemia in familial obesity. Lancet 1: 1043-1046.

37. Jung RT and James WPT (1980). Is obesity metabolic? Br J Hosp Med 24:503-509.

38. Jung RT, Shetty PS, James WPT, Barrand M and Callingham BA (1979). Reduced thermogenesis in obesity. Nature 279:322-323.
39. Karmarkar MG, Kapur J, Deodhar AD and Ramakrishnan CV (1959). Studies on human lactation. Indian J Med Res 47:344-351.
40. Karmarkar MG, Rajalakshmi R and Ramakrishnan CV (1963). Studies on human lactation. I. Effect of dietary protein and fat supplementation on protein, fat and essential amino acid contents of breast milk. Acta Paed Scand 52:473-480.
41. Keys A, Brozek J, Henschel A, Mickelson O and Taylor HL (1950). "The Biology of Human Starvation." Minnesota: Univ. Minnesota Press.
42. Kopelman PG, White N, Pilkington TRE and Jeffcoate SL (1979). Impaired hypothalamic control of prolactin secretion in massive obesity. Lancet 1:747-750.
43. Larson BA, Sinha YN and Vanderlaan WP (1976). Serum growth hormone and prolactin during and after the development of the obese hypoglycaemic syndrome in mice. Endocrinology 98:139-145.
44. Lechtig A, Habicht J-P, Yarborough C, Delgado H, Guzman G and Klein RE (1972). Influence of food supplementation during pregnancy on birth weight in rural populations of Guatemala. Proc. 9th Int Congr Nutr, Mexico, 2:44-52.
45. Lifson N and McClintock R (1966). Theory of use of the turnover rates of body water for measuring energy and material balance. J Theoret Biol 12:46-74.
46. Lunell NO, Persson B and Sterky G (1969). Dietary habits during pregnancy. Acta Obstet Gynecol Scand 48:187-194.
47. Lunn PG, Prentice AM, Austin S and Whitehead RG (1980). Influence of maternal diet on plasma prolactin levels during lactation. Lancet 1:13-14.
48. Maletnlema TN and Bavu JL (1974). Nutrition studies in pregnancy. I. Energy, protein and iron intake in pregnant women in Kisorawe, Tanzania. East Afr Med J 51:515-528.
49. Martinez C and Chavez A (1971). Nutrition and development of infants in poor rural areas. I. Consumption of mother's milk by infants. Nutr Rep Int 4:139-149.
50. Mata LJ, Urrutia JJ and Garcia B (1972). Malnutrition and infection in a rural village of Guatemala. Proc 9th Int Congr Nutr Mexico, 2:175-192.

51. Miller DS (1974). In Burland WH, Samuel PD and Yudkin J (eds): "Obesity." Edinburgh: Churchill Livingstone, pp 160-170.
52. Miller DS and Wise A (1975). Exercise and dietary-induced thermogenesis. Lancet 1:1290.
53. Mora JO, de Navarro L, Clement J, Wagner M, de Paredes B and Herrera MG (1978). The effect of food supplementation on the calorie and protein intake of pregnant women. Nutr Rep Int 17:217-228.
54. N.R.C. (1980). "Recommended Dietary Allowances, 9th revised." Washington DC: National Academy of Sciences, National Research Council.
55. Naismith DJ and Ritchie CD (1975). The effect of breast-feeding and artificial feeding on body weights, skinfold measurements and food intakes of forty-two primiparous women. Proc Nutr Soc 34:116A.
56. Nicholls DG (1979). Brown adipose tissue mitochondria. Biochim Biophys Acta 549:1-29.
57. Norgan NG, Ferro-Luzzi A and Durnin JVGA (1974). The energy and nutrient intake and energy expenditure of 204 New Guinean adults. Phil Trans R Soc Lond B 268:309-348.
58. Ooman HAPC and Malcolm S (1958). Nutrition of the Papuan child. S Pacific Commission Tech Paper 118. Noumea, New Caledonia.
59. Paul AA and Muller EM (1980). Seasonal variations in dietary intake in pregnant and lactating women in a rural Gambian village. In Aebi H and Whitehead RG (eds): "Maternal nutrition during pregnancy and lactation," Bern: Hans Huber, pp 105-116.
60. Paul AA and Southgate DAT (1978). "McCance and Widdowson's The Composition of Foods." 4th edition. London: HMSO.
61. Pittet Ph, Chappins Ph, Acheson K, de Techtermann F and Jequier E (1976). Thermic effect of glucose in obese subjects studied by direct and indirect calorimetry. Br J Nutr 35:281-292.
62. Prentice AM (1980). Variations in maternal dietary intake, birthweight and breast milk output in the Gambia. In Aebi H and Whitehead RG (eds): "Maternal Nutrition During Pregnancy and Lactation," Bern: Hans Huber, pp 167-183.
63. Prentice AM, Lunn PG, Watkinson M and Whitehead RG (1983a). Dietary supplementation of lactating Gambian Women. II. Effect on maternal health, nutritional status and biochemistry. Human Nutr:Clin Nutr 37C:65-74.

64. Prentice AM, Whitehead RG, Roberts SB and Paul AA (1981). Long-term energy balance in child-bearing Gambian women. Am J Clin Nutr 34:2790-2799.
65. Prentice AM, Whitehead RG, Roberts SB, Paul AA, Watkinson M, Prentice A and Watkinson AA (1980). Dietary supplementation of Gambian nursing mothers and lactational performance. Lancet 2:886-888.
66. Prentice AM, Whitehead RG, Watkinson M, Lamb WH and Cole TJ (1983b). Prenatal dietary supplementation of African women and birth weight. Lancet 1:489-492.
67. Rajalakshmi R (1971). Reproductive performance of poor Indian women on a low plane of nutrition. Trop Georgr Med 23:117-125.
68. Rattigan S, Ghisalberti AV and Hartmann PR (1981). Breast milk production in Australian women. Br J Nutr 45:243-249.
69. Rivlin RS and Wolf F (1969). Diminished responsiveness to thyroid hormone in riboflavin-deficient rats. Nature 223:516-517.
70. Roberts SB, Paul AA, Cole TJ and Whitehead RG (1982). Seasonal changes in activity, birth weight and lactational performance in rural Gambian women. Trans Roy Soc Trop Med Hyg 76:668-678.
71. Schoeller DA and van Santen E (1982). Measurement of energy expenditure in humans by doubly labelled water method. J Appl Physiol: Respirat Environ Exercise Physiol 53:955-959.
72. Scholander PF, Hannel HT, Hart JS, Le Messurier DH and Steen J (1958). Cold adaptation in Australian Aborigines. J Appl Physiol 13:211-218.
73. Schutz Y, Lechtig A and Bradfield RB (1980). Energy expenditure and food intakes of lactating women in Guatemala. Am J Clin Nutr 33:892-902.
74. Shetty PS, Jung RT and James WPT (1979). Reduced dietary-induced thermogenesis in obese subjects before and after weight loss. Proc Nutr Soc 38:87A.
75. Shetty PS, Jung RT, James WPT, Barrand M and Callingham BA (1981). Post-prandial thermogenesis in obesity. Clin Sci 60:519-525.
76. Sims LS (1978). Dietary status of lactating women. 1. Nutrient intake from food and from supplements. J Am Diet Ass 73:139-146.
77. Smithells RW, Ankers C, Carver ME, Lennon D, Schorah CJ and Sheppard S (1977). Maternal nutrition in early pregnancy. Br J Nutr 38:497-506.

78. Southgate DAT (1969). Determination of carbohydrate in foods. II. Unavailable carbohydrates. J Sci Fd Agric 20:331-335.
79. Thanangkul O and Amatyakul K (1975). Nutrition of pregnant women in a developing country - Thailand. Am J Dis Child 129:426-427.
80. Thomson AM (1958). Diet in pregnancy. 1. Dietary survey technique and the nutritive value of diets taken by primigravidae. Br J Nutr 12:446-461.
81. Thomson AM, Billewicz WZ, Thompson B and McGregor IA (1966). Body weight changes during pregnancy and lactation in rural African (Gambian) women. J Obstet Gynaecol Br Cwlth 73:724-733.
82. Thomson AM, Hytten FE and Billewicz WZ (1970). The energy cost of human lactation. Br J Nutr 24:565-572.
83. Trayhurn P, Douglas JB and McGuckin MM (1982). Brown adipose tissue thermogenesis is 'suppressed' during lactation in mice. Nature 298:59-60.
84. United Nations University (1979). "Protein-energy Requirements under Conditions Prevailing in Developing Countries: Current Knowledge and Research Needs." Tokyo: UNU.
85. Venkatachalam PS (1962). Maternal nutritional status and its effects on the newborn. Bull WHO 26:193-201.
86. Whichelow MJ (1976). Success and failure of breast feeding in relation to energy intake. Proc Nutr Soc 35:62A.
87. Whitehead RG, Paul AA, Black AE and Wiles SJ (1981). Recommended dietary amounts of energy for pregnancy and lactation in the United Kingdom. UNU Food and Nutr Bull suppl 5:259-265.
88. Whitehead RG, Paul AA and Rowland MGM (1980). Lactation in Cambridge and in The Gambia. In Wharton BA (ed): "Topics in Paediatrics," Tunbridge Wells: Pitman Medical, 2, pp 22-33.
89. Whitehead RG, Rowland MGM, Hutton M, Prentice AM, Muller EM and Paul AA (1978). Factors influencing lactational performance in rural Gambian mothers. Lancet 2:178-181.
90. Widdowson EM (1947). A Study of Individual Children's Diets. Med Res Council Special Rep Series No. 257. London: HMSO.
91. Wyndham CH and Morrison JF (1958). Adjustment to cold of bushmen in the Kalahari Desert. J Appl Physiol 13:219-225.
92. Zahorska-Markiewicz B (1980). Thermic effect of food and exercise in obesity. Europ J Appl Physiol 44:231-235.

Energy Intake and Activity, pages 33–55
© 1984 Alan R. Liss, Inc., 150 Fifth Avenue, New York, NY 10011

MARGINAL INTAKE AND MATERNAL ADAPTATION:
THE CASE OF RURAL TAIWAN

Linda S. Adair

Department of Anthropology
Rice University
Houston, Texas

INTRODUCTION

Many populations throughout the world live with marginal protein and energy intakes but must, nevertheless,
maintain high levels of activity to meet subsistence needs.
Pregnancy and lactation constitute a significant challenge to
the energy balance mechanisms of these populations. By
examining changes in maternal body composition during
pregnancy and lactation, along with birthweights and parameters of post-natal child growth, insight can be gained into
the ways in which such populations continue to demonstrate
reasonable reproductive success in the face of seemingly
marginal intakes. This paper describes changes in maternal
body weight and skinfold thicknesses during pregnancy and
lactation in a rural, marginally nourished population of
Taiwan. Despite caloric intakes considerably below those
recommended in international standards, the population
maintained relatively stable body weights over a long period
of time, and produced healthy offspring with adequate
post-natal growth.

STUDY SITE, DESIGN AND METHODS

The Taiwan data is derived from a longitudinal nutritional intervention field study whose original objective was to
assess the effects of protein supplementation during pregnancy and lactation on the intrauterine and post-natal
growth of offspring. This was a double blind experiment in
which a nutrient dense supplement or placebo could be

provided on a daily basis to a population with a marginal nutritional intake.

The study was carried out by the late Dr. Bacon Chow of the Johns Hopkins School of Hygiene from 1967 to 1973. A group of villages comprise the 27 square mile study site of Suilin township located about 180 miles south of Taipei in west central Taiwan. The climate in the coastal plain area is marked by hot humid summers with maximum temperatures and rainfall in June, July and August, followed by short, mild winters with minimal temperatures and rainfall in December, January and February (Hsieh 1964). Rice agriculture predominates in this economically distressed area. The first annual rice planting takes place in January, and the crop is harvested in June. A second crop is planted in early July and harvested in October or November. Other crops include sweet potatoes (an important winter crop and dietary staple), sugar cane, and peanuts.

Meat is generally not included in the local diet. A preliminary food survey conducted in 1965 found daily protein intakes of 30 to 40 grams from mostly vegetable sources. Caloric intakes were estimated to be in the 1600 to 2000 Kcal range but, based on weighed intakes measured during the course of the study, this may represent an overestimate.

A sample of 294 women was selected from 14 of the Suilin villages. All had previously given birth to at least one child, and planned to have additional children. They ranged in age from 19 to 30 years, had no frank nutritional deficiencies, but had daily protein intakes of less than 40 grams.

Recruitment into the study occurred during the last trimester of pregnancy. Subjects were randomly assigned to groups which were to begin receiving either a nutrient dense supplement (A) or placebo (B) 3 weeks after delivery of the first study infant. A nurse stationed in each of the study villages oversaw the delivery and measured consumption of 2 cans of supplement per day. The A group could potentially receive 800 Kcal and 40 grams of protein from the supplement daily, while the B group received a maximum of 80 Kcal per day. Details of supplement contents have been published elsewhere (McDonald et al. 1981). Each mother gave birth to 2 infants during the study. Mother's weights, triceps, and subscapular skinfolds were measured at regular intervals from the time of recruitment until 15 months after delivery of the second study infant. This design allows for comparison of the outcome of a supplemented and unsupplemented pregnancy in the same woman and for comparisons between the A and B supplement groups.

The following analyses are based on 225 cases selected from the original 294. Subjects were eleminated if they did not give birth to 2 infants over the course of the study, if they moved away, refused the supplement, refused to allow nitrogen balance studies to be performed on their infants, or as a result of infant death. The dropped cases are equally distributed among the A and B groups.

RESULTS

Anthropometric Status of the Population Relative to Standards

Compared to NCHS standards (1966) for women aged 24 to 35, Suilin mothers are small; 23% fell below the 10th centile one month after birth of the first study infant, and only 10% fell above the 50th centile. There seems to have been an overall improvement in the status of both A and B groups with time: 13% of mothers fell below the 10th centile 1 month after the second infant, while 17% were above the 50th.

Caloric Intake

Home dietary assessments became a regular part of the study during the second pregnancy. To measure caloric intake, nurses paid unexpected visits to the participants' homes at meal times once during each trimester of pregnancy and lactation. They weighed the portions of food to be consumed by mothers and took duplicate samples for laboratory analysis of protein, carbohydrates and fat. No inter-meal food consumption data are available. Table 1 presents mean caloric intake from home food and from supplement. The data available does not provide the necessary information to ascertain why all subjects were not surveyed in each trimester. Home food intake values represent 3 meal totals from one day per time period. Supplement intake was calculated from daily intake measurements averaged over the entire time period in question. Caloric intake from the

TABLE 1
MEAN DAILY CALORIC INTAKE (KCAL) FROM HOME FOOD[1] AND
SUPPLEMENT[2] DURING PREGNANCY AND LACTATION

Pregnancy		Group A		Group B		Lactation		Group A		Group B	
		Mean	S.D.	Mean	S.D.			Mean	S.D.	Mean	S.D.
Trimester 1	Home food	1117	344	1211	379	0-2 Months	Home food	1134	299	1319	322
	Supplement	489	184	6	9		Supplement	691	92	24	29
	Total	1606	416	1217	381		Total	1825	330	1343	324
Trimester 2	Home food	1123	318	1228	368	3-5 Months	Home food	1125	322	1288	371
	Supplement	543	190	8	11		Supplement	659	112	29	30
	Total	1666	383	1235	369		Total	1884	357	1316	376
Trimester 3	Home food	1123	312	1151	304	6-8 Months	Home food	1222	327	1366	409
	Supplement	554	178	16	24		Supplement	655	134	37	32
	Total	1678	340	1167	307		Total	1877	377	1403	411
						9-11 Months	Home food	1287	356	1398	410
							Supplement	637	135	37	32
							Total	1924	377	1435	412
						12-15 Months	Home food	1262	324	1269	382
							Supplement	616	173	41	30
							Total	1878	377	1311	389

[1]Estimates based on weighed samples from meals, 1 day per time period
[2]Volume of supplement consumed, measured and recorded twice daily

supplement is, of course significantly higher in the A group
at all times. This accounts for the highly significant A-B
differences in total intake throughout the second pregnancy
and lactation periods. In addition, group B mothers consumed significantly more calories at meals sampled in the
period from birth to 2 months and from 6 to 8 months post-
partum. There is no information on the extent to which the
supplement may have replaced foods usually consumed at
other times of the day. However, the values for total
caloric intakes presented here are comparable to intakes
reported for other pregnant women living in similar economic
circumstances in Taiwan (Table 2). For example, a survey
of Taichung county revealed intakes of 1668 to 1768 kcal per
day (Kao 1980).

TABLE 2

AVERAGE CALORIC INTAKE IN SELECTED AREAS OF TAIWAN

1971	Taipei City	average	2001	Huang et al. (1973)
1974	Taipei City	pregnant ♀	2022	Wu (1974)
1975	Tainan County	♀ age 51	1608	Wang et al. (1977)
1979	Taichung City	pregnant ♀	1768	Kao (1980)
1979	Taichung County	pregnant ♀	1668	Kao (1980)
1977	Taichung County	average	2054	Chiu and Chwang (1978)

Intergroup Comparisons

There are no significant intergroup differences in mean maternal weight, triceps, or subscapular skinfolds at any time during the study. Furthermore, there are no A-B differences in pregnancy weight gain or skinfold changes, nor were there significant differences in weight or skinfold changes during lactation (see Adair et al. 1983b for further details).

Although there are no detectable effects of supplementation on maternal anthropometry, there is evidence of significant supplement effects on pre-natal growth of the offspring. For example, group A second study male offspring weighed 161 g. more than their first study siblings (McDonald et al. 1981). Further evidence of a sex mediated supplementation effect can be seen by comparing sibling-sibling anthropometric correlations in the A and B groups. In the A supplement group, when the second-born member of a sibling pair was male, sibling correlations of weight, length, head circumference, and skinfold thicknesses were low and not statistically significant, while the same correlations in the B groups were on the order of .5. Environmental covariation of siblings due to supplementation of the mother during the gestation of the second study male infants may account for the lack of significant correlations in the A group. There is a significant supplement effect on body proportions measured by Rohrer's index $(wt/1^3)$ in both males and females. Rohrer's index may be a more sensitive indicator of pre-natal development compared to simple anthropometric measures (Mueller and Pollitt 1983).

Thus it appears that the benefits of nutritional supplementation to offspring may accrue without any detectable anthropometric evidence of supplement effects in the mother. The absence of supplement effects on maternal anthropometric variables, and the relatively small effects on offspring, suggest that the Suilin population is well adapted to its marginal energy and protein intakes. To support this assertion, it is necessary to examine evidence of the population's reproductive success. First, mothers gained about 15 to 16% of their pre-pregnant body weight during the second study pregnancy. Such gains are intermediate between women of a frankly malnourished Indian population who gained only about 13% of prepregnant body weight (Venkatchalam et al. 1960), and well nourished British women who gained about 18% of prepregnant body weight (Hytten 1980). Second, infant birth measurements and post-natal growth patterns indicate that the population is doing reasonably well: the mean birth weight of first study male infants (groups A and B combined) was 3070 g, female infants 3025 g. For second study infants: males weighed 3188 g, females 2997 g. Birthweights ranged from 1800 to 4445 g. for first study infants, and from 1590 to 4030 g. for second infants. Only 6 to 7% of infants weighed less than 2500 g. at birth. Post-natal growth shows a pattern typical of marginally nourished populations. Early growth tends to be comparable to the 50th centile of U.S. standards, then begins to fall off by about 6 months of age. This profile of Suilin infants does not, however, represent a severely compromised population.

More can be learned about the nature of the adaptation to low intakes in this population by an examination of maternal anthropometric changes throughout consecutive pregnancy and lactation periods. Since we found no significant A-B differences in maternal anthropometry at any time during pregnancy or lactation, the groups have been combined for the analyses that follow.

PREGNANCY

Due to the high frequency of missing data for the pregnancy period, the maximum sample size representing women with both pre-pregnant measurements and measurements taken close to the time of delivery is 125. There is no reason to suspect that the excluded cases differ in any way from the cases analysed. Pregnancy changes are described for the second study pregnancy only since no pre-pregnant data is available for the first. It is possible however, to make inter-pregnancy comparisons for the 2 months prior to delivery.

Mean pregnancy weight gain, from the last pre-pregnant measurement to within 30 days of delivery was 7.63 kg. Weight velocity, .31 kg/month in the first trimester, reached a maximum of 1.46 kg/month in the second trimester, then declined slightly to 1.11 kg/month in the final trimester. Maternal factors significantly correlated with pregnancy weight gain include pre-pregnant weight, height, and relative weight assessed by the Quetelet index. Weight gain was not significantly related to maternal age, parity, or gender of the fetus being carried. These relationships can be illustrated in another way: the 64 mothers who gained in excess of the mean weight (7.63 kg) were 1.7 cm taller, weighed 1.6 kg more immediately after delivery, and gave birth to infants weighing 258 grams more than mothers who gained less than the mean. However, the mothers who gained more weight during pregnancy had lower mean pre-pregnant weight for height. These differences are all significant at the .05 level or less.

Inter-pregnancy (P1-P2) comparisons show that weights one month prior to the delivery of each study infant are highly correlated, but mothers weighed 2.09 kg more prior to the birth of the second infant than prior to the birth of the first.

Some of the components of pregnancy weight gain can be estimated (Table 3). For example, mean second study

TABLE 3

COMPONENTS OF PREGNANCY WEIGHT GAIN

	Suilin		"Average"[1]	
Age	28.6		24	
Pre-pregnant weight	48.7kg		54kg	
Height	154.7cm		158cm	
Pregnancy weight gain (PWG)	7.63		12.5kg	
Components:	Value	% PWG	Value	% PWG
Fetus (birthweight)	3.095	40.6	3.300	26.4
Placenta	.535	7.0	.650	5.2
Fluids lost at birth	1.082[2]	14.1		
			8.55*	68.4
Maternal tissue	2.592[3]	34.0		
*maternal stores			3.5	28
tissue fluid			1.3	10.4
blood			1.5	12
uterus + breasts			1.1	8.8

1. From Hytten (1980)
2. Weight loss at birth - (fetus + placenta)
3. Post-partum weight - pre-pregnant weight

infant birth weights represent about 40.6% of the total weight gain. Placental weight (mean=535 g) accounts for an additional 7%. Maternal tissue weight increases can be estimated as the difference between pre-pregnant weight and the first post-partum measurement taken within 48 hours of delivery (2.59 kg, or 34% of pregnancy weight gain). The difference between total weight loss at birth and weight of the fetus plus placenta most probably represents maternal fluid losses at birth. Comparison with Hytten's (1980) well nourished "average" woman (who, based on cumulated hospital records, is 24 years of age, weighs 54 kg prior to pregnancy, and gains 12.5 kg during pregnancy) shows that the biggest difference between the 2 populations is primarily in the amount of maternal tissue accumulated during pregnancy, most probably in the form of adipose tissue.

Maternal skinfold changes during pregnancy reveal more about adipose tissue reserves. Skinfold measurements showed a wide range of individual variability (Figure 1);

Figure 1 Mean maternal skinfold thicknesses during pregnancy and lactation (Adair et al. 1983a).

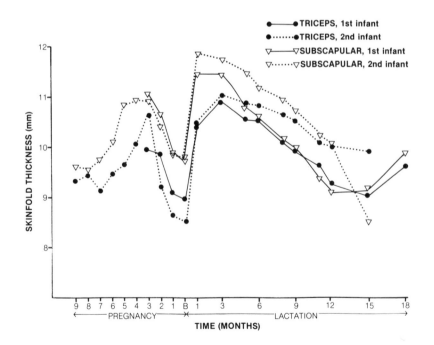

generally they increased early in pregnancy, then declined in the last trimester. Net increases in skinfold thicknesses during pregnancy were associated with higher pregnancy weight gains, but less subcutaneous fat prior to pregnancy. These observations are in accord with those of Taggert et al. (1967) who found larger skinfold increases among women who were underweight very early in pregnancy rather than overweight.

LACTATION

The usual duration of lactation in the Suilin population is 15 months. The overall pattern of weight change during lactation is illustrated in Figure 2 which shows mean maternal weights throughout the study. Patterns of change are remarkably similar during the first (L1) and second (L2) lactation periods, but there is a consistent and significant weight difference of 1.2 to 1.6 kg. The magnitude of the L1-L2 increases was the same in mothers who received the A

Figure 2 Mean maternal weights during pregnancy and lactation (Adair et al. 1983a).

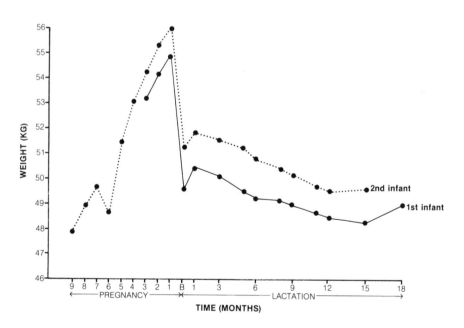

supplement or the placebo. The increase cannot be explained by age or parity of the mother. A breakdown of
maternal weights one month after the birth of the first study
infant and again 15 months after the birth of the second
infant revealed that there is a significant secular trend in
weight: mothers who entered the study later weighed more.
This trend may well be due to improvements in the overall
socioeconomic status of rural Taiwanese populations during
the time covered by the 6 year study.

Returning to patterns of weight change during lactation: there was a consistent weight gain among mothers in
the first post-partum month, followed by weight loss during
lactation. Weight velocities were maximal 3 to 6 months after
birth (when women lost about .3 kg/month), then declined to
the end of lactation. Net weight loss from birth to 15
post-partum months was significantly greater in L2 (1.93 kg)
compared to L1 (1.23 kg).

By looking at mean weights, important individual patterns of weight change are obscured. About one-third of
the mothers gained rather than lost weight during lactation.
Accordingly, weight gain and loss groups were defined based
on net changes during the first 12 post-partum months.
The 12 month time period was chosen to avoid the confounding effects of weaning in the 12 to 15 month period. Figure
3 shows mean weights at 1,3,6,9 and 12 months among women
who lost or gained weight in L1 or L2. As indicated by the
nearly parallel loss or gain lines, L1 changes are replicated
in L2. The magnitude of weight gains experienced by 32% of
mothers during L1 and 36% of mothers during L2 is about
1.6 kg. Net weight gains were achieved by more substantial
increases in the first 3 post-partum months, followed by a
plateau throughout the remainder of lactation. The more
frequent pattern, however, was weight loss. Mothers with
net weight losses had smaller immediate post-partum gains
followed by more precipitous weight losses from 1 to 15
months after birth. Furthermore, these mothers lost significantly more weight during L2 compared to L1.

Sixty-nine percent of mothers replicated their own L1
weight change patterns during L2. The most frequent
pattern was weight loss during both L1 and L2, but it is
interesting to note that 18% of mothers gained weight during
both L1 and L2. Compared with mothers who gained weight
in both L1 and L2, mothers who lost weight in both lactation

Figure 3 Mean maternal weight among women who lost vs. gained weight during 12 months of lactation (Adair et al. 1983a).

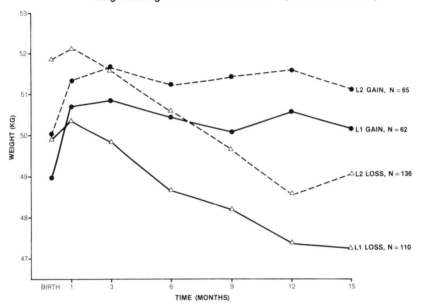

periods had significantly lower pre-pregnant weight-for-heights, but higher pregnancy weight gains. The groups are not differentiated by maternal height, age, parity, or relative weight immediately after birth.

Skinfold changes generally paralleled weight changes (Figure 1). Minimum skinfold thicknesses were achieved at both triceps and subscapular sites immediately after birth, and were followed by a dramatic increase in skinfolds be-tween 2 and 30 post-partum days. Maximum skinfold thick-nesses occurred between 1 and 3 months after birth, then declined slowly thereafter. But, as with weight, not all mothers lost subcutaneous fat during lactation. In fact, during L1, 56% of mothers experienced net gains in triceps fat and 46% gained subscapular fat between birth and 12 post-partum months. During L2, 80% gained triceps and 52% gained subscapular fat. All mothers initially increased skinfold thicknesses in the first 3 post-partum months, but those with net triceps fat losses lost fat at a greater rate from 3 to 12 post-partum months. A similar pattern was seen at the subscapular site. Initial increases were largely limited to the first post-partum month, followed by a plateau or slight decline among mothers with net skinfold thickness gains, and a sharper decline in the net loss group. Correlations between triceps and subscapular skinfolds during lactation ranged from .6 to .7, while skinfold-weight correlations were in the .3 to .5 range.

Lactation weight, triceps and subscapular changes were negatively correlated with pregnancy changes, i.e. mothers who accumulated more adipose tissue during pregnancy lost more during lactation.

FACTORS WHICH INFLUENCE MATERNAL ANTHROPOMETRIC CHANGES

Many other investigators have reported seasonal differences in body composition related to cycles of agricultural activity, food availability, and morbidity. For example, Prentice et al. (1981) found that their lactating subjects in the Gambia gained weight during the dry season, but lost weight during the rainy season when food shortages are common.

Seasonal effects are important determinants of anthropometric changes in the Taiwanese population as well (Adair and Pollitt 1983). Tests for seasonality included a comparison of mean monthly weights or skinfold thicknesses by a one way ANOVA using pooled data from consecutive years, and t-tests of measurements taken relative to warm or cold season births. The "cold" season comprises the 4 consecutive months with mean monthly temperatures below 21°C (December-March), while the "warm" season includes the 4 consecutive months with mean monthly temperatures above 27°C (June-September).

There is no apparent birth season in the population. Although the number of births per month ranged from 12 to 21, there is no significant deviation from an expected uniform distribution.

Birth weights of first and second study infants by month of the year are shown in Figure 4 with mean monthly temperature and rainfall data for Taiwan, the closest city in the same ecozone for which published data are available. For first study infants, there were both monthly differences

Figure 4 Top: Mean monthly temperature and rainfall for Tainan. Bottom: Mean infant birthweights by month of the year (Adair and Pollitt 1983).

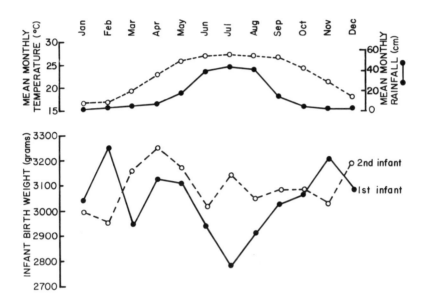

in birth weight (F=2.01, p=.03) and differences in birth weight between infants born during warm vs cold seasons (t=2.27, p=.025). The lowest mean birthweights occurred during the hot, rainy summer months. Furthermore, a significantly disproportionate number of infants who weighed less than one standard deviation (380 g) below the mean birthweight (3050 g) were born between May and October. There were no significant seasonal differences among second study infants.

Although there were no differences in birth length, infants born during the warm season had a significantly lower relative weight (assessed by Rohrer's) than those born during the cold season (t=4.49, p<.01). No significant effects of season on birthweight, birth length or Rohrer's index were apparent among second study infants.

Turning to seasonal differences in maternal variables, it was found that weight and subcapular (but not triceps) skinfolds measured within 30 days prior to delivery of first study infants differ significantly by season of birth. Just prior to the second pregnancy, seasonal differences were significant only at the subscapular site. In general, mothers were fatter prior to cold season births than prior to warm season births, but total pregnancy weight gain did not vary by season of birth.

Figure 5 Top: Mean monthly temperature and rainfall for Tainan. Bottom: Mean maternal weights by month of the year (Adair and Pollitt 1983).

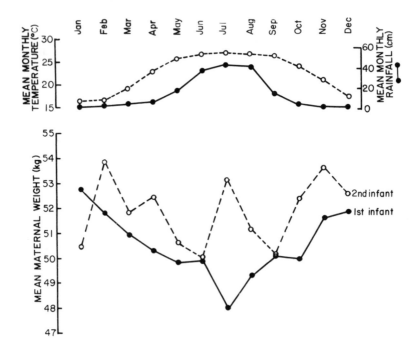

After birth, there are clear seasonal differences in maternal weight and skinfold thicknesses: Figure 5 shows mean maternal weight one month after delivery along with temperature and rainfall data. Mothers weighed more and also had thicker triceps and subscapular skinfolds during the colder months, irrespective of their stage of lactation (Table 4). To follow changes in weight that occur during

TABLE 4

MATERNAL ANTHROPOMETRY RELATIVE TO WARM VERSUS COLD
SEASON BIRTHS

	First Infant				Second Infant			
	Warm		Cold		Warm		Cold	
	n	X	n	X	n	X	n	X
MATERNAL WEIGHT (kg)								
pre-delivery	45	53.40	54	56.04*	33	55.13	41	56.67
birth	66	48.84	66	50.51**	57	50.94	69	51.59
1 month	67	49.39	64	51.87*	57	51.64	68	51.98
3 months	67	49.53	67	51.21	56	51.93	67	51.76
6 months	65	49.87	66	48.79	55	51.81	63	50.69
9 months	62	49.46	64	49.75	54	50.50	65	50.30
12 months	52	47.63	56	49.75*	53	48.87	62	50.35
WEIGHT CHANGES (kg)								
birth-1 month	66	.56	64	1.33*	57	.69	68	.31
1-3 months	67	.14	64	- .60*	65	.23	67	- .30
3-6 months	65	.52	66	-2.45**	55	- .28	63	-1.16*
6-9 months	62	- .68	64	.35**	54	-1.20	63	- .33*
9-12 months	52	-1.72	56	.51**	53	-1.65	62	.08**
birth-12 months	51	-1.01	55	- .74	53	-2.08	62	-1.28
pregnancy					33	7.72	41	7.43
TRICEPS (mm)								
pre-delivery	44	8.7	54	9.4	33	8.3	41	9.4
birth	66	8.6	65	9.5	57	7.9	69	8.7
1 month	66	10.0	63	11.2*	57	9.8	68	10.5
3 months	67	10.5	65	11.3	55	10.8	66	11.0
6 months	64	11.3	66	9.7**	55	11.3	63	10.5
9 months	62	10.5	64	9.6	54	10.2	65	10.5
12 months	52	8.7	56	10.0*	52	9.0	62	10.5*
SUBSCAPULAR (mm)								
pre-delivery	44	9.1	54	10.8**	33	9.0	41	10.9**
birth	66	8.8	65	10.5**	57	9.0	69	10.2*
1 month	66	11.1	63	12.5*	57	11.0	68	12.1*
3 months	67	11.0	65	12.6**	55	11.5	66	12.0
6 months	64	11.5	66	10.1*	55	11.3	63	11.2
9 months	62	10.7	64	9.7	54	10.5	65	11.0
12 months	52	8.8	56	10.0*	54	8.8	62	11.2**

*T-test (warm vs. cold season) $p<.05$ ** $p<.01$

lactation, Figure 6 plots mean maternal weights 1,3,6,9 and 12 months after births which occurred either during warm or cold seasons. During L1, mothers who gave birth during the warm season weighed significantly less just after birth and at 1 and 3 months post-partum compared to women who gave birth during the cold season. Following warm season

Figure 6 Mean maternal weight 1, 3, 6, 9 and 12 months after warm or cold season births (Adair and Pollitt 1983).

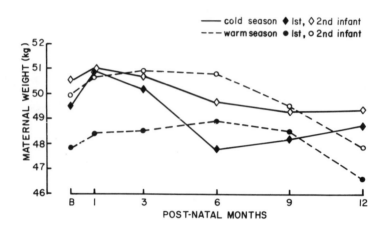

births, mothers gained weight through the first 6 post-partum months (as they moved into the cold season), then began to lose weight, reaching a minimum in the next warm season 12 months after the birth. In contrast, following cold season births, mothers lost weight over the first 6 post-partum months, reaching a minimum, for them, during the warm season. They then gained weight from 6 to 12 months post-partum (moving back into the cold season). Net changes for the entire 12 month post-partum period were not significantly different following warm versus cold season births.

Similar trends were apparent for L2. Although differences in attained weight were not significant following warm versus cold season births, weight changes during lactation did differ significantly by season, following the same pattern described for L1 (Table 4). Seasonal differences are also apparent at triceps and subscapular skinfold sites in both L1 and L2, lending support to the notion that seasonal changes in weight represent altered maternal energy stores. It is apparent that seasonal factors contribute significantly to maternal body composition changes during pregnancy and lactation, and also influence infant birth weights. Regardless of lactation status, mothers weighed more and had thicker triceps and subscapular skinfolds just before and up to 3 months after cold season compared to warm season births. Moreover, infants born during the colder, winter months weighed significantly more than those born during the summer.

Effects of season during the second pregnancy and lactation period are less striking. This may be due, in part, to a sampling bias. The July second study sample (n=12) is smaller than most other months, and taller mothers are disproportionately represented in this group. This may account for the relatively high mean maternal weights and infant birthweights in that month relative to either adjacent months or first study sample data. In addition, the population may have become less susceptible to environmental effects in the latter years of the study. A secular trend in weight was documented earlier: mothers who entered the study later weighed more. Furthermore, overall nutritional stratus of the population improved with time, as judged by the decreasing number of women whose weights-for-height fell below the NCHS 10th centile (Adair et al. 1983a).

Clearly, seasonal variables consititute a significant challenge to the energy balance mechanisms of the Suilin population, though the challenge may vary in magnitude and effect from year to year. The underlying factors which can best account for seasonal maternal and infant body composition changes include:

1. Seasonal changes in energy expenditure due to the demands of the agricultural cycle. Increased work output is required during harvesting and planting of rice and sweet potatoes.
2. Changes in food availability and quality. Winter harvests of sweet potatoes and other vegetables could significantly improve diets during the winter months while, for example, supplement consumption remained constant year round.
3. Changes in morbidity, particularly gastrointestinal illnesses, can both increase nutrient needs and impair nutrient utilization. Although no published data on seasonal differences in morbidity for the Sui Lin area has been found, analogy with other published data leads to a prediction of a higher incidence of gastrointestinal illness during the

rainy season (Poskett 1972; Waldmann 1973; Chen et al. 1979; Trowbridge and Newton 1979).

Data from the Sui Lin Study do not answer these specific questions, but the study clearly documents the impact of seasonality on maternal energy reserves during pregnancy and lactation and on intrauterine growth.

Another important factor found to determine the course of maternal anthropometric changes in Suilin mothers during lactation is growth of their infants. There is a consistent tendency for higher infant weight and length velocities to be associated with higher maternal weight at the beginning of lactation, and weight gains or only small weight losses during lactation. For example, correlations between maternal weight changes from 6 to 9 and from 9 to 12 post-partum months and average infant weight velocity in those same trimesters fall between .25 and .35.

In light of the Frisch hypothesis (Frisch and McArthur 1974; Frisch 1978), there was also interest in investigating the relationship between fatness and birth intervals in the Suilin population. The mean birth interval was 758 + 163 days, and ranged from 392 to 1445 days. Birth interval was positively correlated with mother's age at the birth of the second infant, but unrelated to parity. In general, fatter mothers had longer birth intervals. This is shown by the significant correlation between birth interval and maternal relative weight just after the birth of the second infant and by the fact that maternal weight increments from one lacta-tion period to the next were higher in mothers with long (upper tercile) versus short (lower tercile) birth intervals. This relationship may be most simply explained by suggest-ing that the longer a mother has without the stress of pregnancy and lactation, the more likely she is to establish a positive energy balance and thus gain weight.

SUMMARY AND CONCLUSIONS

To summarize the major points presented thus far:

1. Based on weighed food intakes from 3 meals per day, the Suilin population is marginally nour-ished, consuming fewer calories and less protein

than is recommended in international standards for pregnant and lactating women.

2.   Suilin mothers have low weight for height relative to U.S. NCHS standards.

3.   Substantial seasonal variation in maternal weight, skinfold thicknesses, and infant birthweights further attest to the stressful nature of the environment in which the population lives.

4.   Despite their size and marginal dietary intakes Suilin women:

   a.   show no effects of nutrition supplementation on body weight or skinfold thicknesses;

   b.   do not show the weight losses with age or parity that are typical of more severely malnourished populations;

   c.   experience moderate increases in weight and skinfold thicknesses over the course of the 2 studied pregnancy and lactation periods; and

   d.   tend to return to their non-stressed states over time. For example, greater pregnancy weight gains, and thus higher energy reserves at the onset of lactation, are associated with greater losses of weight and skinfold thickness during lactation. Furthermore, weight and subcutaneous fat loss during the summer months are regained during the cooler, dryer winters.

5.   The population exhibits reproductive success as evidenced by the low incidence of low birth weight infants, low child mortality, and adequate child growth performance.

Conclusions based on these observations are that the population is well adapted to its marginal nutrient intakes, and individuals are able to maintain long term energy balance. The adaptation appears to be characterized by a degree of opportunism made possible by hormonal and metabolic changes that are characteristic of pregnancy and lactation. For example, skinfold thicknesses increased early in pregnancy when the metabolic demands made by the developing fetus were relatively low. Then maternal fat losses characterize the last trimester of pregnancy when the fetus lays down its own body fat reserves. Laboratory studies have shown that fat deposition is facilitated by the high progesterone levels typical of pregnancy. During the last trimester, rising estradiol levels act antagonistically, and fat deposition decreases (Naismith 1980). Furthermore, human placental lactogen is secreted in increasing amounts through pregnancy, and serves to stimulate fat mobilization (Strange and Swyer 1974; Williams and Coltart 1978) and promote peripheral resistance to insulin (Grumbach et al. 1968).

Following a precipitous drop in skinfold thicknesses at birth, there is a marked increase in both skinfolds and weight during the first post-partum month. These changes have also been observed in well nourished populations, but are not as dramatic. The basis of rapid puerperal changes is poorly understood. Although tissue hydration and compressability may vary immediately after birth, these factors alone cannot account for the observed increases in weight and skinfolds. Rather, this may be another period of opportunism resulting in rapid subcutaneous fat deposition. Mothers may have developed a high degree of metabolic efficiency late in pregnancy when fetal and placental demands are high. Immediately after birth, mothers no longer need to meet the metabolic demands of the placenta, early milk production is low, and total energy intake is increased relative to the third trimester of pregnancy. These factors, along with rapid hormonal shifts, could favor rapid fat deposition in the first post-partum month. Then, as the demands of lactation increase, these stores could be called upon. It is interesting to recall that it was primarily the changes in the first post-partum month that determined the course of weight and skinfold changes during lactation. Furthermore, child growth rates were related to maternal weight at the beginning of lactation. For marginally nourished populations, then, this early, rapid, post-natal accumulation of fat could be highly significant in the context of adaptation.

What lessons does the Suilin study hold for those interested in the study of energy balance in human populations? First, there is an increasing body of literature which points to the ability of marginally nourished populations to maintain energy balance over long periods of time despite changes associated with pregnancy, lactation and seasonality. The excellent work of Prentice (1981) and his colleagues in the Gambia and of J.V.G.A. Durnin (1980) in New Guinea has been central to the recognition of this phenomenon. The Suilin data, although originally collected to test a different set of hypotheses, show strong parallels with the Gambia data and further substantiate hypotheses about long term adaptation to marginal food intake. Furthermore, the existence of marked effects of seasonality in a climate like that of the Taiwanese coastal plain illustrate the importance of considering season whenever energy balance studies or nutrition supplementation protocols are carried out.

Second, recognizing the ability of populations like those in Taiwan and the Gambia to develop effective adaptations to marginal food intake may result in changed conceptions of what constitutes populations nutritionally at risk. Caloric intakes in the range of 1200-1800 kcal/day in the Suilin population were capable of supporting pregnancy and lactation without excessive infant mortality or poor growth.

Third, the Taiwan study with its large sample size and longitudinal design provides an excellent data base for the analysis of changes which occur over the course of several pregnancy and lactation periods in the same woman. Body weight and skinfold thicknesses provide clear evidence of long term energy balance mechanisms at work. This type of data base is important for the generation of new hypotheses about the exact nature of the energy balance mechanisms central to the adaptations of marginally nourished populations.

REFERENCES

1. Adair LS, Pollitt E and Mueller WH (1983a). Changes in maternal anthropometry during pregnancy and lactation. Hum Biol (In press).
2. Adair LS, Pollitt E and Mueller WH (1983b). The Bacon Chow Study: Effect of nutritional supplementation on maternal anthropometric changes during pregnancy and lactation. Brit J Nutr (In press).
3. Adair LS and Pollitt E (1983). Seasonal variation in maternal body dimensions and infant birthweights. Am J Phys Anthr (In press 62:00).
4. Chen LC, Chowdhury AKMA and Huffman SF (1979). Seasonal Dimensions of Energy-Protein Malnutrition in Rural Bangladesh: The Role of Agriculture, Dietary Practices, and Infection. Ecol Food Nutr 8:75-87.
5. Chiu CH and Chwang LC (1978). Dietary survey in the endemic mottled enamel area of central Taiwan. J Chinese Nutr Soc 3:29.

6. Durnin JVGA (1980). Food consumption and energy balance during pregnancy and lactation in New Guinea. In Aebi H and RG Whitehead (eds): "Maternal Nutrition During Pregnancy and Lactation." Bern: Hans Huber. p. 86.
7. Frisch RE and McArthur J (1974). Menstrual cycles: Fatness as a determinant of minimum weight for height necessary for their maintenance or onset. Science 185:949-51.
8. Frisch RE (1978). Population, food intake and fertility. Science 199:22-30.
9. Grumbach MM, Kaplan SL, Isciarra JJ and Burr IM (1968). Chorionic growth hormone-prolactin (CGP): secretion, disposition, biologic activity in man and postulated function as the "growth hormone" of the second half of pregnancy. Ann N.Y. Acad Sci 148:501-31.
10. Hsieh CM (1964). Taiwan Ilha Formosa: A geography in perspective. Washington: Butterworths.
11. Haung PC, Wei SN and Hung MH (1973). Food consumption survey in Yen-Pin section, Taipei City. J Formosan Med Assn 72:427.
12. Hytten FE (1980). Nutritional aspects of human pregnancy. In Aebi H and Whitehead RG (eds). "Maternal Nutrition During Pregnancy and Lactation." Bern: Hans Huber. p. 27.
13. Kao MD (1980). Application of the EGR assay in evaluating riboflavin nutritional status of pregnant women in the central part of Taiwan. J Chin Nutr Soc 5:41.
14. McDonald EC, Pollitt E, Hsueh AM and Sherwyn R (1981). The Bacon Chow Study: Maternal nutritional supplementation and the birthweight of offspring. Am J Clin Nutr 34:2133-44.
15. Mueller WH and Pollitt E (1983). The Bacon Chow Study: Effects of nutrition supplementation on sibling-sibling anthropometric correlations. Human Biol 54:455-60.
16. Naismith DJ (1980). Endocrine factors in the control of nutrient utilization during human pregnancy. In Aebi H and Whitehead RG (eds): "Maternal Nutrition During Pregnancy and Lactation." Bern: Hans Huber, p. 16-26.
17. National Center for Health Statistics (1966). Weight by height and age of adults. Vtl Hlth Stat Series 11, No. 14.

18. Poskett EM (1972). Seasonal variation in infection and malnutrition in a rural pediatric clinic in Uganda. Trans R Soc Trop Med Hyg 66:931-936.
19. Prentice AM, Whitehead RG, Roberts SB and Paul AA (1981). Long term energy balance in childbearing Gambian women. Am J Clin Nutr 34:2790-99.
20. Strange RC and Swyer GIM (1974). The effect of human placental lactogen on adipose tissue lypolysis. J Endocrinol 61:147-52.
21. Taggert NR, Holliday RM, Billewicz WZ, Hytten FE and Thomson AM (1967). Changes in skinfolds during pregnancy. Brit J Clin Nutr 21:439-51.
22. Trowbridge FL and Newton LH (1979). Seasonal changes in malnutrition and diarrheal disease among pre-school children in El Salvador. Am J Trop Med Hyg 28:135-141.
23. Venkatachalam PS, Shankar K and Golapan G (1960). Changes in body weight and body composition during pregnancy. Ind J Med Research 48:511-17.
24. Waldmann E (1973). Seasonal variation in malnutrition in Africa. Trans R Soc Trop Med Hyg 67:431-4.
25. Wang CM, Chwang LC, Chiu CH, Lin CC and Yang TH (1977). Dietary survey in the endemic blackfoot disease area. J Chinese Nutr Soc 2:13.
26. Williams C and Coltart AM (1978). Adipose tissue metabolism in pregnancy: the lypolytic effect of human placental lactogen. Br J Obstet Gynaecol 85:43-46.
27. Wu TH (1974). Dietary Intake of Pregnant Women in Taipei City, Annual Report, Nat Sci Council Vol. 43.

Energy Intake and Activity, pages 57–76
© *1984 Alan R. Liss, Inc., 150 Fifth Avenue, New York, NY 10011*

AUTO-REGULATORY PROCESSES TO MAINTAIN ENERGY BALANCE IN THE INDIVIDUAL*

Sheldon Margen

Public Health Nutrition Program
University of California at Berkeley
Berkeley, California

HISTORICAL PERSPECTIVE

The primary question considered in this paper is how most adult animals and humans are able to maintain constant weight and body composition over prolonged periods of time, in spite of relatively free access to food and activity. Stated another way, how is it possible for energy balance to equal zero over long periods of time in the absence of growth, pregnancy, and lactation? The author believes that the answer lies in understanding the theory of auto-regulatory processes to maintain energy balance.

It is clear that scientific thinking and hypothesis building are dynamic processes whereby one builds upon his own discoveries and those of colleagues from other disciplines. This has certainly been true with regard to the theory of the autoregulatory, homeostatic nature of energy balance. The seeds of this theory were planted almost at the beginning of "nutritional science" and, over time, questions and answers about it and other theories have contributed to the body of knowledge available today.

---

*This is a shortened version of the original paper. In order to fully understand the hypothesis presented, the reader may request a copy of the unabridged version from the author.

Mott-Smith reviewed the history of the concept of energy in an exciting book published in 1934. In 1902 Max Rubner published an important monograph based on his brilliant conceptualization and experimentation and pointed out that either protein, fat, or carbohydrate could be used for heat production in the body. He also calculated the exact caloric equivalent per gram of each foodstuff. At about the same time, Neumann, another physiologist, was attempting to explain his observation that weight could apparently be maintained on two different levels of energy intake (Neumann 1902). He proposed that the mechanism involved converted excess energy intakes directly into heat and he named this phenomenon luxuskonsumption. Although his data might not be particularly convincing today, his explanation for many of the observed phenomena is extremely important in the evolution of theories of energy balance. In fact, it was the work of Rubner and Neumann that finally led Miller (1967) to propose the term 'dietary induced thermogenesis' which, at least in his initial concept, included both specific dynamic action and luxuskonsumption.

By the turn of the century it was agreed that the law of conservation of energy not only covered the transfer of electrical energy into heat, but that radiant energy, chemical energy, work, and virtually any other type of energy were also transformed into heat by the animal organism. This led to the classic equation which states that energy intake (E_i) is equal to energy output (E_o); ($E_i = E_o$) and E_o equals BMR (or RMR) + activity + dietary induced thermogenesis (DIT). Most investigators believed that DIT included only specific dynamic action, but a few others continued to accept the addition of luxuskonsumption to this concept. Since the basal or resting metabolic rate could be determined quite easily, and it appears that the DIT did not contribute a great deal to the intake/output equation (although many authors have used DIT to account for otherwise unexplained variations), much of the physiological work turned to defining the efficiency of work.

The most significant initial work in this area was that of Atwater and Benedict (1903) who measured heat production in men working on bicycle ergometers inside a respiration calorimeter. In these experiments the efficiency of human work, expressed by the ratio of work performed to "chemical energy" spent, ranged from 13-21%.

Since 1913, and particularly since World War II, there has been a tremendous resurgence of interest in human energy metabolism and one of the primary questions has been whether or not it is "regulated." Passmore (1971) was one of the first to conclude that, based upon more general considerations, human body weight must be regulated; however, this was by no means a universal point of view. In a symposium held in the early 1970's, the participants were unable to conclude whether or not energy was a regulated phenomenon in humans (Vigy et al. 1973). The question is probably misphrased because of the loose use of the word 'regulation.' Perhaps the real issue is whether an adequate theoretical basis exists for understanding how adult body weight is maintained. Obviously body weight can be maintained in only one of two ways: either by alteration of intake or by alteration of output. But what is the empirical and theoretical evidence to explain weight maintenance, and the fact that body weight does not change in a linear manner when calories are added or removed, but rather in a curvilinear fashion that indicates some type of adaptation is taking place due to alterations in caloric intake? It is these phenomena which this paper attempts to reconcile.

THEORETICAL AND STATISTICAL CONSIDERATIONS

The model proposed for the "explanation" of the regulation of energy balance in man is based upon newer probability (stochastic) theory, rather than the deterministic model previously attempted (but found wanting). Space does not allow the development of these concepts but the reader is referred to three excellent books on the subject (Box and Jenkins 1976; Howard 1971; Chatfield 1975).

In examining the model, we find a phenomenon of co-variance between two values z_t and z_{t+k}, separated by k units of time (called the auto co-variance at lag k). This is known as auto-correlation and its presence indicates that one is dealing with a regulated process. This helps to determine the nature and extent of the regulation.

PRIOR MODELS USED TO EXPLAIN ENERGY BALANCE

Examination of all the models which have been suggested to explain the constancy of weight gain or the regulation of energy balance would go far beyond the purpose of this paper. However, a few important theories will be considered and some of their limitations discussed. One of the first and most important papers written was by Durnin (1961). In his study of 69 individual subjects, he measured intake and expenditure of energy during 7 consecutive days. The correlation coefficient was determined for (1) the intake and expenditure of calories for the same day; (2) the intake and expenditure of the previous day; and (3) the energy expenditure of two days previously. The significance of the difference between the mean daily calorie intake and expenditure over 7 days was also analyzed. The results indicate that the then-current theory of appetite being a regulator in humans was unlikely to be true since there was no significant correlation between any of the above factors. Durnin stated that "the factors regulating this control from day-to-day would seem to be much more gross in action" (1961, p305). This exploded some prior work which had suggested that there were correlations, but that they were separated by up to a week.

The following year, Miller and Payne (1962) demonstrated that weight maintenance could be achieved in rats and pigs over a wide range of caloric regimens. It was concluded, therefore, that food energy may be converted directly into heat. They did not actually build a model however, and much of the discussion had to do with the role of protein in regulation.

Because of the lack of correlation, some investigators began to question whether the constant weight really represented energy balance or whether this apparent balance was achieved at the cost of unrecognizable changes in body composition. This led to consideration of the contrast between body fat and fat-free body mass which was discussed in a paper by Pitts (1979).

The first clear approach to modeling, in an attempt to explain energy balance, is seen in the paper of Payne and Dugdale (1977). They suggest a homeostochastic model for energy balance and homeostasis. At the time their paper was published, there was no adequate theoretical basis for understanding how adult body weight is regulated. They agreed that weight in normal individuals, even when averaged over periods of days or weeks, may remain fairly constant even though energy intake and expenditures are not balanced. They recognized that regulation might occur but stated that the problem is further complicated by the fact that:

> Even among people in similar occupations, there is a wide range of food intakes (Edholm, Adam, Healy, Wolff, Godlsmith and Best, 1970) and of body weights and compositions; all of which seem to be relatively stable. Nevertheless, overfeeding and underfeeding experiments have shown that individuals can achieve a new equilibrium after considerable changes in food intake, while in some developing countries the poor people have stable body weights on intakes well below those which are common in richer countries. The homeostatic mechanisms relating energy balance to body weight and composition obviously allow considerable variability between persons as well as a wide range of individual adaptability (p 525).

Their thesis is very close to the one set out in this paper, but the models they develop are somewhat unclear. Although Payne and Dugdale state that their models were stochastic in nature (having a mean and a given variability, and being subject to a degree of uncertainty) they assume that all the models are based upon a simple equation. At the end of each day the tissue metabolism and activity energy are subtracted from food energy intake to arrive at energy balance. If the balance is positive, the energy is stored; if negative, the energy will be withdrawn. In either case, at the end of the day the body weight will be changed. The models are not mathematical, but rather are compartments with a set of rules for transfer of energy between those compartments. They have apparently used a digital computer to test their model and have begun with a simple two compartment (fat/non-fat) configuration. The two compartment model was then broken down into three, and ultimately four compartments. The models do not possess a specific type of regulatory mechanism but they do predict that, within certain limits, changes in food intake would lead to new equilibrium.

Payne and Dugdale realize the limitations of their model. Among these they indicate that "no account is taken of possible differences in efficiency of energy deposition for diets of varying compositions" (1977, p. 533). In addition, although they tend to predict certain effects of diet on body composition, they address neither the reasons why the body maintains equilibrium at different levels of energy input and output, nor the potential nature of the regulation.

The model which comes closest to that developed by Sukhatme and Margen (1982) is one designed by Garby (1982a; 1982b). With particular reference to the control of energy intake and expenditure in the regulation of energy balance, Garby's model utilizes the conventional observations that energy is exchanged between the body and its surroundings, and that it is transformed within the body. The most important assumption is that the processes underlying these transactions can be controlled so that, in spite of external perturbations, one or several of the manifestations are regulated to within relatively constant values. Garby builds an interesting and elaborate series of control and feedback systems. He states that:

> Perhaps the most important consequence of the model is the prediction that, if the local feedbacks are important, regulation of the potentials takes place by varying the efficiency of the energy transaction process.

He goes on to say:

> The model does not predict that food energy intake is under precise control or, which amounts to the same thing, that the set point elements are critical for the functioning of the model. The model does not contain explicit mechanisms for regulating the body energy content and does not explain how or where the regulation might take place.

AUTO-REGULATORY HOMEOSTATIC NATURE OF ENERGY BALANCE

The data upon which the theory of the auto-regulatory homeostatic nature of energy balance is based is examined in the paper by Sukhatme and Margen (1982). Since there is insufficient space to develop this further here, the reader must refer to this article in order to understand the rationale behind the model.

Nutrient requirements have been defined traditionally as averages which are applicable to a specific category of individuals. Within each category requirements may differ from person to person, but everyone is assumed to have his own fixed level of necessary intake. In fact, although not explicitly stated, it is often inferred that this is genetically determined. An analysis by Sukhatme and Margen suggests that adaptations do occur as a result of changes in efficiency of energy utilization, and that, over time they may be as significant for the maintenance of individual weight equilibrium as are genetics. These concepts bring into question the theory of fixed requirements.

Current Theory

The current theory, at least one widely accepted among nutritionists, is that adults of the same age, sex, and body composition, who share similar lifestyles, ecological settings and activity patterns, have similar energy requirements. Obviously, there is some inter-individual variation which is generally accounted for on a genetic basis. The energy requirements for adults are presumed to be determined by three components: (1) the energy needed for maintenance; (2) the extra energy needed for physical activity; and (3) the relatively small increment which is due to dietary induced thermogenesis. The latter usually implies only the specific dynamic action of food, but some investigators believe it can be further influenced by a food-activity interaction. According to this theory, therefore, if such individuals have different energy intakes they must be engaged in different levels of activity in order to maintain constant weight and body composition. As a corollary, individuals engaged in similar activities, but with different energy intakes, will show changes in weight, although most observers believe that after a period of time many will assume a new weight equilibrium. Thus, a healthy adult who is engaged in similar activities from day-to-day and who is maintaining body weight and composition, should have a nearly constant requirement equal to his/her habitual intake (children and pregnant and lactating women are excluded from this model and discussion). Moreover, energy requirements can be calculated by measuring the habitual energy intakes of healthy individuals in specified categories of age, sex, and activity level. Some individuals may need more and others less than the tabulated average, depending upon deviations of physical activity from the prescribed level, variations in body weight, special growth and physiological needs, and possibly some genetic factors. According to the 1973 FAO/WHO Report the requirements of a given individual may vary over time, but this will be negligible relative to variation between individuals. In this sense the requirements of all individuals are fixed.

Contraindications in the Present Theory

In 1947 Widdowson observed that in a healthy, active population of specified age and sex, engaged in similar work, two individuals out of every 40 will exhibit a mean daily intake twice as large as the others. This implies a coefficient of variation for mean weekly intake of about 16 percent. Thus, the moderately active reference adult, according to the latest FAO/WHO standards, weighs approximately 65 kilograms and "requires" 3000 kilocalories per day. Therefore, within a group of so-called reference men, the intakes would vary from 2,520 to 3,480 calories at one standard deviation, and at two standard deviations the range would increase to 2,060 to 3,960 calories. Her explanation for the discrepancy is that some individuals are apparently more efficient machines than others.

More recently, studies have attempted to combine simultaneous measurements of intake and expenditure. The most extensive and objective of these was carried out by Edholm, et al. (1970). These noted British investigators used the best available measurement techniques on young army recruits during the second, fifth and eighth weeks of a nine week training period at six different depot centers in the United Kingdom. This study confirmed Widdowson's observation that intake varied much more widely than expenditure in subjects engaged in similar work, but it raised an even more serious question. It was observed that even when averaged over a week, with allowances made for variation in body weight over time, the intake did not balance expenditure in individual subjects. In addition, there was no correlation between daily intake and expenditure.

In a communication to Nature, Durnin et al. (1973) interpreted these and other data to mean that either the errors in intake and expenditure measurement were too large to permit comment on balance in the same individual, or that the human requirement for energy was unknown given the present state of knowledge. The possibility that the answer could lie in the stationary stochastic nature of energy requirements obviously was not considered.

The Nature of Errors in Energy Balance

The usual view, that energy intake in an adult who is maintaining body weight must equal energy expenditure in some direct deterministic fashion, assumes that measurement errors are primarily chance or random and that successive observations are independent. The data reported by Edholm et al. (1970) do not support this. Table 1 shows a reconstruction of data from Edholm's original record for five of the six depots. The implication of this finding is that even when the daily intake is averaged over several days, a difference from week to week in the same individual continues to be large. In particular, the coefficient of variation of mean weekly intake is about 15 percent. If day-to-day variations were random, resulting from errors of measurement, the coefficient of variation should be much smaller. It cannot be assumed, therefore, that the variations over time in the same individual are random. Instead, the data must be accepted as indicating that successive observations of intake, in humans maintaining body weight, are correlated. Unlike intake, the difference in energy expenditures from week to week is small; the coefficient of variation is approximately 7-8%.

Clearly, even when intake has been averaged over several days, the totals are such that part of the variation which Widdowson ascribed to differences in efficiency between individuals must be regarded as a result of individual variation in intake. In other words, Edholm's data (1970) do not support the assumption that an average week's intake is equal to habitual or usual intake in humans who are maintaining body weight, and who are engaged in similar activities from day to day. Rather, they suggest

Table 1

Analysis of Variance of Weekly Calorie Intake and
Expenditure per kg of Body Weight

Source	d.f.	Intake kg/day		Expenditure kg/day	
		M.S.	Estimated true variance	M.S.	Estimated true variance
Depot Centers A, B, & C					
Between subjects within centers	14	93.3	14.2	25.2	4.5
Within subjects	34	50.8	50.8	11.7	11.7
Depot Centers D & E					
Between subjects within centers	7	115.7	22.6	15.0	0
Within subjects	18	48.0	48.0	16.0	16.0

that the body regulates its energy balance by adjusting either intake or expenditure or both and that, consequently, the requirements cannot be considered as fixed and equal to habitual intake.

Similar conclusions can be reached by examining the data reported by Acheson et al. (1974; 1980) even though these authors interpreted the errors as random. Their study was conducted on six subjects at Haley Bay in Antarctica. In this unique setting the individuals lived free lives which were, nevertheless, so similar and controlled that they closely simulated laboratory conditions. Of the six subjects, number 4 was studied daily for intake and expenditure for 315 days, while the others were studied for 7 consecutive days every month. In Table 2 the standard deviation of daily intake is compared with a standard deviation of weekly means on subject 4. The table also includes the standard deviations obtained from the second, third and fourth weekly means. Although the standard deviation

Table 2

Standard Deviations of Daily Intake and Expenditure
in kcal/day Compared with Those of Daily Means
Based on 1,2,3, and 4 Weekly Periods

	Daily	1 week	2 weeks	3 weeks	4 weeks
Intake	646	370	286	259	243
Expenditure	725	441	303	262	233

calculated from weekly means is reduced, it is much larger than would be expected if the successive observations were independent. The data again confirm that the so-called customary weekly food intake and expenditure have a coefficient of variation approximately equal to 12%.

In an unpublished thesis (1984) Acheson demonstrated a certain rhythm characteristic of auto regulation. Unfortunately, since the daily data were unavailable, it is not clear whether this entire process was regulated. One might ask whether there was any other evidence, similar to that reported, for the magnitude of the inter-individual variation.

Although Widdowson thought the weekly intake represented a fairly reliable estimate of habitual intake, Yudkin (1951) reported that individuals varied markedly in their intake from week to week, even when maintaining body weight and level of activity. Chappell (1955) observed the same phenomenon. The question arises as to why Edholm and Acheson found no relationship between energy intake and expenditure if the successive values of balance are correlated. The answer lies in the data situation and in the method of analysis, which is different from that visualized in the calculation of coefficients of variation. Determining intake and expenditure for any day is difficult and involves measurement errors which are too large to be made negligible relative to the true differences between successive days. For this reason, the problem is to separate regulatory messages (if any) from underlying errors (noise), using what are known as stationary stochastic processes developed in the theory of communications.

The energy balance study reported by Edholm et al. (1970) is limited to 3 non-continuous weeks. It does not, therefore, permit a direct study of autocorrelations and how they evolve over time. Edholm's data on energy balance must, therefore, be interpreted to mean that, although intake may not be equal to expenditure even when averaged over a week, humans are probably in balance every day with varying intervals between peaks and troughs and varying amplitudes in daily balance. For this reason, the data cannot be expected to show the fixed period that Edholm (1955) and Durnin (1961) have been seeking. However, Edholm's et al. limited analysis and the analogy to the longer N balance data (Edmundson 1980) suggest also that balance will be distributed around zero, within limits which we call homeostasis and which are independent of time.

This does not mean that the first law of thermodynamics has been violated, as suggested in the statement made by Durnin et al. (1973). In living biological systems, a time lag must be expected in balancing intake with expenditure. Periods of stress may modify the time lag, but there is always movement towards balance through built-in auto-regulatory mechanisms. The fact that the distribution of energy balance is stochastic insures that the expected balance value is zero and that the standard deviation is independent of time.

Since Edholm's data are of insufficient length, they cannot be utilized to work out an autocorrelegram. They can be examined for autocorrelation, however, by computing variance of the mean balance when daily balance is averaged over two, three or more successive days. The variance of the mean balance is not inverse to the length of the period, but decreases slowly, thus confirming that the successive values are serially correlated. It seems perfectly plausible, then, that the daily balance is distributed in a stochastic stationary manner of the same Markovian type observed with nitrogen, with serial correlation of the first order.

Although the same model described in the Sukhatme and Margen (1978) paper on nitrogen balance cannot be used, it appears that the process is autoregressive (AR), which again must be interpreted to mean that energy balance exhibits a regulatory homeostatic character. Actually, what is relevant is the value of r in the pattern of energy balance in men engaged in specified activities. In terms of the regulation, we do not know whether it is due to an adjustment of intake, expenditure or both. In the brief series, intake seemed to show autocorrelation and expenditure did not. In view of the paucity of data, it is only possible to speculate on the source(s) of regulation. This serves to emphasize that habitual intakes of healthy men who are maintaining body weight and who are engaged in specified levels of activity are not constant as is currently assumed.

Another argument which can be raised is that the consolidated figures tend to obscure the true picture. Examination of the data from each subject, however, shows that the energy balance varies considerably from day to day and week to week, and from day to day within weeks. The subjects did not obtain balance at the end of any observed week or period. Some subjects did show overall balance at the end of the three periods, but these are not continuous weeks. For most subjects in other depots, the cumulative balances not only vary considerably from one period to the other, but also are often all positive or all negative to the extent of several thousand kilocalories each. The only inference to be drawn is that energy intake is used with variable efficiency by means of some homeostatic mechanism and, in the process, body weight is controlled. If it had been otherwise, the men would have gained or lost up to 5 kilograms during periods as short as 6-8 weeks.

The real controlling variable in the homeostatic process is not energy balance, but fluxes such as pressure, concentration, body temperature, environments, etc. Thus the dissipated heat, as a controlling variable requiring both input and output characteristics, increases as intake and energy balance increase, and the opposite occurs as intake and energy balance decrease. This gives a wide, though strictly limited, range to the energy intake. However, it is important to realize that a point is reached in intake below which the body is not able to maintain itself, and it is then forced to part with its fat and protein. This point of undernutrition is also called the lower threshold value of the homeostatic range for maintaining the nutritional state of the body. It must be concluded, therefore, that if intra-individual variation is a fundamental source of variation, it is because the variation over time appeared to stabilize as the period of observation increased from one day to seven days. This means that as the individual advances in time he becomes a different individual. The specialized environment in which he is being brought up apparently interacts with the genetic component to keep the variance constant. Although the genetic contribution to these effects will not be discussed in detail, it is possible to confirm the hypothesis that nutritional status is a process in which genetic entities interact with environment.

In the author's opinion newer data, such as that of Edmundson (1979; 1980) and Whitehead's group (Prentice 1984) can be interpreted only according to the above model.

Significance of Intra-Individual Variation

Edholm's data also illustrate that, even over a week, intra-individual variance accounts for the largest part of the total variance (Table 1). An important implication of this finding is that the differences observed by Widdowson et al. (1947) were not due to mixed inter-individual differences. Rather, they could be due to intra-individual differences and are a reflection of the fact that energy is used with variable efficiency in an attempt to regulate body stores.

When intra-individual variation in energy balance is the fundamental source of variation, and the successive values can be generated by an AR process such as Markoff, it also means that there is no absolute energy requirement for any day or period. The individual is in homeostasis and his/her requirement is controlled by a regulated system, the nature of which is not presently understood. Viewed this way, intra-individual variation would appear to reflect the capacity to adapt (or regulate) intake and expenditure in such a way that the expected value of daily energy balance is zero and the co-variance between daily energy balance K days apart is constant over time. One certainly cannot visualize a "calorie counter" at the input level measuring energy intake of food consumed and then telling the individual to stop eating. Not only would this be absurd but, as we have seen, balance is maintained in a probablistic and not absolute sense. On the other hand, metabolic mechanisms which may lead to variation in energy utilization are known and it seems more likely that the body regulates its energy balance by varying the efficiency of energy utilization.

When discussing variable efficiency of energy utilization, it is easier to understand mechanisms for energy wastage than for increased energy efficiency. We know little of how energy utilization for work may be varied (especially increased) and mechanisms for such have not been sought. It appears that at least 50% of the food energy is dissipated as heat without work, but even this statement may be questioned because the total requirements for maintaining body functions, including temperature, are still unknown.

In the case of wastage, a healthy individual increases intake when the wastage is larger and decreases intake when it is lower. This is done without altering body weight and level of physical activity: thus homeostasis is maintained within certain limits. Large changes in physical activity may also influence balance and regulation, as does food, although the magnitude of this latter effect is open to question (Atwater and Benedict 1971).

Apfelbaum's work (1971) also confirms that within the range of intra-individual variation, RMR increases as intake increases, and vice versa, without changing body weight or physical activity. It is apparently the autoregressive mechanism in daily expenditure which enables individuals to adapt requirements without affecting net energy needed for maintenance and physical activity. All this suggests that energy requirements of humans, or the efficiency with which energy consumed is used, varies greatly over the range of intra-individual variation.

At the lower threshold value of 1900 kcal, an individual may function with maximum efficiency (50%); at 2550 kcal, which is the "average rerequirement" for adult Indian males, the efficiency of utilization would be 37% and at 3200 kcal would drop to 30%. It would be interesting to know the maximum amount of energy from food which could be available for essential anabolic processes and physical activity.

CONCLUSIONS

The significance of intra-individual variation described above has important implications for defining requirements. It was stated earlier that "requirement" is a dynamic (not static) concept because in a healthy, active individual engaged in specific tasks, balance will vary around zero as a matter of course. In statistical jargon, energy balance will vary with stationary variance without implying under-or-over nutrition. A person must be considered in balance whenever his intake falls within homeostatic limits determined by the stationary distribution for balance. It is only when the balance "exceeds" the homeostatic mechanism that an individual is under stress from inadequate or excessive intake.

The validity of the procedures described in the literature for evaluating the nutritional status of individuals must be judged with this in mind. While it may be valid to compare the average intake of a population with a reference standard such as described by FAO/WHO, great care must be exercised in this regard. Even if one assumes a normal distribution of the population, intake estimates against FAO/WHO or other standards can be misinterpreted. A glaring example of such misuse is found in a World Bank study on the dimensions of malnutrition and poverty (Reutlinger and Selowsky 1976). The authors of the study estimate that 44% of the population in Brazil is malnourished because this population (consisting principally of low income groups) has an intake less than the average FAO/WHO recommendations for the region.

If the people with intakes below these recommendations are to be classified as malnourished, then the 56% above the poverty line must be considered as overnourished and at risk of obesity. If the dividing line between under- and overnutrition is the average level of recommendation, one must conclude that the more serious problem for Brazil is overnutrition. Simple as the logic is, it has been ignored in describing the nutrition situation in developing countries.

During the early years of FAO, this method was used to conclude that two-thirds of the world was under- and malnourished (FAO 1952). Still earlier, Bowley (Wright 1966) used the same method to suggest that half the British population was undernourished because they had intakes below the average requirement for Great Britain. However, this was 40 years ago when the concept of energy require- ment had not developed to a point where its full implications could be grasped. To adopt the same method today for comparing intake with requirement, one which was discarded by Great Britain decades ago, is to ignore the knowledge that has been gained in understanding the concept of physiological requirement.

That such assessments are misleading can also be seen from the findings of Ferro-Luzzi, Norgan and Durnin (1975). Thus, a nutritional survey of 1000 children in New Guinea has shown that a high proportion of nutritionally inadequate diets, assessed using FAO standards, does not match physiological or clinical signs and symptoms of malnu- trition. Less than 3% of the children examined were clini- cally malnourished in contrast to the 50% placed in that category on the basis of comparison of intake with require- ments suggested by the World Bank and frequently by other economists (Dandekar 1971). If such exaggerations persist the benefits of nutrition programs will be seized by those who need them least, while the really poor and un- dernourished will continue to suffer.

None of this should detract from concern about the serious deprivation which can occur when an individual's requirements exceed the limits of homeostasis because of heredity, work, or ecological setting. Those people most clearly at risk are laborers, landless peasants, urban slum dwellers, and the children of these individuals. For those living on the lower borderline of homeostasis, acute ecologi- cal changes, i.e., drought and other losses of food produc- tion capacity and/or income, can rapidly precipitate severe malnutrition. Conditions such as these are also prevalent in the developing world among individuals in the lower economic classes who are relatively isolated from the main- stream of society. They have already made the maximum adaptation to deprivation and cannot adjust to a loss of equilibrium. History shows that the failure of emergency feeding programs is frequently influenced by the occurence of disasters. These can strike so rapidly that interventions are often subverted to external forces, and those at the bottom limits of homeostasis cannot survive long enough to be helped.

Analysis has shown that the actual prevalence of "malnutrition" is lower than previously estimated. Although poverty and malnutrition are closely correlated, everyone below the poverty line is not malnourished. The claim that the developing countries do not have the resources to cope with the problem of malnutrition is not true. Virtually every developing country can solve the problem of malnutrition once they realize that the magnitude of the problem is not as great as had been indicated by improper assessment of the information. The primary etiology of malnutrition is not insufficient food, but socially induced maldistribution and exploitation.

REFERENCES

1. Acheson KJ (1974). The assessment of techniques for measuring energy balance in man. Unpublished Ph.D. thesis. London: Queen Elizabeth College, University of London.
2. Acheson KJ, Campbell IT, Edhold OG, Miller DS and Stock MJ (1980). A longitudinal study of body weight and body fat changes in Antarctica. Am J Clin Nutr 33:972.
3. Apfelbaum M, Bostarron J and Lacatis D (1971). Effect of calorie restriction and excessive caloric intake on energy expenditure. Am J Clin Nutr 24:1405.
4. Atwater WD and Benedict (1971). Experiments on the metabolism of matter and energy in the human body. U.S. Dept of Agri OH Exp Sta Bull 136:1-357.
5. Bowley Lord A (1966). Quoted in Wright NC. Book Review of Sukhatme PV "Feeding India's Growing Millions." Popul Studies 19:201.
6. Box GE and Jenkins GM (1976). "Time Series Analysis: Forecasting and Control." San Francisco: Holden-Day.
7. Chappell GM (1955). Long-term individual dietary surveys. Brit J Nutr 9:323.
8. Chatfield C (1975). "The Analysis of Time Series: Theory and Practice." London: Chapman and Hall.
9. Dandekar VN and Rath M (1971). Poverty in India. Bombay: Econ and Pol Wkly 6:parts 1 and 2.
10. Durnin JVGA (1961). 'Appetite' and the relationship between expenditure and intake of calories in man. J Physiol 156:294.

11. Durnin JVGA, Edholm OG, Miller AS and Waterlow JE (1973). How much food does man require? Nature 242:418.
12. Edholm OG, Adam JM, Healy MJR, Wolff HS, Goldsmith R and Best TW (1970). Food intake and energy expenditure of army recruits. Brit J Nutr 24:1091.
13. Edholm OG, Fletcher JG, Widdowson EM and McCance RA (1955). The energy expenditure and food intake of individual men. Brit J Nutr 9:286.
14. Edmundson W (1979). Individual variation and basal metabolic of mechanical work in efficiency in East Java. Ecol of Food Nutr 8:189.
15. Edmundson W (1980). Adaptation to undernutrition. How much food does man need? Soc Sci and Med 14:119.
16. The Second World Food Survey (1952). Rome: FAO.
17. Ferro-Luzzi A, Norgan NT and Durnin JVGA (1975). Food Intake, its relationship to body weight and age and its apparent nutritional adequacy in New Guinean children. Am J Clin Nutr 28:1443.
18. Garby L (1982a). Control of energy intake and expenditure in the regulation of energy balance. Unpublished ms.
19. Garby L (1982b). Principles and problems in human energy exchange. Unpublished ms.
20. Howard RA (1971). "Dynamic Probabilistic Systems Vol 7. Markon Models." N.Y.: John Wiley & Sons, Inc.
21. Miller DS (1975). Overfeeding in man. In Bray G (ed): "Obesity in Perspective," Washington, DC: U.S. Government Print Office, p. 137.
22. Miller DS, Mumford PM and Stock MJ (1967). Gluttong 2. Thermogenesis in overeating man. Am J Clin Nutr 20:1223.
23. Miller DS and Payne PR (1962). Weight maintenance and food intake . J Nurtr 78:255.
24. Mott-Smith M (1934). "The Story of Energy." NY: D. Appleton Century Co.
25. Neumann RD (1902). Experimentelle Beitrage zur Lehre von den tagliehen Nahrungs bedarf des Menschen unter besondenh Berucksichtigung der notgendigen Eiweissmeng. Arch Hyg 45:1.
26. Passmore R (1971). The regulation of body weight in man. Proc Nutr Soc 30:122.
27. Payne RR and Dugdale AE (1977). A model for the prediction of energy balance and body weight. Ann Human Biol 4:525.

28. Pitts GC (1979). Physiologic regulation of body energy storage. Metabolism 27:460.
29. Prentice Andrew M (1984). Adaptations to long-term low energy intake. In Pollitt E and Amante P (eds): "Energy Intake and Activity," NY: Alan R. Liss, Inc. (In Press).
30. Reutlinger S and Selowsky M (1976). Malnutrition and poverty. World Bank Occasional Paper No. 23.
31. Rubner M (1968). die Geetz des energie ver brauchs die der ernohrung, Fran Deuticke, eipz'q Und Wien, 1902. (Ed and trans by Joy RJT, US Army Inst of Env Med) Natick, Mass.
32. Sukhatme PV and Margen S (1982). Auto-regulatory homeostatic nature of energy balance. Am J Clin Nutr 35:355.
33. Sukhatme PV and Margen S (1978). Models for protein deficiency. Am J Clin Nutr 31:1237.
34. Vigy M, Appelbaum M and Miller DS (ed) (1973). Energy Balance in Man. General Discussion. Paris: Masson et cie.
35. Energy and Protein Requirements. Report of a Joint FAO/WHO Ad Hoc Expert Committee. WHO Technical Report Series No. 522. (FAO Nutrition Meetings Report Series No. 52).
36. Widdowson EM (1947). A study of individual children's diets. Special Report Series. Med Res Council No. 257, 1947.
37. Yudkin J (1951). Dietary surveys: variation in the weekly intake of nutrients. Brit J Nutr 5:177-194.

METHODOLOGY–ADULTS

Energy Intake and Activity, pages 79–99
© 1984 Alan R. Liss, Inc., 150 Fifth Avenue, New York, NY 10011

ENERGY INTAKES AS PREDICTORS OF ENERGY BALANCES
IN FREE-LIVING POPULATIONS

Anna Ferro-Luzzi

National Institute of Nutrition

Via Ardeatina 546, 00179 Rome, Italy

INTRODUCTION

The title of this paper refers to a controversial and insufficiently explored field and supplementary information, seldom collected or reported in dietary surveys, would be necessary to deal with it properly. It is common to infer, on the basis of assumptions which are reasonable but without strong supporting evidence, that at least in the long term, energy intake equals energy expenditure for the great majority of people. This assumption rests on three critical preliminary stipulations:

a) that mean daily energy intakes, as currently assessed, represent true mean intakes;

b) that intakes recorded over a given period are representative of habitual intakes; and

c) that observed energy intakes bear a fixed relationship to energy expenditure.

Each of these points deserves attention and the paper is organized to examine and discuss them individually. On the first point some methodological aspects concerning, but not limited to, the dietary survey technique as an instrument shall be considered. The impact of intra- and inter-individual variability in eating behavior on the accuracy of estimated energy intakes will be considered in connection with the second point. To explore the third point, data on energy balance of free-living subjects will be presented and compared with similar data from the literature, and the correlation between energy balance and a number of relevant variables will be discussed.

Data on energy intakes often are obtained by means of dietary surveys. Although surveys necessarily cover only limited fractions of time (days or weeks), and are carried out on samples of the target group, it is common practice to draw wider conclusions from the assembled data.

DIETARY SURVEYS AS MEASURES OF "TRUE MEAN" INTAKE

The question here is the reliability and validity of dietary survey methodology. Reliable, accurate, and representative data on energy intake are fundamental prerequisites for any discussion of this topic. The dietary survey method, like any other scientific instrument, needs to be tested and calibrated regularly, both before and during use. Dietary surveys are expensive procedures and investigators often adopt one of the simplified versions of the precise weighing technique. The tendency has been to use these variants without determining their reliability. In particular, two relatively inexpensive variants based on the interview technique, the dietary history and the 24-hr recall, have been used widely to assess individual dietary intakes. The subjective component of these interview techniques is so large that regular validation should be mandatory. In practice, this is seldom done; in most cases it is assumed that the validations described in the literature apply universally, and that no further controls for the specific study conditions are needed. If the literature is properly read, however, there is ample evidence that methodological errors differ with the age, sex, cultural background, etc. of the respondents. Even when the surveyed groups are comparable to those on whom the literature reports the validation, interviewers themselves are a potential source of further variation, one which needs to be assessed and taken into account in each case.

Several valuable studies and reviews of the validity and reliability of various methodological variants of the dietary survey technique have been published over the past 4 decades (Balogh et al. 1971; Beaton et al. 1979; Chalmers et al. 1952; Marr 1971; Morgan et al. 1978; Young et al. 1952). Some relevant points will be illustrated briefly here. The ability of the respondents to recall the exact amount of food consumed during the previous 24 hours or more, to estimate and quantify portions sizes, and to average them through time is the basic element in the accuracy of the information collected by interview. That this ability is not a fixed characteristic, and that it may vary with age, sex, cultural background, time span covered, existence of a definite eating pattern, etc., has been established by several studies. For example, children's ability to recall their dietary intakes appears to be age-dependent (Emmons and Hayes 1973); elderly men and women from a rural area in Southern Italy have been found (Sette et al., In preparation) to differ from each other in the extent to which they over and under recall what they ate in the previous 24 hrs. The interviewer's ability to probe subjects deeply enough, without eliciting the phenomenon of retroactive interference (Osgood 1953), has been revealed as another, usually neglected, source of unreliability. Table 1 illustrates the effects of sex, age, and environment on dietary recall (Campbell and Dodds 1967). Interviewers themselves also constitute a potential source of methodological error. Since it is common to use different interviewers in a survey, and it is inevitable that they will be different in different surveys, it is crucial that the impact of the interviewer on the outcome of the interview should be assessed regularly. Beaton et al. (1979) in an accurately designed analysis of the source of variance in 24-hour dietary recall, conducted under controlled and standardized conditions on 60 subjects, found no consistent differences between three certified nutritionists. In contrast, Church et al. (1954) and Dawber et al. (1962) showed differences on the order of 1 to 8% between interviewer estimates of energy intake. At present the evidence is insufficient to demonstrate that interviewers with similar background and training invariably produce similar data. It is clear that additional studies are needed.

Table 1   Percent energy contributed by the probe to total energy assessed by 24-hr recall (Adapted from Campbell and Dodds 1967).

	In institutions				At home	
	young		old		old	old
	men	women	men	women	men	women
Energy %	21	13	35	28	18	13

The ability to evaluate portion size is another critical factor in the interview technique. A group of 9 trained dietitians and 6 untrained observers were tested for the ability by viewing 40 odd pieces of familial portions and food items and estimating the weight of each (Alicino et al., In preparation). The results, shown in Table 2, indicate that formally trained dietitians were no more successful than untrained persons is assigning weights, and that underestimation of weights prevailed. The slope of the regression lines revealed a tendency to underestimate heavier items. Translated into measures of energy content, the incorrect weight estimation affected the results in a variable and unpredictable way depending on the nutrient composition of the item.

Table 2 Estimate of portion sizes and carry-over effect on energy content by trained and untrained observers (Alicino et al.).

Observer		Weight		Energy	
		Estimated as % or measured	Correlation r	Estimated as % or measured	Correlation r
Trained	(n = 9)	-15 ± 17	0.87	-13 ± 16	0.84
Untrained	(n = 6)	-12 ± 16	0.80	+ 2 ± 12	0.82
Total	(n = 15)	-14 ± 16	0.84	- 7 ± 16	0.83

Forty different food items were observed sequentially and weight estimates given within 30 sec. of inspection for each item.

Differences between interviewers have been reported even at the stage of interpreting and calculating the same dietary records. These differences are influenced by the nutritionists' ability to interpret the descriptive terms and the approximate measurements reported in the dietary records, the tables of food composition used, and the judgements exercised by the nutritionist in substituting for a dietary item not existing as such in the tables. This type of error was assessed by Eagles et al. (1966) and a significant difference (573 kcal; 4% in terms of SE) was reported. The study was conducted under the relatively simple conditions of a metabolic ward, and the authors warn that the differences they found are likely to represent the minimum to be expected from such exercise. In the study by Beaton et al. (1979) the variance introduced by the coding and computational procedures was negligible, but these authors also recognize that this step is a potentially important source of error unless special care is exercised.

Replicability of the data obtained in two separate sittings on the same subjects may be used as a measure of the reliability of the method. When this procedure was applied to 24-hr recall and dietary history data, the results were discouraging. In a sample of children 5 to 13 years of age, Rasanen (1979) found approximately a 2% mean difference between energy intakes recalled on two separate occasions. He showed a 25% difference between two replicated dietary histories, and a 35% difference when 24-hr recalled energy intakes were compared to the energy intakes obtained by means of the dietary history. Correlation coefficients between the values from the first and the second survey were low, ranging from r = 0.42 for calories from recall to r = 0.59 for calories from dietary history. Balogh et al. (1971) compared the dietary history findings on energy intakes with those obtained by 24-hr recall (average of 8 or more interviews), obtaining for energy a correlation coefficient of r = 0.69. They state that "...with correlation coefficients in this range we were likely to get substantially different results in epidemiological studies concerned with classifying individuals....(p. 307)." Dawber et al. (1962) obtained higher correlation coefficients, r = 0.84, between dietary histories collected 4 yrs apart than when the time lapse was 2 years, r = 0.92. Karvetti and Knuts (1981) report an interclass correlation coefficient of r = 0.56 for energy intake assessed by 4 different interview methods. In that study the energy intake assessed by the history method produced the largest value (2330 kcal) while the 24-hr recall produced the smallest (1802 kcal).

Young et al. (1952) compared 7-day records with dietary histories and 24-hr recall. The mean percentage difference in energy intakes ranged from + 28 to - 9% between dietary history and 7-day record, while there was a rather good agreement, 1 to 7%, between 24-hr recall and 7-day record. However, the regression analysis between the energy intakes assessed by the two methods suggested that the recall tended to underestimate the extremes (regression coefficient [b]<1.0). Other authors (Gersovitz et al. 1978; Madden et al. 1976) have confirmed this tendency of the interview methods to over-report low intakes and under-report high intakes, a pattern known as the 'flat slope' syndrome.

The author's experience suggests that the 'flat-slope' syndrome may not be a universal finding. In a study where dietary intakes of 20 elderly peasants of southern Italy were simultaneously assessed by the precise weighing and the 24-hr recall method, it was found that while women had a slope not significantly different from 1, at least for energy (b = 1.24), the men showed a slight but significant 'steep-slope' (b = 1.44). Average differences between energy intakes assessed by the recall and by the precise weighing technique were + 8% and - 4%, respectively for women and for men (Sette et al., In preparation).

Even the precise weighing method is not immune to criticism; it has been blamed for inducing the so called Hawthorne effect whereby "the act of being measured influences behavior and reporting of behavior, and does so to varying degrees and in different ways for different individuals" (Liu et al. 1978, pp. 409-410). The author has been unable to find in the literature any experimental evidence to support this hypothesis. In a study carried out on a group of 150 adult males, in which the 7-day weighing of all food was carried out almost exclusively by dietitians (Norgan and Ferro-Luzzi 1978), the analysis of variance did not reveal any evidence of a day-of-the-survey effect (F = .917; p < .05), but did demonstrate the presence of a day-of-the-week effect (F = 13.328; p < .000). This suggests that, even if the subjects were not totally oblivious to the presence of an intruder weighing all their food, such presence did not disturb their spontaneous weekly cycle of eating behavior.

In conclusion it appears that while carefully conducted precise weighing method surveys are likely to measure energy intake reliably, the outcome of the simplified version, the interview-based technique, depends on scrupulously incorporating validations of factors which are potential sources of methodological error. Unfortunately, these validations are seldom carried out, thus leaving ample room for doubt and criticism, especially when bizarre values are obtained and reported.

ASSESSMENT OF "HABITUAL" INTAKE

The variability of energy intake affects the reliability with which the habitual intake of the individual can be estimated. Most people eat different foods and/or different quantities of the same foods on different days. This pattern is usually reflected in a day-to-day variation in energy intake. Energy intake also varies between individuals. Several authors report a surprisingly wide range in inter-and intra-individual and group energy intake (Ashworth 1968; Durnin 1979; Edholm et al. 1955; Edholm et al. 1970; Widdowson 1962; Widdowson 1974). These studies suggest that some individuals subsist on approximately half the energy consumed by other individuals or groups of similar age, sex, size and even occupation. These findings should alert us to the difficulties associated with estimating 'true' habitual intakes. Hallfrisch et al. (1982), for example, found that only 4 of 24 subjects were able to maintain their body weight when fed the same amount of energy they had themselves reported having consumed during one week. It appears obvious that extravagantly low or high energy intakes assessed by simplified versions of the more rigorous weighed survey may be of questionable validity.

The same interpretation would not apply to findings obtained by more careful studies conducted with appropriate methodology. In two such studies (Ashworth 1968; Durnin 1979), the previously recorded habitual food intakes were shown experimentally to have been grossly underestimated. The amounts were inadequate to maintain the body weights of the subjects when they were fed the same amount under strictly controlled laboratory conditions. Inter- and intra-individual variance in these cases may be an important element in the degree of reliability of the dietary survey findings, i.e. the ability to correctly and consistently classify individuals according to their estimated energy intakes. Beaton et al. (1979) and Liu et al. (1978) have pointed out that the presence of high intra-individual variability is a major source of potential difficulty in understanding the results of dietary surveys, and that it interferes with the consistency of the classification of individuals within a group.

While data on inter-individual variability are regularly reported in the literature, considerably less is published about intra-individual variability in energy intake. Estimates have been reported and analyzed by Balogh et al. (1971), Beaton et al. (1979), Ferro-Luzzi (1982), Liu et al. (1978), and Marr (1971). The author has calculated estimates of intra-individual variability in energy intake from published data. Studies were selected in which the procedures for dietary intake assessment offered the guarantee of low methodological error, and where individual data presentation allowed the calculation of the intra-individual coefficient of variation (CV) for energy intake. The analysis has been limited to adult males because different variabilities may be associated with differences in age and sex. The data shown in Table 3 indicate that the degree of variance in energy intake, expressed as coefficient of variation (σ/mean), is large and variable. It ranges from 16 to 30%, and the highest variance is associated with the subsistence farming environment of two New Guinean groups. Documentation from developing countries is almost non-existent for intra-individual variance in dietary intakes. As a result, very little is known about the day-to-day variation in the eating behavior of people living in areas where low income, seasonal food availability, and the reputedly high prevalence of malnutrition may control dietary intake and significantly affect its variability.

Table 3: Intra-individual variability of energy intake.

	CV_i	% Deviation		No. days for % Dev. ≤ 10%
		1 day	7 days	
Developed Countries				
British Cadets (Edholm et al. 1955)	16	31	12	10
Univ. Students (Passmore et al. 1952)	16	31	12	10
Australian School Boys (McNaughton and Cahn 1970)	17	33	13	12
Heavy Industry Workers (Ferro-Luzzi 1982; Norgan and Ferro-Luzzi, 1978)	17	33	13	12
Mean	17	33	13	11
Developing Countries				
New Guinea Kaul Farmers (Norgan et al. 1974)	30	59	22	36
New Guinea Lufa farmers (Norgan et al. 1974)	27	53	20	28
Mean	29	56	21	32

Estimated coefficients of intra-individual variation (CV_i) of energy intake and 95% range (expressed as % deviation) of observed individual values (D) from true means with 1 and with 7 replicas.

One day survey data has been analyzed for developed countries and, using the calculation method suggested by Beaton et al. (1979), the 95% confidence limit for the percent deviation between observed and true mean intakes of sub- jects is approximately ± 33%, for a mean CV_i of 17%. Using the same CV_i, but a 7 day survey, and assuming that each of these days varies independently from the others, the 95% confidence limits of the percent deviation from the true mean is ± 13%. Expressed in terms of kcal/day this is the equiva- lent of saying that, for an average intake of approximately 3200 kcal/day, the observed energy intake of any individual may fall between 2800 and 3600 kcal/day. This is a rather wide range if energy intake data is to be used to evaluate the energy balance of individuals. To maintain the deviation at no more than 10% of true intake, 10 to 12 days of survey would be needed, a duration that is seldom attained in field studies for a number of practical reasons. These results are not encouraging when related to the ability to correctly interpret currently available energy intake data on individu- als, and could explain some of the extreme values reported in the literature. New Guineans, given their unusually high CV_i, would require 32 days of measurements to achieve the same degree of accuracy, i.e. ± 10% at 95% confidence limits.

To illustrate the practical implications of this observa- tion it is worth noting that the two studies mentioned previ- ously (Ashworth 1968; Durnin 1979) were conducted on subjects from developing countries. Data is not available on the internal variability of eating patterns for either Jamai- cans or Ethiopians but, if it is assumed that their CV_i is similar to that recorded for the New Guineans, it would be expected that observed energy intake for the 7-day survey would show a ± 22% deviation from true mean intakes, i.e. would fall between 2626 and 1644 kcal for the Ethiopians and between 2100 and 1350 for the Jamaican men. This range may provide at least a partial explanation of why several subjects went into negative energy balance on those amounts. In other words, as Durnin (1979) pointed out, their "normal" energy intakes were obviously not the "real normal".

ENERGY INTAKE AND ENERGY BALANCE UNDER FREE-LIVING CONDITIONS

Consideration of the relationship between energy intake data and energy balance necessitates some overlap into the area of energy expenditure. Indeed, unless the state of body energy stores during the time span of the survey is known, it is impossible to discuss energy balance without entering the field of energy expenditure.

This topic is confronted with some reluctance. The area is not clearly defined nor are the data sufficient for reaching solid general conclusions. Moreover, the real problem with energy metabolism does not concern the ability to diagnose energy equilibrium by measuring dietary intake, but with defining the functional and biological cost of achieving energy equilibrium when food availability is chronically or periodically restricted. A related and contrasting problem is to define the energy requirements for optimum performance in terms of health, productivity, fitness, reproductivity, etc. Common sense indicates that the majority of people must be in long term energy equilibrium, whether or not they are in medium-or short-term equilibrium. It seems pointless to question whether or not the state of the energy balance for a given individual can be predicted on the basis of energy intake data. The answer must be that it is not possible unless intakes are equal to, or below, either basal metabolic rate (BMR) or perhaps BMR multiplied by a minimum, or maintenance factor. A subject or group may be deliberately observing a religious fast or a hunger strike, be affected by anorexia nervosa, abstain from food in order to be slim, or simply be the unwilling victim(s) of famine. Similar situations may be encountered, but they are obviously uncommon in practice (except for the recurrence of famines in various areas of the world) and, by definition, temporary. If food intake is zero or close to zero and if the situation is prolonged, death will be the inevitable outcome. Except for such extreme situations energy intakes alone, no matter how large or small, are not sufficient to allow any conclusions about the state of energy balance. Negative energy balances can exist at intakes as high as 4250 kcal/day (Edholm 1977) and apparently equilibrium can be achieved with intakes as low as 1500 kcal/day (Durnin 1979).

Energy intake data alone do not define the state of energy balance during the short-term, where large day-to-day fluctuations are a normal occurrence; nor are they sufficient for medium-term observations where the currently available field methods are not accurate enough to capture the small imbalances in energy equilibrium that are at the basis of cyclical fluctuations in body energy stores. The most obvious, and also the least expensive and simplest way to approach the issue, would be to check bodyweight changes during the period of dietary survey. This measurement is not commonly performed because it would be done connection with measurements of food intake, and the latter are usually done over a period of one week at most. Normal day-to-day fluctuations of body weight are such that any consistent trend in gain or loss of body energy stores would be obscured by this schedule. Weight changes of up to 1kg from one day to the next have been reported in normal healthy people by several authors (Durnin 1961; Edholm 1961; Taggart 1962) and fluctuations of approximately 0.5 kg are a common occurrence. These changes have been shown to reflect mainly alterations of the body water compartment (Taggart 1962). Because of this peculiarity, a negative or positive energy balance of about 300 to 400 kcal/day, producing a loss or gain in body weight of less than 0.5 kg in a week, would be likely to escape detection. Another approach for appraising the state of energy balance is to measure simultaneously both energy intake and expenditure for an adequate length of time. This approach, which is very costly and technically complex, is seldom used.

Man in free-living conditions neither requires nor achieves energy equilibrium on a daily basis. For example, British recruits and cadets, at the individual level, took about 14 days to equilibrate intake and expenditure (Edholm et al. 1955; Edholm 1961), but no data exist to indicate whether this 'energetic' behavior applies equally to all people and to different, more natural, environments. Seasonal body weight fluctuations in primitive agricultural societies (Spencer and Heywood In press; Prentice et al. 1981) suggest that cycles of energy imbalance may last longer than 14 days, and that they occur in associaiton with scarcity of food resources, as a consequence of bouts of intense physical activity, or as a combination of the two. On purely technical grounds, then, conventional 7 day dietary surveys do not permit determination of the state of energy balance of the individual. Intra-individual variability in energy intake is such that true habitual intake cannot be estimated accurately; therefore, energy intake as currently assessed (over

Table 4   Energy intake and energy balance in selected groups from developing and developed countries.

	Subj. N	Age yrs	Energy Intake kcal/d		kcal/kg	Energy Balance kcal/d	
			M̄	SD	M̄	M̄	SD
Developing Countries (LDC)							
Farmers Kaul (Norgan et al. 1974)	42	32	2037	504	36	-324	542
Farmers Lufa (Norgan et al. 1974)	40	28	2530	487	44	-41	554
Farmers Upper Volta (Bleiberg et al. 1981)	11	45	2148	613	38	+18	508
Farmers Guatemala (Viteri et al. 1971)	18	30	3555	712	59	-138	765
Farmers Philippino (DeGuzman et al. 1974a)	9	28	2471	509	48	-836	830
Jeepney drivers, Philippino (DeGuzman and Kalaw et al. 1974c)	10	30	2634	397	48	-142	361
Shoemakers, Philippino (DeGuzman et al. 1974b)	10	30	2595	386	46	-118	414
Clerk-typists, Philippino (DeGuzman et al. 1978)	10	28	2352	369	44	+161	440
Total	150	31	2483	683	44	-154	606
Developed Countries (DC)							
Heavy Ind. Workers It. (Ferro-Luzzi 1982; Norgan Ferro-Luzzi 1978)	149	37	3242	612	43	+96	499
Army Cadets UK (Edholm et al. 1955)	12	20	3433	361	49	+17	446
University Students UK (Durnin and Brockway 1959; Passmore et al. 1962)	9	22	3343	490	47	-13	306
School boys Australia (McNaughton and Cahn 1970)	5	18	2903	388	41	+318	361
Antarctic Exped. team (Acheson et al. 1980)	12	24	3009	424	42	-107	653
Total	187	34	3235	562	43	+79	508

a one week period) cannot be guaranteed to represent true 'habitual' intake. In practice this means that if the survey findings show, as they usually do, that intake and expenditure do not match in the same individual over the time span of the observation, there is no basis on which to judge the state of his energy balance. It can be seen however, that group data provide a different picture, especially if the group is large and relatively homogeneous. Usually a near-equilibrium situation is observed over seven days.

The utility of studies on energy intake and expenditure has been questioned by Rivers and Payne (1982, p 97) who stated that: "...intake studies in conjunction with simultaneous studies of energy expenditure do not improve the quality of the evidence, at best it (sic) provides an extremely tedious and inaccurate confirmation of the first law of thermodynamics." Studies of this type usually are conducted to address two separate questions which are independent and self-contained and which are relevant to different, if related, fields of interest. Two totally separate sets of information are acquired. Fortunately, as a by-product, they also provide insight into the reciprocal behavior of energy intake and expenditure under ordinary living conditions; unfortunately, few such studies exist. Screening the literature as far back as the 1940's allowed the selection of a number of studies conducted on adult males (Table 4) in which the assessments were performed according to reliable techniques (3 to 7 days or more of weighed intakes, time-and-motion studies in conjunction with indirect calorimetry) and for which individual data were available. Examination and discussion of these data should indicate whether it is possible to draw from them any general conclusions about energy intake in relation to energy balance under free-living conditions.

A large variety of environmental, dietary, occupational and age and body weight situations are represented in these studies. They include subsistence farmers in tropical environment (Bleiberg et al. 1981; De Guzman et al. 1974a; Norgan et al 1974), Antarctic expedition components (Acheson 1980), university students (Durnin and Brockway 1959; Passmore et al. 1952), army personnel (Edholm et al. 1955), and heavy industry workers (Norgan and Ferro-Luzzi 1978). Mean group intake varies between 2037 and 3555 kcal/day for the developing country groups, averaging 2483

± 683 kcal/day, or 44 kcal/kg body weight for the pooled
sample of 150 men. The 187 men of the developed country
group had an average intake of 3235 ± 562 kcal/day or 43
kcal/kg. The 95% confidence range of energy intake falls
between 2374 and 2592 kcal/day for the pooled individuals
from the developing countries, and between 3154 and 3316
kcal/day for individuals from the developed countries.
Energy balances for developing countries range between -836
kcal/day and + 161 kcal/day, with an average of -154
kcal/day. Energy balances for the developed countries
range between -107 and +318 kcal/day with an average of +79
kcal/day. Standard deviations are very high for both
groups.

The correlation coefficient between average individual
intake and balance is r = 0.33 for the developed countries
and r = 0.60 for the developing countries. Both are highly
significant, but intakes explain only 10% of the variance of
energy balance in the developed country groups and 36% in
the developing country groups. The 95% confidence limits
for energy balance are -251 and -57 kcal/day for the developing countries and +6 and +152 kcal/day for the developed
nations. A very low order correlation (r = 0.25) between
energy balance and body weight was obtained for the total
sample of 187 men from developed countries. No correlation
exists between the same parameters for the 139 men from the
developing countries groups. Low order correlations for the
two groups also have been obtained between energy intake
and body weight, while energy intake and energy expenditure correlate significantly (r = 0.55) in both groups. The
correlation between energy intake and expenditure was not
improved by expressing energy expenditure as energy in
excess of BMR.

A more detailed study of the dynamics of short term
energy balance regulation was made using the three groups
for whom individual energy expenditure and intake data were
available on a daily basis. The mean group energy intake
for New Guinean subsistence farmers (Norgan et al. 1974)
was less than expenditure, thus leading to a markedly
negative energy balance, while the Italian shipyard workers
(Ferro-Luzzi 1982; Norgan and Ferro-Luzzi 1978) showed a
slight positive energy balance. An analysis of the individual
daily values during the progression of the observation period
reveals that the New Guinean farmers reduced the negativity
of the energy balance in the village of Kaul, or even

achieved a positive one in Lufa, either by increasing their energy intakes during the last days of the survey period (Kaul) or by decreasing their energy expenditure (Lufa). Such a day-of-the survey effect, in the absence of a day of the week effect, suggests that in these two communities the fact of being observed may have induced a systematic modification of the spontaneous eating and activity patterns. Energy balance did not correlate with either energy intake or energy expenditure.

With the exception of a slight negativity of the energy balance on the first day of observation, the Italian shipyard workers do not show any evidence of a day-of-the survey effect, but a very definite weekly trend of energy balance is present (Ferro-Luzzi 1982; Norgan and Ferro-Luzzi 1978). Their energy balance correlates positively with energy intake ($r = 0.74$) and negatively with energy expenditure ($r = 0.39$) indicating that on the days when energy intake is high, energy expenditure is low (positive energy balance) and, conversely, that high energy expenditure days are not followed by a proportional increase in energy intake on the following day. This trend becomes even more conspicuous and diversified when the group is divided into three categories according to the characteristics of the job. Table 5 illustrates that the positive week-end (rest days) energy balance is the outcome of the combined effect of a pronounced decrease in physical activity and a moderate gorging, with the moderate and heavy workers compensating for the negative energy balance of the working days by consuming approximately 500 kcal in excess of their needs over the weekend. The sedentary group, which is in positive energy balance throughout the week, does not appear to adjust over the weekends, and an average excess of 166 kcal/d results. This suggests, for subjects who were free from external constraints of food availability, the existence of some adaptive or regulatory mechanism which operates on a weekly basis to redress a negative, but not a positive, energy balance. As neither body weight nor body fat were significantly correlated with energy balance, however, it is also possible that sedentary workers are able to regulate their energy balance in the long-term, perhaps on a seasonal basis.

Table 5   Infra-week variation in energy intake and balance in three
groups of industry workers (Ferro-Luzzi 1982; Norgan and
Ferro-Luzzi 1978).

Work Category	N	Work days		Rest days		Weekly Total	
		Intake kcal/d	Balance kcal/d	Intake kcal/d	Balance kcal/d	Intake kcal/d	Balance kcal/d
Light	38	2963	+110	3162	+295	3021	+166
Medium	36	3201	-45	3309	+404	3236	+94
Heavy	75	3294	-185	3475	+670	3357	+61
Total	149	3187	- 76	3335	+510	3242	+96

SUMMARY

Energy intake data is collected for a variety of purposes and therefore, may require different levels of precision, reliability and representativity. If food consumption data are employed to evaluate the state of individual energy balance, rigorous methods of assessment are required, and techniques free of systematic methodological bias (e.g. "flat-slope" syndrome) should be used.

It is reasonably safe to assume that, with notable exceptions such as growing children, the great majority of the world's population is in long-term energy equilibrium. This equilibrium apparently results from a succession of cycles of energy imbalance which are more or less periodic, reciprocally compensatory, and of variable duration. Thus, over an appropriate period of time, the energy intake of most individuals may be equal to their energy expenditure, while over shorter periods the balance varies and energy intake alone cannot provide an indication of the state of energy balance. Given the long-term energy equilibrium of populations and an appropriate time-frame, then, energy intake data can be expected to relate to energy expenditure by means of a complex multimodal distribution.

Day-to-day energy equilibrium appears to be the exception in subjects under free-living conditions, but more documentation is needed on intra-individual variability of energy balance. This is especially true in situations where free access to unrestricted food is not guaranteed and where peaks in energy output are expected to occur.

There is also insufficient documentation on how energy balance is achieved in the mid-term. Certain groups have been found to keep food intake constant while varying the level of energy expenditure (e.g. Italian shipyard workers), while others are likely to adjust food intake to energy expenditure, either simultaneously or after a lag of variable duration.

Body weight fluctuations over time remain the simplest approach to diagnosing the dynamics of energy balance. Simultaneous measure of food consumption can provide supplementary information on the levels of energy intake at which equilibrium is achieved in energy metabolism. Neither of these, however, represents a complete and meaningful set of data. The major issue in free-living conditions is not whether energy equilibrium is achieved or not at a given energy intake level, but the determination of which activities are curtailed in order to re-equilibrate a negative energy balance. This determination can be achieved only by the simultaneous, global assessment of food intake, time allocation, energy spent on various activities, and the economic, social and functional relevance of these activities.

REFERENCES

1. Acheson KJ, Campbell IT, Edholm OG, Miller DS, and Stock MJ (1980). The measurement of daily energy expenditure; an evaluation of some techniques. Am J Clin Nutr 33:1155-1164.
2. Alicino G, Barison E, Sette S, Scaccini C, and Ferro-Luzzi A (In preparation). Potential erros in dietary survey methodology: 1. Estimate of portion sizes in the 24-hr. recall technique.
3. Ashworth A (1968). An investigation of very low calorie intakes reported in Jamaica. Br J Nutr 22:341-355.
4. Balogh M, Kahn HA, and Medalie JH (1971). Random repeat 24-hour dietary recalls. Am J Clin Nutr 24:304-310.
5. Beaton GH, Milner J, Corey P, McGuire V, Cousin M, Stewart E, de Ramos M, Hewitt D, Grambsch PV,

Kassim N, and Little JA (1979). Sources of variance in 24-hour dietary recall data: implications for nutrition study design and interpretation. Am J Clin Nutr 32:2546-2559.

6. Bleiberg F, Brun TA, Goihman S, and Lippman D (1981). Food intake and energy expenditure of male and female farmers from Upper-Volta. Brit J Nutr 45:505-515.

7. Campbell VA and Dodds ML (1967). Collecting dietary information from groups of older people. J Am Dietet Assoc 51:29-33.

8. Chalmers FW, Clayton MM, Gates LO, Tucker RE, Werts AW, Young CM, and Foster WD (1952). The dietary record-how many and which days? J Am Dietet Assoc 18:711-717.

9. Church HN, Clayton MM, Young CM, and Foster WD (1954). Can different interviewers obtain comparable dietary survey data?. J Am Dietet Assoc 30:777-779.

10. Dawber TR, Pearson G, Anderson P, Mann GV, Kannel WB, Shurtleff D, and McNamara P (1962). Dietary assessment in the epidemiologic study of coronary heart disease: the Framingham study II. Reliability of measurement. Am J Clin Nutr 11:226-234.

11. De Guzman MaPE, Dominguez SR, Kalaw JM, Buning MN, Basconcillo RO, and Santos VF (1974a). A study of the energy expenditure, dietary intake and pattern of daily activity among various occupational groups. I. Laguna rice farmers. Phil J Sci 103:53-65.

12. De Guzman MaPE, Dominguez SR, Kalaw JM, Buning MN, Basconcillo RO, and Santos VF (1974b). A study of the energy expenditure, dietary intake and pattern of daily activity among various occupational groups. II. Marikina Shoemakers and Housewives. Phil J Nutr 27:21-30.

13. De Guzman MaPE, Kalaw JM, Tan RH, Recto RC, Baconcillo RO, Ferrer VT, Tumbokon MS, Yuchingtan GP, and Gaurano AL (1974c). A study of the energy expenditure, dietary intake and pattern of daily activity among various occupational groups. III. Urban Jeepney Drivers. Phil J Nutr 27:182-188.

14. De Guzman MaPE, Cabrera JP, Basconcillo RO, Gaurano AL, Yuchingtan GP, Tan RM, Kalaw JM, and Recto RC (1978). A study of the energy expenditure, dietary intake and pattern of daily activity among various occupational groups. V. Clerk-Typist. Phil J Nutr 31:147-156.

15. Durnin JVGA and Brockway JM (1959). Determination of the total daily energy expenditure in man by indirect calorimetry: assessment of the accuracy of a modern technique. Brit J Nutr 13:41-53.
16. Durnin JVGA (1961). Calorie balance in man. Proc Nutr Soc 20:52-67.
17. Durnin JVGA (1979). Energy balance in man with particular reference to low intakes. Biblthca Nutr Dieta 27:1-10.
18. Eagles JA, Grant Whiting M, and Olson RE (1966). Dietary appraisal. Problems in processing dietary data. Am J Clin Nutr 19:1-9.
19. Edholm OG, Fletcher JG, Widdowson EM, and McCance RA (1955). The energy expenditure and food intake of individual men. Brit J Nutr 9:286-300.
20. Edholm OG (1961). Energy expenditure and calorie intake in young men. Proc Nutr Soc 20:71-83.
21. Edholm OG, Adam JM, Heavy JR, Wolff HS, Goldsmith R, and Best TW (1970). Food intake and energy expenditure of army recruits. Brit J Nutr 24:1091-1107.
22. Edholm OG (1977). Energy balance in man. J Hum Nutr 31:413-431.
23. Emmons L and Hayes M (1973). Accuracy of 24-hr recalls of young children. J Am Dietet Assoc 62:409-415.
24. Ferro-Luzzi A (1982). Meaning and constraints of energy-intake studies in free-living populations. In Harrison GA (ed): "Energy and Effort, Symposia of SSHB," London: Taylor and Francis, pp. 115-137.
25. Gersovitz M, Madden JP and Smiciklas Wright H (1978). Validity of the 24-hr dietary recall and seven-day record for group comparison. J Am Dietet Assoc 73:48-55.
26. Hallfrisch J, Steele P, and Cohen L (1982). Comparison of seven-day diet record with measured food intake of twenty-four subjects. Nutr Res 2:263-273.
27. Karvetti RL and Knuts LR (1981). Agreement between dietary interviews. J Am Dietet Assoc 79:654-660.
28. Liu K, Stamler J, Dyer A, McKeever J, and McKeever P (1978). Statistical methods to assess and minimize the role of intra-individual variability in obscuring the relationship between dietary lipids and serum cholesterol. J Chron Dis 31:399-418.

29. Madden JP, Goodman SJ, and Guthrie HA (1976). Validity of the 24-hr recall. J Am Dietet Assoc 68:143-147.
30. Marr JW (1971). Individual dietary surveys: purposes and methods. Wld Rev Nutr Diet 13:105-164.
31. McNaughton JW and Cahn AJ (1970). A study of the energy expenditure and food intake of five boys and four girls. Br J Nutr 24:345-355.
32. Morgan RW, Jain M, Miller AB, Choi NN, Mathews V, Munan L, Burch JD, Feather J, Howe GR, and Kelly A (1978). A comparison of dietary methods in epidemiologic studies. Amer J Epid 107:488-498.
33. Norgan NG, Ferro-Luzzi A, and Durnin JVGA (1974). The energy and nutrient intake and the energy expenditure of 204 New Guinean adults. Philos Trans R Soc Lond B 268:309-348.
34. Norgan NG and Ferro-Luzzi A (1978). Nutrition, physical activity, and physical fitness in contrasting environments. In Pariskova J and Rogozkin VA (eds): "Nutrition, Physical Fitness, and Health; Int. Series Sport Sci.," Baltimore: University Park Press, pp. 167-193.
35. Osgood CE (1953). "Method and Theory in Experimental Psychology." New York: Oxford Univ Press, pp. 550-597.
36. Passmore R, Thomson JG, Warnock GM, Dixon CM, Kitchin AH, Smith G, Vaughan MC, and Watt JA (1952). A balance sheet of the estimation of energy intake and energy expenditure as measured by indirect calorimetry, using the Kofranyi-Michaelis calorimeter. Br J Nutr 6:253-164.
37. Prentice AM, Whitehead RG, Roberts SB, and Paul AA (1981). Long-term energy balance in child-bearing Gambian women. Am J Clin Nutr 34:2790-2799.
38. Rasanen L (1979). Nutrition survey of Finnish rural children. VI. Methodological study comparing the 24-hour recall and the dietary history interview. Am J Clin Nutr 32:2560-2567.
39. Rivers JP and Payne PR (1982). The comparison of energy supply and energy need: a critique of energy requirements. In Harrison GA (ed): "Energy and Effort, Symposia of SSHB," London: Taylor and Francis, pp 85.
40. Sette S, Minnucci D, Scaccini C, and Ferro-Luzzi A (In preparation). Potential errors in dietary survey meth-

odology: 2. The validation of the 24-hr. recall technique in elderly persons.

41. Spencer T and Heywood P (In press). Seasonality, subsistence agriculture and nutrition in a Lowlands Community of Papua, New Guinea. Ecol Food Nutr.

42. Taggart N (1962). Diet activity and body-weight. A study of variations in a woman. Brit. J. Nutr 16:223-235.

43. Viteri FE, Torun B, Galicia JC, and Herrera E (1971). Determining energy costs of agricultural activities by respirometer and energy balance techniques. Am J Clin Nutr 24:1418-1430.

44. Widdowson EM (1962). Nutritional variation. Proc Nutr Soc 21:121-135.

45. Widdowson EM (1974). Spc Rep Ser Med Res Coun no. 257.

46. Young CM, Chalmers FW, Church HN, Clayton MM, Tucker RE, Werts AW, and Foster WD (1952). A comparison of dietary study methods. I. Dietary history vs. seven-day-record. J Am Dietet Assoc 28:124-128.

Energy Intake and Activity, pages 101–113

SOME PROBLEMS IN ASSESSING THE ROLE OF PHYSICAL ACTIVITY IN THE MAINTENANCE OF ENERGY BALANCE

J.V.G.A. Durnin

Institute of Physiology
University of Glasgow

INTRODUCTION

Energy balance is defined as a state of equilibrium between energy intake and energy expenditure. This balance can occur at any one of a range of body weights for the individual; i.e., it may be attained within some 'desirable' range of body mass, or it may exist at body weights lower or higher than the norm. As an illustration of this, many young women in so called 'developed' countries maintain, sometimes semi-permanently, body weights at levels which are low relative to their stature because their fat mass is minimal. This results from long-continued low food intakes, and it is accompanied by the physiological adaptations to semi-starvation, i.e., loss of body mass in the initial stages, (usually) low levels of physical activity, and perhaps the most important adaptation - a fall in the basal metabolic rate (BMR).

At the other extreme is the state of moderate obesity where individuals are fatter than is desirable for health or welfare, but where body mass and composition can remain stable for long periods of time. Most of the evidence seems to indicate that little metabolic adaptation takes place here other than the increase in metabolic rate which ensues because of the larger total body mass.

ACTIVITY AND FATNESS

At energy balances where body mass is either very small or very large, physical activity is usually low - in the

one case because the total food intake may not allow sufficient energy for exercise, and in the other because obesity
is often accompanied by relative inactivity. This last relationship has been shown in several populations. Data from a
study on middle-aged men and women and on adolescent girls
(Durnin 1967) (Table 1) shows a clear inverse relationship
between body fatness and the duration of physical activity.

TABLE 1

Mean time (min/d) in 'moderate' physical
activity of middle-aged men and women
and of adolescent girls
related to body build.

	Middle-aged Men	Women	Adolescent girls
Thin	143	99	91
'Normal'	101	57	93
Moderately Obese	87	36	63

In later studies on adolescents, Durnin et al. (1974)
(Table 2) found that energy intake was much lower in the
fattest adolescent girls than in the thinnest, and McKillop
and Durnin (1982) showed the same phenomenon in infant
girls. While different metabolic rates may contribute, it is

TABLE 2

Energy intake (kcal/d) of fattest and
thinnest (highest 10% and lowest 10%
of the population) adolescent
girls and infants

	Thinnest	Fattest
14y girls	2207	1690
infant girls (3 months to 2y)	946	867

almost certain that the fattest groups expended considerably less energy in physical activity. Similar inverse relationships between physical activity and obesity have been described by Rand and Stunkard (1974), Bromwell et al. (1980), and Baeke et al. (1983). However, Lincoln (1972) and Saris (1982) did not report the same findings, so there is no absolute consensus on this issue.

METABOLIC ADAPTATIONS TO ENERGY IMBALANCE

Some of the problems associated with consciously restricted low food intakes are illustrated in a small but lengthy experiment carried out on a middle-aged woman during about 20 months. Physical activity was held constant at the usual level, but energy intake was varied considerably (Ghali and Durnin 1977). During separate periods, each of about 4 weeks duration, the daily intake of energy was varied, more or less randomly, to either 700 kcal above or below the control level. Intake returned to 'normal' during intervening periods. The design of the experiment is shown in Fig. 1.

Figure 1

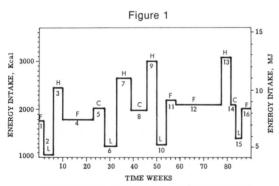

Design of the study, arrangement of the different periods and
level of energy intake at each
F = free, L = low, H = high, C = control

During the undereating phases the BMR decreased. This adaptation has been well documented in the past (Keys et al. 1950; Grande et al. 1958). When the body weight increased during the overeating stages, the BMR rose again.

An unexpected finding appeared, however, in that with repeated periods of undereating the BMR seemed to become reduced to progressively lower levels (Fig. 2) so that at the end of the 20 months of the experiment, although the body weight had returned to its original control value, the BMR was 15% lower than initially. In this case, the physiological adaptation to low food intakes had resulted in a situation where, in the absence of physical activity, energy balance was difficult to maintain since the energy requirements for balance at the original body weight had become so reduced.

Figure 2

CHANGE IN METABOLIC RATE IN UNDER- AND OVER-FEEDING

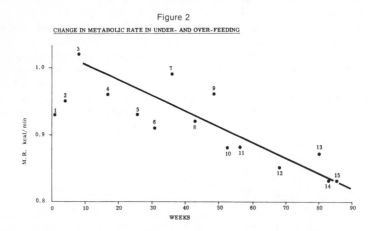

METHODOLOGICAL PROBLEMS

The methods used to measure energy balance under free-living conditions present a problem of considerable magnitude. It is possible to assess energy balance solely on the basis of the maintenance of a constant body weight. That phenomenon will be informative about the existence of energy balance, but will not tell us at what level it is occurring or what adjustments in intake or expenditure have occurred. Therefore, unless energy balance is being assessed at a very superficial level, measurements of both energy intake and energy expenditure are required.

Some of the problems connected with the measurement of energy intake have been discussed in this volume by

Ferro-Luzzi and they are impressively difficult. The complexities of measuring energy expenditure may well be even worse. It is not the intention of this paper to present details of the various methodologies, some of which have been described and analysed elsewhere (Durnin 1978) and some of which also are the concern of other chapters in this volume. However, some possibly contentious conclusions can be drawn from the author's recent data. These conclusions, not previously documented, have become evident because of the unusual nature of the study - a series of repeated measures of all the factors concerned in energy balance in a group of pregnant women studied longitudinally.

There may be considerable discrepancy between energy intake and expenditure of individuals, or even of groups, when these are measured during several consecutive days. Durnin (1961) showed that only 5% of a group of 69 men and women had intakes of energy which were closely related to expenditures on a daily basis. On a weekly basis, about 60% of the individuals reached agreement between the two. The remainder demonstrated no relationship between intake and expenditure of energy during 7 days. There are also notorious and unexplained examples of marked discrepancy in mean intake and energy expenditure between groups. Norgan et al. (1974) in a study of 2 village populations in New Guinea, one coastal and one highland, obtained very similar results for energy intake and expenditure for both men and women in the highland group, but observed a difference of about 500 kcal/d between the two sets of measurements in both men and women in the coastal village. The methodology was exactly the same in both situations and there seems to be no adequate explanation for the discrepancy on the basis of season, work, food availability, changing body weight, etc.

These incompatibilities between intake and expenditure have been a source of concern to investigators, but usually have been shrugged off as reflecting the probability that measurements on an individual (or on groups of individuals), carried out during short periods of time, may reflect normal variability in both daily food intake and physical activity. The methodology in this field is too imprecise to detect the resulting small alterations in body mass and body composition caused by these short-term energy imbalances.

OBJECTIVES OF ENERGY EXPENDITURE MEASUREMENTS

Measurements of energy expenditure by indirect calorimetry have relevance in two broad categories. First, they attempt to quantify the energy expended during short periods of time, often of only some minutes duration. These periods might be related to specific activities concerned with work, leisure, sport, or home. The second category is concerned with the assessment of the total energy expended during longer periods of time, perhaps a full 24 hour day, an 8 hour work shift, or something similar. The assumption is that intermittent measurements of the energy expended in specific activities, together with a timed record of the pattern of activities, will provide a reasonably accurate assessment of the total energy expended during the period. An accurate validation of this second category has almost never been done under field conditions. An exception, however, is some recent work by Webb using an ingenious version of a direct calorimeter (Webb et al. 1980).

POSSIBLE MEASUREMENT ERRORS

Several studies described recently (Durnin et al. 1982) suggest cause for concern about the use of and limitations on the measurement of energy expenditure. A series of experiments recently carried out in Glasgow (Durnin et al. 1982) on pregnant women has allowed, possibly for the first time, a reasonably well-grounded value to be attached to one side of the equation involved in energy balance, thus providing a comparison for energy expenditure estimates. Measurements have been made on a group of 22 women, beginning in early pregnancy (6-10 weeks) and repeated approximately once every 6 weeks throughout pregnancy, i.e. performed 5 to 6 times on each woman. The measurements consisted of 5 consecutive days of weighed food intake using the individual inventory method; energy expenditure during the same 5 days determined by a combination of an activity diary and indirect calorimetric measurements of the important activities; BMR measured in the laboratory; anthropometric measures of skinfolds, limb circumferences, skeletal diameters, height and weight; body fat measured by densitometry using the underwater weighing method; exercise test on the treadmill; and weekly body weights. There are various reasons why this particular situation should allow a better assessment of the validity and accuracy of moderate to long-term energy expenditure estimates. This study provided more than a straight comparison between energy intake and energy expenditure, each measured during a few days. Almost without exception, all previous measurements of energy intake and expenditure in free-living individuals have been done in a state of equilibrium. That is, the measurements have been done on groups of farmers, house-wives, office clerks, or shop workers, etc. during a limited period of time (usually 5-7 consecutive days for each indi-vidual person), when these people have been in a more or less stable state. For almost all the groups, mean energy intake and mean energy expenditure have agreed to within about ± 10% of each other and this has been assumed to give an indication of the approximate error of the method. Even when the relevant values for individual men or women have not agreed, this has often been regarded as only a tempo-rary aberration of either intake or expenditure.

In the present instance, the subjects are not in energy equilibrium. Over an interval of some months, changes have occurred in the energy equilibrium which have resulted in a measurable increase in the total energy mass of the individu-al woman. She has produced a baby whose weight was known exactly, and whose body composition could be estimat-ed with an unimportant small error. The placenta was weighed at the time of delivery; the size of the uterus could be estimated to levels which would involve inaccuracies of no importance in energy balance. The change in body weight and in body fat of the mothers was measured, again with an error which, as discussed below and as shown in Tables 3 to 6, is not relevant to the main conclusions.

Table 3

Subject A.P.

Energy Balance During Pregnancy

Periods (Weeks)	Wt (kg)	Fat (kg)	Energy Cost of Gain (Kcals)				E.I. (Kcals/d)	E.E. (Kcals/d)	E.I.-E.E. (Kcals/d)	Energy Balance Over Period (Kcals)
			Fat Gain (Kcals)	Foetus + Placenta + Uterus + Breast, Etc.		Total (Kcals)				
				Protein (Kcals)	Fat (Kcals)					
(1)	(2)	(3)	(4)	(5)	(6)	(7)	(8)	(9)	(10)	(11)
11-16	1.6	0.43	4730	325	55	+ 5110	2326	2160	+166	+ 5810
16-24	3.5	2.20	24200	920	480	+25604	2295	2137	+158	+ 8848
24-30	2.0	1.22	13420	990	660	+15070	2662	2025	+637	+26754
30-37	1.0	0.30	3300	1505	2849	+ 7654	2270	2146	+124	+ 6076
37-40	3.5	1.05	11550	645	1221	+13416	2324	2212	+112	+ 2352
Total	11.6	5.20	57200	4385	5269	+66850				+49840

Initial Body Wt: 56.90 kg.
Birth Wt: 3.06 Kg.
Placenta: 600 g.

Table 4

Subject E.W.

Energy Balance During Pregnancy

Periods (Weeks)	Wt (kg)	Fat (kg)	Energy Cost of Gain (Kcals)				E.I. (Kcals/d)	E.E. (Kcals/d)	E.I.-E.E. (Kcals/d)	Energy Balance Over Period (Kcals)
			Fat Gain (Kcals)	Foetus + Placenta + Uterus + Breast, Etc.		Total (Kcals)				
				Protein (Kcals)	Fat (Kcals)					
(1)	(2)	(3)	(4)	(5)	(6)	(7)	(8)	(9)	(10)	(11)
13-18	1.60	0.60	6600	325	55	+ 6980	2480	1735	+745	+26075
18-24	3.20	1.20	13200	790	460	+14450	1954	1882	+72	+ 3024
24-31	3.20	2.00	22000	1205	1067	+24272	2466	1885	+581	+28469
31-37	2.20	0.80	8800	1290	2442	+12532	2608	1849	+759	+31878
Total	10.20	4.60	50600	3610	4024	+58234				+89446

Initial Body Wt: 71.90 kg
Birth Wt: 2.78 kg
Placenta Wt: 627 g.

Table 6

Subject S.H.

Energy Balance During Pregnancy

Periods (Weeks)	Wt (kg)	Fat (kg)	Energy Cost of Gain (Kcals)				E.I. (Kcals/d)	E.E. (Kcals/d)	E.I.-E.E. (Kcals/d)	Energy Balance Over Period (Kcals)
			Fat Gain (Kcals)	Foetus + Placenta + Uterus + Breast, Etc.		Total (Kcals)				
				Protein (Kcals)	Fat (Kcals)					
(1)	(2)	(3)	(4)	(5)	(6)	(7)	(8)	(9)	(10)	(11)
13-19	6.50	+3.60	39600	390	79	+40069	1857	2005	-148	- 6216
19-25	5.75	+3.50	38500	890	68	+39458	1803	1953	-150	- 6300
25-31	-0.55	-0.20	-2200	1040	462	- 698	2484	2016	+468	+19656
31-37	4.25	+1.50	16500	1290	2442	+20232	*1342	2104	-762	-16002
37-40	0.80	+0.35	3850	645	1221	+ 5716	2396	1969	+427	+ 8967
Total	16.75	8.75	96950	4255	4272	+104777				+ 105

Initial Body Wt: 67.00 kg
Birth Wt: 3.64 kg
Placenta Wt: 800 g.

* 3 weeks dieting; calculated as 21 days at - 762 Kcal/d

Table 5

Subject A.F.

Energy Balance During Pregnancy

Periods (Weeks)	Wt (kg)	Fat (kg)	Energy Cost of Gain (Kcals)				E.I. (Kcals/d)	E.E. (Kcals/d)	E.I.-E.E. (Kcals/d)	Energy Balance Over Period (Kcals)
			Fat Gain (Kcals)	Foetus + Placenta + Uterus + Breast, Etc.		Total (Kcals)				
				Protein (Kcals)	Fat (Kcals)					
(1)	(2)	(3)	(4)	(5)	(6)	(7)	(8)	(9)	(10)	(11)
13-18	2.40	1.90	20900	325	66	+21291	2271	2267	+4	+ 140
18-25	4.15	1.90	20900	955	576	+22431	2502	2141	+361	+17689
25-31	1.70	0.50	5500	1040	957	+ 7497	2127	2279	-152	- 6384
31-39	3.10	1.00	11000	1720	3256	+15976	2310	2188	+122	+ 6832
39-40	-	-	-	-	-	-	2411	2221	+190	+ 1330
Total	11.35	5.3	58300	4040	4855	+67195				+19607

Initial Body Wt: 57.65 kg
Birth Wt: 3.35 kg
Placenta Wt: 600 g.

Using these measures, it was possible to calculate the overall energy required to effect these changes (the energy costs of depositing the protein and the fat components were calculated separately). Food intake was measured by the woman herself, each individual weighing all items of food eaten or drunk during each period of 5 days. With modern electronic scales, incorporating a zeroing button and a large digital read-out, it became a simple and almost automatic procedure for the women, especially since this was done 5 or 6 times during the pregnancy. The impression of the investigators is that the individual subjects undertook this task with high levels of accuracy.

The study indicates that the energy intakes and the separate energy costs of pregnancy were calculated with relatively small errors. Therefore, if energy expenditures could have been assessed similarly, there should have been reasonable agreement between both sides of the energy equation, i.e. the differences between energy intake and energy expenditure should have equalled the total energy costs of pregnancy. Tables 3 to 6, however, provide some examples, for individual cases, of the very considerable disagreement between the theoretical requirements and the measured energy imbalance.

Column 7 in each of these tables indicates the energy costs for subject's fat gain and for the increase in weight of the fetus, placenta, uterus, and breasts. Column 11 shows the calculated total of energy difference for each measurement period (energy difference multiplied by number of days in period). The overall totals of the two columns represent combined figures for the pregnancy and should be approximately equal.

In fact, in Table 3 there is a disagreement of -17010 kcal, in Table 4 of +31212 kcal, in Table 5 of -47588 kcal and in Table 6 of -104672 kcal. Apart from Table 3, most of these disagreements are considerable and would markedly influence the calculation of the supposed energy need of pregnancy. (The 4 tables show results which are more or less proportionately typical of the group of 22 women measured in Glasgow). There are several possible explanations for these large discrepancies, of which the most likely are errors in the measurement and estimated energy cost of the increased body mass, and errors in the energy intake and energy expenditure measurements. Long experience with these techniques in the laboratory suggests that the measurements of body mass, by repeated estimations using both body density and skinfold thicknesses, will have been in error by one to two kg at the most. The total amount of fat gained is usually on the order of 4-5 kg, so an error of 1-2 kg represents ± 20-40% - a large and unlikely error indeed!

There seems little scope for error in the energy cost of laying down the fat mass. The energy value of fat is 9 kcal per g, or 9000 kcal per kg. The cost of depositing this in the body is rated as 11000 kcal (which includes the energy content of the fat). It is almost impossible that an error of more than about ± 1000 kcal can occur here. One is almost compelled to assume, therefore, that by far the largest source of error is either in the measurement of food intake or of energy expenditure. Food intake seems an improbable source of consistent or large bias in assessing energy intake, as has been briefly discussed above. Energy expenditure, on the other hand, because of the notorious difficulty in applying the rather primitive methodology in field conditions, is the most likely source of a consistent and important error. For example, if energy expenditure were overestimated by as little as 200 kcal per day (which is about a 10% error and would be tolerated, normally) it would be equivalent to 56000 kcal over the 280 days of pregnancy.

CONCLUSION

The conclusion appears to be that energy expenditure measurements, as they are carried out at present, can be of little assistance in assessing energy balance under free-living conditions. This is not to say that the measurements do not have wide-ranging uses: they provide information on the energy cost of single activities which may be helpful in determining the stress of work situations; they are of interest, and perhaps of medical importance, in sport; they are useful in giving advice about the prevention or treatment of obesity; they can be utilized in measuring mechanical efficiency of different body movements, or of differing designs of work tools. Valid assessment of physical activity can give us critically important information in marginally nourished or flagrantly malnourished populations. However, the errors are of such magnitude when these measurements are applied to the assessment of total energy expenditure over large parts of a day, or as the average over several complete days, that the interpretation of such information must have very serious limitations.

There are several reasons for the potential errors. One of the most important is uncertainty about the validity of the value obtained when the measure is applied in real situations. It is clear that in these cases the actual energy expended could vary considerably. For example, the average of even several measurements of 'sitting' or 'walking' may not represent the average energy expended in such highly variable activities. On the other hand, the estimate of total energy expenditure is seldom essential in the context of energy balance. A general indication of the level of physical activity and of its fluctuations in normal everyday life is often useful in situations where energy balance is being investigated, e.g. in rural populations whose nutritional status may be marginally adequate. However, reasonably satisfactory information can usually be obtained by a few measurements of the energy expended in some specific activities, coupled with an approximate breakdown of the duration of the varying activities for an average day. There is no need - and it is probably invalid in any case - to attempt an accurate estimation of the average total 24 hour energy expenditure.

In most cases total energy intake, which is more easily and exactly measured, coupled with data on changes in body weight and body composition, will provide satisfactory data on energy expenditure and energy balance. The basic information can be obtained from measurements of energy intake, repeated on more than one occasion (e.g., a 5-day survey repeated after an interval of several weeks), combined with long-term measurements of fluctuations in body weight. A regression line plotted over a course of several months, for weekly or biweekly weights of an individual, will easily show whether or not body weight is stable. The energy intakes will indicate at what level the stability is occurring.

Of necessity, most surveys of this kind would be done on small numbers of individuals. This is a disadvantage, but it is better to accumulate, even though slowly, more of this important information than to continue with the acquisition of data which is not only very difficult to obtain in field conditions, but which also has very limited usefulness. One can criticize, in the same fashion, the likely advantages of some of the newer techniques of determining oxygen consumption over long periods - several days - by carbon and oxygen labelling; such techniques may well end up simply as temporarily interesting and expensive ways of validating energy intake measurements. What will be obtained will be an estimate of total oxygen consumption, allowing total energy expenditure to be calculated. However, there is still the problem of knowing how representative is that total value of energy expenditure relative to the normal long-term pattern of the individual. And no breakdown of the activity pattern will have been obtained.

There are several areas within the subject of energy balance which could be explored profitably and some of them require only simple methodology. For example, long-term measurements of body weight on various populations, particularly those nutritionally at risk, would provide evidence on existence of or fluctuations in energy balance. Repetitive measurements of food intake on those populations could supply valid evidence on the level of energy intake at which energy balance does (or does not) exist. Physical activity patterns, particularly in leisure time, could give an indication of whether a population might be in apparent energy balance but still have insufficient food energy available to allow for active leisure pursuits.

It is astonishing that reliable data on these subjects is so scarce, particularly when their nutritional and socio-anthropological importance for much of the world's population is so evident.

REFERENCES

1.   Baecke JAH, van Staveren WA, and Burema J (1983). Food consumption, habitual physical activity, and body fatness in young Dutch adults. Am J Clin Nutr 37:278-286.

2. Bromwell KD, Stunkard AJ and Albaum JM (1980). Evaluation and modification of exercise patterns in the natural environment. Am J Psychiat 137:1540-l545.
3. Durnin JVGA (1961). 'Appetite' and the relationships between expenditure and intake of calories in man. J Physiol 156:294-309.
4. Durnin JVGA (1967). Activity patterns in the community. Can Med Ass J 96:882-886.
5. Durnin JVGA (1978). Indirect calorimetry in man: a critique of practical problems. Proc Nutr Soc 37:5-12.
6. Durnin JVGA, Lonergan ME, Good J, and Ewan A (1974). A cross-sectional nutritional and anthropometric study with an interval of 7 years on 611 young adolescent children. Br J Nutr 32:169-179.
7. Durnin JVGA, McKillop FM, Grant S and Fitzgerald G (1982). Studies on the energy requirements of human pregnancy and lactation - Glasgow. Proc Nutr Soc 41:146a.
8. Ghali N and Durnin JVGA (1977). A study of the energy balance of a woman on varying energy intakes during 14 months. Proc Nutr Soc 36:91a.
9. Grande F, Anderson JT and Keys A (1958). Changes of basal metabolic rate in man in semi-starvation and refeeding. J Appl Physiol 12:230-235.
10. Keys A, Brozek J, Henschel A, Mickelsen A, and Taylor HL (1950). The Biology of Human Starvation. Minneapolis: University of Minnesota Press.
11. Lincoln JE (1972). Caloric intake, obesity and physical activity. Am J Clin Nutr 25:390-394.
12. McKillop FM and Durnin JVGA (1982). The energy and nutrient intake of a random sample (305) of infants. Hum Nutr: App Nutr 36a:405-421.
13. Norgan NG, Ferro-Luzzi A and Durnin JVGA (1974). The energy and nutrient intake and the energy expenditure of 204 New Guinean adults. Phil Trans R Soc Lond B 268: 309-348.
14. Rand C and Stunkard AJ (1974). Obesity and psychoanalysis. Am J Psychiat 135:547-551.
15. Saris WHM (1982). Aerobic power and daily physical activity in children. Thesis of Catholic University of Nijmegen, Holland.
16. Webb P, Annis JF and Troutman SJ (1980). Energy balance in man measured by direct and indirect calorimetry. Am J Clin Nutr 33: 1287-1298.

Energy Intake and Activity, pages 115–129
© 1984 Alan R. Liss, Inc., 150 Fifth Avenue, New York, NY 10011

APPROPRIATE METHODOLOGY FOR ASSESSING PHYSICAL
ACTIVITY UNDER LABORATORY CONDITIONS IN
STUDIES OF ENERGY BALANCE IN ADULTS

Edward S. Horton

Metabolic Unit
University of Vermont College of Medicine
Burlington, Vermont   05405

INTRODUCTION

When considering appropriate methodology for assessing
energy expenditure due to physical activity, it is important
to view the energy costs of performing work in the context
of both total energy balance and the other processes which
contribute to energy expenditure in man. Energy expenditure can be divided conveniently into four major compartments consisting of the resting metabolic rate, the thermic
effect of food, the thermic effect of physical exercise, and
the phenomenon of adaptive thermogenesis (Horton and
Danforth 1982). The resting metabolic rate (RMR) refers to
the energy expended when an individual is resting quietly in
a comfortable environment several hours after significant
physical activity or the ingestion of a meal. Although
slightly higher than the true basic metabolic rate, it is a
good measure of the energy consumed for maintenance of
normal body functions such as a cardiorespiratory activity,
maintenance of metabolic homeostasis, and other biochemical
processes within the body. There is also a small component
related to sympathetic nervous system activity and to the
thyroid hormones. For an average 70 kg male the RMR is
approximately 1500 kcal/day and comprises 60-70% of total
daily energy expenditure.

The thermic effect of food refers to the extra heat
produced following ingestion of a meal. All three major food
stuffs (carbohydrates, fats and proteins) produce an increase in the metabolic rate which lasts for several hours.

The magnitude of the thermic response to a given meal depends on several factors including the caloric content and composition of the meal itself, and the nutritional state and antecedent diet of the individual. It can be accounted for largely by the energy required for the digestion, absorption, transport, metabolism, and storage of the ingested food; however, other factors, such as activation of the sympathetic nervous system, may contribute as much as 25-50% of the thermogenic response. On average, the thermic effect of food usually accounts for approximately 10% of ingested calories.

Of all the compartments of energy expenditure, the energy cost of performing physical work is the most variable. In man, as in other animals, the metabolic efficiency of performing physical work is approximately 30% and the daily energy requirements for physical work depend on both the intensity and duration of the activities performed. Changes in diet or nutritional status, which may have major effects on the resting metabolic rate, appear to have little or no effect on the thermic effect of exercise.

The final compartment of energy expenditure, adaptive thermogenesis, refers to changes in the resting metabolic rate which are the result of adaptations to changes in ambient temperature, food intake, emotional stress, or other environmental conditions. Good examples of this are the increases in RMR which occur in cold adapted animals or in response to overfeeding, and the decrease in RMR which occurs during food restriction. The mechanism by which adaptive thermogenesis occurs is not yet fully understood although there is now good evidence that activity of the sympathetic nervous system, and changes in circulating concentrations of thyroid hormones and other thermogenic hormones, such as insulin, all may play a role. Adaptive thermogenesis probably never accounts for more than a 10-15% change in the resting metabolic rate, but over along periods of time this may be important in maintaining energy balance under a variety of environmental conditions.

Taken in the context of total energy balance, it is the purpose of this paper to discuss a number of methods that are available to investigators to quantitate energy expenditure associated with physical activity in a laboratory setting. The advantages and disadvantages of the various methods will be discussed with regard to their accuracy, complexity, versatility, availability, and cost. It is also important to consider the manner in which data are to be expressed. It is now customary to express energy expenditure as kcal or joules per unit time or as watts, the latter being the most common in studies of physical activity. Rates of oxygen consumption, carbon dioxide production and calculation of the non-protein respiratory quotient may be converted to any of the above units. When reporting data, however, it is important that investigators provide enough information to allow others to make conversions to more familiar units or to compare one study with another. It is also important to provide information regarding the accuracy of the method used as well as the range of observations and standard errors of the data.

A frequent problem in studies of energy expenditure is to decide what to use as the denominator in calculating the data. Should it be per individual, per kilogram body weight, per kilogram of lean body mass (or fat free mass), or as some function of weight and height such as weight $^{0.75}$, weight $^{0.67}$, weight/height^2 or "ideal body weight"? In studies of energy balance, or when body composition is not known, it seems preferable to express the data per individual. When comparing data from groups of individuals it is best to relate energy expenditure to lean body mass or fat free mass since these give the best approximation of the respiring tissue mass. When there is a limited range of factors, such as body size, body composition, age or sex, affecting metabolic rate it is acceptable to express data per kilogram body weight, and little or no advantage is achieved by using a function of weight and height. However, in assessing energy expenditure in a laboratory setting, every attempt should be made to measure body composition and express the data per kilogram lean body mass or fat free mass.

METHODS OF MEASURING ENERGY EXPENDITURE DURING PHYSICAL ACTIVITY

Direct Calorimetry

Ever since the pioneering experiments of Atwater and Benedict (1905) direct calorimetry has provided the "gold standard" for measuring energy expenditure over fairly long periods of time. Subsequently, several more modern chambers have been constructed (Garrow 1978; Pittet 1981) but none of them have exceeded the accuracy achieved in the early studies where the errors of measurement were as low as 1%. There are many drawbacks, however, to the use of direct calorimetry for studying the energy costs of physical activity. Direct calorimetry chambers are complex, expensive to build, and require a highly trained staff for their successful operation. Consequently, only a few chambers are currently in use and, although some are equipped with a cycle ergometer, they are small, do not allow a wide range of types of physical activity, and are unsuited for measuring energy expenditure of daily, real life activities. The response time is usually too slow and stored heat is not measured until it is dissipated in the chamber environment. Thus, direct calorimetry is best suited for long-term measurements of energy expenditure in which short-term changes in metabolic rate are integrated over a longer time. It does provide, however, an extremely valuable resource for obtaining highly accurate, standardized data on energy expenditure in humans.

In an attempt to increase the versatility of direct calorimetry for studies of energy expenditure during daily activities, Webb, Annis and Troutman (1980) have developed a "space suit" type direct calorimeter which gives excellent results when compared to measurements of energy expenditure by indirect calorimetry. However, this apparatus is somewhat cumbersome, is no more accurate than indirect calorimetry, and must still be considered experimental.

Indirect Calorimetry Methods

In recent years, the use of indirect calorimetry to measure energy expenditure in human studies has become increasingly popular. Energy expenditure can be calculated if one knows the rate of oxygen consumption and the relative proportions of carbohydrates, lipids, and proteins that are being oxidized. The latter can be estimated from the non-protein respiratory quotient which is derived from measurements of CO_2 production, O_2 consumption, and urinary N_2 excretion.

There are several techniques that have been used to measure O_2 consumption and CO_2 production during physical activity in humans. They vary in complexity, versatility, availability, cost, and accuracy, but over the years most of them have provided excellent data on the energy expenditure associated with physical activity and continue to be the best methods available today. Some of the advantages and disadvantages of the various techniques are discussed below.

Portable respirometer. Portable respirometers employ a face mask with valves that direct expired air through collection tubes to a respirometer carried on the subject's back. This contains a flowmeter and a sampling device so that an aliquot of expired gases is collected for analysis at a later time (Kofranyi and Michaelis 1940; Wolff 1956). The accuracy of this method depends on the accuracy of the gas flow meter, the loss of oxygen and carbon dioxide by diffusion through the collection bag, leaks about the face mask and collection system, and the accuracy of the gas analyses (Orsini and Passmore 1951). With proper calibration of the flowmeter, modern materials, and good techniques the error is approximately 2-5%. Portable respirometers provide a relatively simple method of indirect calorimetry. Their portability makes them versatile in measuring energy expenditure across a wide range of physical activities, including many recreational or occupational tasks (Passmore and Durnin 1955). There is relatively minor interference with physical activity, but the wearing of a tight fitting face mask limits the duration of observation and is somewhat unpleasant. The apparatus is fairly lightweight and carrying it adds little to the total energy expenditure during physical activity. Drawbacks of this method are that there is an inherent delay in obtaining results and the rates of energy expenditure during work performance are integrated over the entire periods of gas collection. Nonetheless, the method is relatively inexpensive and easily adapted to field conditions.

Stationary Respirometers. In contrast to the portable versions, stationary respirometers collect all expired gases. This is accomplished with either an inflatable bag (Douglas bag) or a displacement respirometer (Douglas 1911). The total volume of gas is measured and mixed and an aliquot is analyzed for O_2 and CO_2 content. The accuracy is somewhat better than that with a portable apparatus since total expiratory volume is measured directly and gas analysis can often be done immediately after collection. The major sources of error are those due to leaks in the system and the extra work performed by subjects using a mouthpiece (Shephard 1955). For studies of energy expenditure during exercise, a cycle ergometer, treadmill, or other stationary work device is usually used. The versatility and cost of this method are excellent for relatively short-term measurements of energy expenditure in a fixed location. Stationary respirometers are used in many laboratories thoughout the world, both to collect primary data and to calibrate the variety of non-calorimetric methods of estimating energy expenditure which are commonly used in field work.

Ventilated Hood Systems. Instead of collecting expired gases by a mouthpiece or face mask, ventilated hoods have been developed in which the subject is fitted with a transparent hood equipped with a snugly fitting collar. Fresh air is drawn into the hood via an intake port and expired air is drawn out of the hood by a motorized fan. The flow rate is measured by a pneumotachograph, and aliquots of the outflowing air are analyzed for O_2 and CO_2 after adjusting temperature and water vapor content. Oxygen consumption and CO_2 production are calculated from the differences in their concentrations in the inflowing and outflowing air and the flow rate (Ashworth and Wolff 1969; Consolazio and Johnson 1971; Jequier 1981). The accuracy achieved with this method is similar to that of stationary respirometers although it is necessary to have very accurate O_2 and CO_2 analyzers, particularly the latter which must be sensitive and linear at CO_2 concentrations of 0-1%. The flow rate through the hood should be adjusted to maintain a CO_2 concentration of approximately 0.5-1.0% in order to allow accurate measurements and avoid ventilatory changes due to CO_2 retention. The most convenient ventilated hood systems are those that interface measurements of flow rate, O_2, and CO_2 concentration with a computer to provide continuous measurements of O_2 consumption, CO_2 production, respiratory quotient (RQ), and energy expenditure.

Ventilated hood systems are excellent for both short and long-term measurements of energy expenditure in the laboratory. They are particularly useful in studying resting metabolic rate and the thermic effect of food, since continuous measurements can be made over a period of many hours. They are also very useful for studies of mild to moderate exercise, but are less well suited to studies of heavy exercise in which the hood may be uncomfortable for the subject and there is a problem with dissipation of perspiration and water vapor. Many laboratories are now using ventilated hood systems instead of, or along with, stationary respirometers. The cost of the apparatus is moderate and they are relatively easy to construct and operate.

Respiration Chambers. In recent years, some laboratories have built large respiration chambers which operate on the same principal as the ventilated hood system (Jequier 1981; Ravussin et al. 1982). A large, airtight room is constructed in which temperature and humidity are controlled. Fresh air is drawn into the chamber and allowed to mix. Simultaneously, air is drawn from the chamber, the flow rate is measured, and it is analyzed continuously for O_2 and CO_2 content. The size of the room allows the subject sufficient mobility to sleep, eat, exercise, and perform normal daily routines, thus allowing detailed measurements of energy expenditure over a period of several hours or several days.

The accuracy of energy expenditure measurements made in a properly designed large respiration chamber is equal to that of other indirect calorimetry methods, i.e., the error range being approximately 2-5%. To achieve this, respiration chambers must be carefully designed and constructed and utilize very accurate gas analyzers and data processing systems. It is probably the best method currently available for conducting detailed long-term studies of energy expenditure in humans where one wishes to measure resting metabolic rate, the thermic effect of food, energy expenditure due to physical activity, and adaptive thermogenesis. To facilitate the separation of total energy expenditure into its various compartments, the respiration chamber at the University of Lausanne, Switzerland, has been equipped with a radar device which uses a Doppler effect to record movement in the chamber (Schutz et al. 1982). The radar system has a sensitivity level of 7.5 cm/sec. and is activated by movement of the subject within the chamber. As with other movement recording devices, it does not quantitate the intensity of physical activity. In long-term studies, however, there is excellent correlation between "percent activity" and energy expenditure in the chamber. When the correlation line is extrapolated to 0% activity, the residual energy expenditure compares closely with the resting metabolic rate in fasting subjects or to the resting metabolic rate plus the thermic effect of food in fed subjects. Thus, this method is particularly well suited to long-term studies of energy expenditure and allows one to separate the components of resting metabolic rate, thermic effect of food, and energy expenditure during exercise. It is less well suited to short-term measurements of physical activity because of the lag time due to mixing of expired air in the large chamber volume. For such short-term measurements use of a stationary respirometer with a mouthpiece, face mask, or ventilated hood system is preferable. Only a few indirect calorimetry chambers are currently available. They are moderately expensive to construct, but cost much less than a direct calorimeter and have greater flexibility.

Non-Calorimetric Methods

In an attempt to avoid some of the problems associated with use of either direct or indirect calorimetry to measure energy expenditure during physical activity, several less complicated (and consequently less accurate) methods have been devised. Some are used in conjunction with indirect calorimetry measurements for validation or standardization. These methods have recently been reviewed by Schutz (1981) and by Garrow (1978). They may be subdivided into methods employing physiological measurements, observation and records of physical activity, activity diaries or recall, and the use of doubly labeled water.

Pulmonary Ventilation Volume. In situations where direct or indirect calorimetry methods are not practical, other physiological measurements which correlate with oxygen consumption may be substituted. This method is based on the relationship between ventilation volume and O_2 consumption, but is not nearly as accurate as measuring O_2 consumption directly (Durnin and Edwards 1955; Ford and Hellerstein 1959; Malhotra et al. 1962). Since a mouthpiece or tightly fitting face mask and a respirometer must be used to measure ventilation volume, the method has all of the drawbacks of indirect calorimetry. With the general availability of modern gas analyzers this method offers no advantages over indirect calorimetry and should no longer be used for studies of energy expenditure in a laboratory setting.

Heart Rate Recording. There is very good correlation between heart rate and O_2 consumption during moderate to heavy exercise. The correlation is much poorer at low levels of activity, and heart rate may be altered by such things as anxiety or change in posture without significant changes in O_2 consumption. This method has been validated by simultaneous indirect calorimetry measurements and has the advantage of being applicable to field work or measurements over a long period of time (e.g. 2-3 days). However, each subject must be calibrated in the laboratory to relate heart rate to oxygen consumption (Bradfield 1971; Warnold and Arvidsson-Lenner 1977). There are frequently technical problems in recording heart rate (electrode contact and comfort, sensitivity, and electrical artifacts), but for some types of studies this may be the most practical method for measuring energy expenditure in the field or peri-laboratory setting.

Integrated Electromyography. This method was devised to record muscle electrical activity and correlate it with resting metabolic rate (Harding and Sen 1970). It is entirely unsatisfactory for studies of energy expenditure during physical exercise and should not be used for this purpose.

Energy Balance Studies. It is possible to estimate energy expenditure over relatively long periods of time by measuring energy intake and changes in body composition (Acheson et al. 1980). The errors in this method are those inherent in accurate determination of energy intake over several days, weeks, or months, and in the methods available for determination of body composition. While this method could be used for long-term balance studies of free living individuals, the technique is cumbersome and small errors in measuring intake or change in body composition may significantly effect the results.

Time and Motion Studies. Several recording techniques have been used to estimate energy expenditure due to physical activity in real life situations. In time and motion studies, detailed records of physical activity are made by an observer and energy expenditure is estimated from the duration and intensity of work performed. The major problem with this method is that there is marked individual variation in the energy costs of doing a particular task. Some individuals work more efficiently than others and, if the method is to be used at all, the energy costs of specific tasks must be measured in the laboratory for each individual studied. Even with this degree of "calibration" the method is quite inaccurate (Wolff 1959; Consolazio et al. 1963). While somewhat more accurate than the following two methods, the data generated from time and motion studies must be considered only a rough approximation of actual energy expenditure in studies of individuals or groups of individuals.

Activity Diaries. With this method, both the energy costs of different activities and the time spent in each activity are estimated. The necessity of keeping detailed records severely limits this method. Record keeping is often inaccurate and may interfere with the subject's normal activity (Widdowson et al. 1954; Durnin and Passmore 1967).

Activity Recall. Attempts have been made to estimate energy expenditure associated with physical activity by interview or questionnaire techniques (Montoye 1971). This method is extremely inaccurate and is not applicable to studies of energy expenditure in the laboratory setting. In the field, errors in recall and lack of data regarding both the intensity and duration of physical activity as well as the variation of work efficiency of individual subjects makes the method too inaccurate to be worthwhile.

Cine Photography. In an attempt to obtain better documentation of physical activity, various direct means of recording physical activity have been employed. The analysis of physical activity by study of motion pictures has been useful in observing activity patterns of certain groups of individuals, but does not give any quantitative data on actual energy expenditure (Bullen et al. 1964). This technique is useful for studying behavioral patterns as in the comparison of the activity patterns of lean and obese camp girls by Bullen et al. (1964), but is of no real value in measuring the actual amount of energy expended.

Mechanical Activity Meters. Measuring motion by devices such a pedometers or accelerometers may provide an index of physical activity but, like cine photography, does not quantitate energy expenditure (Stunkard 1960; Morris 1973). In some studies, the use of mechanical activity meters has been correlated with measurements of energy expenditure obtained by indirect calorimetry. This improves the accuracy of the technique but not enough to make it useful in detailed studies of energy expenditure.

Radar Motion Recorders. As with the devices described above, radar may be used to record movement in a confined environment by a Doppler effect (Schutz et al. 1982). To date, this method has been used only in conjunction with indirect calorimetry in a respiration chamber. Since motion, rather than energy expenditure, is recorded is it not really applicable to other settings.

The Doubly Labeled Water Method. This method for measuring energy expenditure was first developed for use in small animals and has recently been extended to studies in humans. The principal is that oxygen in respired CO_2 is in rapid equilibrium with the O_2 in body water. Thus, if one administers doubly isotopically labeled water (^2H and ^{18}O), the isotopically labeled oxygen leaves the body as both CO_2 and H_2O whereas the isotopically labeled hydrogen leaves entirely as H_2O. Knowing the differential rates of ^{18}O and ^2H turnover after administration of doubly labeled H_2O, it is possible to calculate the rate of CO_2 production and estimate energy expenditure (Schoeller and Van Santen 1982). The method is relatively simple to use in mobile subjects. Doubly labeled H_2O is administered by mouth and excretion is determined in urine samples. It is quite costly, however, and requires sophisticated analysis using mass spectroscopy. The versatility is potentially very great since the method does not interfere with daily activity and can be used for studying energy expenditure over long periods of time, with 5 to 10 days being optimal. The error range for adults is 6-8%, so the accuracy is not quite as good as that achieved by indirect calorimetry, but the advantages of being able to study individuals in a free living situation and further improvements in technique may overcome this slight disadvantage. Currently, the availability of the method is limited because of the need for access to specialized mass spectroscopy equipment for analysis of the ^{18}O and ^2H enrichment in urine samples, and because of the relatively high cost of obtaining the isotopes. Samples can be collected and shipped for long distances, however, and the development of a centralized analytical facility may make this method particularly valuable for studies of energy expenditure in free living populations throughout the world.

CONCLUSIONS

A number of techniques have been developed and are currently in use for assessing energy expenditure in humans during physical activity. Direct calorimetry is the most accurate method of measuring energy expenditure in the laboratory, but is not suitable for many situations because of the confined space, limits on the types of exercise which can be performed, slow response time, high cost, and lack of availability.

Indirect calorimetry is nearly as accurate as direct calorimetry and the various techniques for measuring O_2 consumption and CO_2 production during physical activity in humans allow a wide range of applications. For field studies, portable respirometers are quite satisfactory. In the laboratory, stationary respirometers or ventilated hood systems allow accurate determinations over a wide range of exercise intensities and durations, but restrict subject mobility and thus limit the types of physical activity that can be monitored. Respiratory chambers allow subjects to be in a more "free living" situation and are excellent for longer term studies of energy expenditure, including measurements of resting metabolic rate, the thermic effect of food, energy exenditure during exercise, and adaptive thermogenesis.

The doubly labeled water method has great promise as a technique for measurement of total energy expenditure in free living individuals over relatively long periods of time, i.e. 5-10 days. It will not dissociate energy expenditure due to physical activity from that associated with the other compartments of energy expenditure and, although its accuracy seems to be nearly as good as that obtained by indirect calorimetry, the method still needs additional testing and validation in human studies. Currently, the cost and limited availability of isotope analysis are obstacles to general adoption of the method.

The various non-calorimetric methods for assessing energy expenditure during physical activity have their primary application to field studies. The best of these methods is heart rate recording since heart rate correlates well with energy expenditure during moderate to heavy physical activity. At low levels of activity, however, the method is less accurate. If one wishes to estimate energy expenditure during specific tasks, it is possible to determine rates of energy expenditure for given heart rates in the laboratory using indirect calorimetry and then to extrapolate these data to heart rate measurements in the field with a reasonable degree of accuracy.

Finally, in all studies of energy expenditure associated with physical activity it is important to express the data in terms that are readily understandable to others in the field. It is also important to provide sufficient information regarding the accuracy of the methods used, the range of observations made, and the standard error, so that others may compare and interpret the results. Unless data are expressed per individual, every attempt should be made to obtain measurements of body composition so that data can be expressed in terms of lean body or fat free mass.

REFERENCES

1. Acheson KJ, Campbell IT, Edholm OG, Miller DS and Stock MJ (1980). The measurement of food and energy intake in man - an evaluation of some techniques. AM J Clin Nut 33:1147-1154.
2. Ashworth A and Wolff HS (1969). A simple method for measuring calorie expenditure during sleep. Pfleugers Arch ges Physiol 306:191-194.
3. Atwater WO and Benedict FG (1905). A respiration calorimeter with appliances for the direct determination of oxygen. Carnegie Institute of Washington, publication 41:193.
4. Bradfield RB (1971). A technique for determination of usual and daily energy expenditure in the field. Am J Clin Nutr 24:1148-1154.
5. Bullen BA, Reed RB and Mayer J (1964). Physical activity of obese and non-obese adolescent girls, appraised by motion-picture sampling. Am J Clin Nutr 14:211-223.
6. Consolazio CF, Johnson RE and Pecora LJ (1963). Physiological Measurements of Metabolic Functions in Man. New York: McGraw-Hill, pp. 326-333.
7. Consolazio CF and Johnson HL (1971). Measurement of energy cost in humans. Fed Proceed 30:1444-1453.
8. Douglas CG (1911). A method for determining the total respiratory exchange in man. J Physiol (London) 42:17P-18P.
9. Durnin JVGA and Passmore R (1967). "Energy, Work and Leisure." London: Heinemann, p.165.
10. Durnin JVGA and Edwards RG (1955). Pulmonary ventilation as an index of energy expenditure. Quart J Exp Physiol 40:370-377.
11. Ford AB and Hellerstein AB (1959). Estimation of energy expenditure from pulmonary ventilation. J Applied Physiol 14:891.

12. Garrow JS (1978). Energy Balance and Obesity in Man. Volume 2. Amsterdam: Elsevier/North Holland, pp. 17-52.
13. Harding RM and Sen RN (1970). Evaluation of total muscular activity by quantification of electromyograms through a summing amplifier. Med Biol Erg 8:343-356.
14. Horton ES and Danforth E Jr. (1982). Energy metabolism and obesity. In Brodoff BN and Bleicher SJ (eds): "Diabetes Mellitus and Obesity," Baltimore: Williams and Wilkins, pp. 261-272.
15. Jequier E (1981). Long-term measurement of energy expenditure in man: direct or indirect calorimetry? In Bjorntorp P, Cairella M and Howard AN (eds): "Recent Advances in Obesity Research: III," London: John Libbey, pp. 130-135.
16. Kofranyi E and Michaelis HF (1940). Ein tragbarer Apparat zur Bestimmung des Gasstoffwechsels. Arbeitsphsiologie 11:148-150.
17. Malhotra MS, Ramaswamy SS, Ray SN and Schrivastav TN (1962). Minute ventilation as a measure of energy expenditure during exercise. J Applied Physiol 17:775-777.
18. Montoye HJ (1971). Estimation of habitual physical activity by questionnaire and interviews. Am J Clin Nutr 24:1113-1118.
19. Morris JRW (1973). Accelorometry: A technique for the measurement of human body movements. J Biomech 6:729-736.
20. Orsini D and Passmore R (1951). The energy expended carrying loads up and down stairs: Experiments using the Kofranyi-Michaelis calorimeter. J Physiol (London) 115:95-100.
21. Passmore R and Durnin JVGA (1955). Human energy expenditure. Physiological Reviews 35:801-840.
22. Pittet PG (1981). Direct calorimeter with fast response time using the radiant-layer principal: Some illustrations of its utilization in human studies. In Bjorntorp P, Cairella M and Howard AN (eds): "Recent advances in obesity research III," London: John Libbey, pp. 146-152.
23. Ravussin E, Bernand B, Schutz Y and Jequier E (1982). 24-hour energy expenditure and resting metabolic rate in obese, moderately obese, and control subjects. Am J Clin Nutr 35:566-573.
24. Schoeller DA and Van Santen E (1982). Measurement of energy expenditure in humans by doubly labeled water

method. J Appl Physiol: Respirat Environ Exercise Physiol 53(4): 955-959.

25. Schutz Y (1981). Use of non-calorimetric techniques to assess energy expenditure in man. In Bjorntorp P, Cairella M and Howard AN (eds): "Recent Advances in Obesity Research: III." London: John Libbey, pp. 153-158.

26. Schutz Y, Ravussin E, Diethelm R and Jequier E (1982). Spontaneous physical activity measured by radar in obese and control subjects studied in a respiration chamber. Int J Obesity 6:23-28.

27. Shephard RJ (1955). A critical examination of the Douglas bag technique. J Physiol (London) 127:515-524.

28. Stunkard A (1960). A method of studying physical activity in man. Am J Clin Nutr 8:595-601.

29. Warnold I and Arvidsson-Lenner R (1977). Evaluation of the heart rate method to determine the daily energy expenditure in disease. A study in juvenile diabetics. Am J Clin Nutr 30:304-315.

30. Webb P, Annis JF and Troutman Jr. SJ (1980). Energy balance in man measured by direct and indirect calorimetry. Am J Clin Nutr 33:1287-1298.

31. Widdowson EM, Edholm OG and McCance RA (1954). The food intake and energy expenditure of cadets in training. Brit J Nutr 8:147-155.

32. Wolff HS (1956). Modern techniques for estimating energy expenditure. Proc Nutr Soc 15:77-80.

33. Wolff HS (1959). Modern techniques for time and motion study in psychological research. Ergonomics 2:354-362.

Energy Intake and Activity, pages 131–156
© *1984 Alan R. Liss, Inc., 150 Fifth Avenue, New York, NY 10011*

PHYSIOLOGICAL MEASUREMENT OF ACTIVITY AMONG
ADULTS UNDER FREE LIVING CONDITIONS

Thierry Brun

Unité de Recherches sur la Nutrition et
l'Alimentation (U.1.INSERM)
Paris, France

INTRODUCTION

Many attempts have been made by nutritionists to
measure the energy expenditure of free living individuals
(Bleiberg et al. 1980; 1981; Bradfield et al. 1969; Brun et
al. 1980; 1981; 1979; Durnin and Passmore 1967;
Ferro-Luzzi and Durnin 1981; Fox 1953; Garrow 1974;
Geissler et al. 1981; DeGuzman et al. 1978; 1974a; 1974b;
1974c; 1979; Keys et al. 1950; Norgan et al. 1974; Passmore
and Durnin 1955; Phillips 1954; Viteri et al. 1971). Energy
expenditure, however, is only one aspect of activity; the
latter term encompasses a wide range of physiological and
non-physiological manifestations. For the purpose of this
discussion, activity is defined as a set of coordinated acts
and their output.

From a biological standpoint, activity is associated with
a variety of physiological and psychological phenomena that
can be observed and often measured in terms of heart rate,
oxygen uptake and CO_2 output, heat output, body
movement, etc. No single method of measurement answers
all questions raised by a large variety of investigators;
therefore, the validity of any single method is determined
by the objectives of specific studies.

The review in this chapter is limited to the assessment
of activity under conditions of low energy intake in developing countries. Commonly used methods will be discussed,
as will methods which are still in the experimental stage.

Some difficulties of validating both present and potential techniques will also be analysed.

MEASURING ACTIVITY IN LOW-INCOME COUNTRIES

Investigators have attempted to measure activity for a variety of reasons. One is to compare energy output to energy requirement and energy intake (Delegation Generale 1980; Norgan et al. 1974). This type of study often reflects the concept of energy deficit, and the assumption that when energy intake is below a theoretical energy requirement, energy out (and in particular work output) may be depressed. The value of this type of study is limited by the fact that the process of adaptation to low energy intake is not well known for populations exposed to long-term chronic food restrictions (Durnin 1979; Edmundson 1977; 1979; 1980; Keys et al. 1950; Norgan 1981; Norgan et al. 1974).

Activity is also measured in order to determine the relationship between activity and a large number of non-nutritional parameters. Investigators have attempted to formulate questions concerning: decreases in work output and/or social activities among farm laborers who are iron deficient or infested by Schistosoma mansoni or other parasites and the degree of anemia or infestation at which it is statistically significant (Basta et al. 1979; Collins et al. 1976); whether the excessive work load during pregnancy of many rural women of West Africa is responsible for the low birthweight of babies born during the rainy season (Briend 1980) and in what way the pattern of activity and the amount of time dedicated to agriculture is affected by the introduction of new technologies such as mechanization (Brun et al. unpublished), animal traction for ploughing (Barett 1982), or mechanical pumping for irrigation.

PRESENT METHODS OF MEASUREMENT

It is clear that research on the questions alluded to above, requires methods of measurement suitable for difficult field conditions. Factors such as isolation from laboratories, unstable electrical supply, heat, humidity, and the fears and expectations of the population involved are of the utmost importance in the selection of the appropriate techniques to assess activity.

While anthropologists, sociologists, agronomists and other investigators have conducted careful observations of workers in both rural and urban environments, the urban, industrial setting has proved more amendable to observation. The use of time has been documented in detail for 30,000 randomly sampled individuals in twelve countries (Szalai 1972).

In industry, time and motion studies have been used extensively to improve work efficiency, reduce fatigue, and increase safety. When the work is repetitive and monotonous, the level of activity on the job can often be assessed by recording the number of items produced or manipulated. Satyanarayana et al. (1977), for example, studied work output measured in terms of the number of fuses produced per day. He also assessed the relationship between work output and anthropometric, biochemical, and socioeconomic parameters among industrial workers. The study showed a positive correlation between work output, work rate, and either body weight or lean body mass. The indirect assessment of activity by energy expenditure measurements in industrial situations does not differ markedly between developing countries and industrialized nations. For a review see Maxfield (1971).

In agriculture, major emphasis has been placed on the assessment of the duration of each task related to a specific production. There is, therefore, a fair amount of data on the number of hours and days per month which is required for soil preparation, sowing, spraying, harvesting, and the processing of each vegetable product (BDPA 1965). These data are used, in turn, to maximize productivity of the labor force of the farm, and to allocate manpower for more profitable activities. For physiologists interested in human energy expenditure, however, they are difficult to use because they are incomplete. For example, it is difficult to reconstruct the use of time by a single category of worker over a period of 24 hours if non-productive activities are not described (BDPA 1965). In addition, the energy cost of some activities cannot be estimated precisely in the absence of actual measurements. For these reasons, the metabolic rates of farmers and farmworkers must be determined by independent time an motion studies.

Investigators concerned with work productivity have often expressed work output in terms of acreage planted or ploughed, the quantity of the product harvested per worker, or other measurable indexes of activity. Spurr et al. (1975) for example, measured activity both in kilograms of cane cut per hour and oxygen uptake during work. Using the daily productivity for each man, they were able to estimate their 8-hour daily energy output while cutting sugar cane. They showed that heavier, taller men were better producers and exhibited greater efficiency. Their data also suggests that the work level involved in manual sugar cane cutting approaches the highest energy expenditure values that can be sustained for an 8-hour day.

Basta et al. (1979) measured the output of workers on a rubber plantation in West Java, in Indonesia, in terms of the weight of latex collected. The output for weeders was measured by the area of trenches dug in parallel rows by each man. The rubber tappers were paid according to their work output and their earnings correlated with hemoglobin levels (45% of them were anemic). Treatment with 100 mg of elemental iron for 60 days resulted in a significant improvement in hematological status and work output.

In addition to the assessment of activity by measuring the amount of time dedicated to each task, and recording work output, there are a variety of instruments which record either movement, heart rate, or oxygen uptake and CO_2 production in field conditions (Consolazio et al. 1963; Durnin and Passmore 1967; Garrow 1974). Pedometers provide an index of activity when used for repetitive activities and when adequately calibrated.

The need for techniques which cause the least possible interference with the usual behavior of the subjects has oriented investigators toward heart rate measurements. The method, based on the relationship between oxygen consumption and heart rate, requires the determination of the relationship between these two parameters for activities performed in different postures, e.g.: sitting, lying, and in upright positions involving large muscle groups. When preparatory work is done correctly, the habitual rate of activity and the variations of daily energy expenditure can be assessed for long periods of time with minimal inconvenience to the subjects. In tropical areas, however, electrodes must be removed every second day because of skin irritation resulting from their use.

Bradfield et al. (1969) further improved the technique of heart rate measurement by coupling the monitoring system worn by the subject to a telemetry unit, thus enabling one to read accumulated heart rate at any moment without disturbing the subject's activity. A simultaneous comparison of the respirometer and heart-rate telemetry technique in each of six activity levels in 24 adult males showed that the standard error in estimation was less than 0.64 kcal per minute in 21 out of 24 subjects. The coefficient of regression (r) was greater than 0.95 for the entire sample.

The equipment most commonly used by nutritionists for counting heart rate of the free-ranging individual is probably the SAMI (Socially Acceptable Monitoring Instrument) manufactured by T.E.M. Sales Ltd. (Crawley, Sussex, England). The method for validating this heart rate monitoring system requires measurement of oxygen consumption. Respiratory samples collected in Douglas bags or on portable respirometers are used to calibrate heart rate counts versus metabolic rates.

The respirometer method of measuring energy expenditure (Consolazio et al. 1963; Durnin and Passmore 1967; Weir 1949) is the one most widely used for the assessment of energy expenditure of subjects under free living conditions. It cannot be worn for long periods of time, however, and it modifies the usual behavior of the subject (Consolazio et al. 1963). Combined with a diary technique, it permits the calculation of energy expenditure over the total duration of the diary record but, whether kept by the subject or by an observer, the diary technique itself is also likely to affect the behavior of the subject. People who are observed or measured tend to increase their activity as compared with a normal situation.

The combined respirometer-diary technique frequently has recorded average energy expenditure significantly higher than energy intake for the same period (Bleiberg et al. 1981; Ferro-Luzzi and Durnin 1981). The amount of weight loss experienced by subjects is not sufficient to account for this discrepancy and suggests that, in field conditions, the respirometer-diary technique overestimates actual energy expenditure. Expenditures higher than intakes also have been obseved in other studies of energy balance in free-living individuals (Durnin and Passmore 1967).

RECENT DEVELOPMENTS IN REPRESENTATIVE MEASUREMENTS OF ENERGY EXPENDITURE

On the basis of a study of the Machiguenga Indians of the Upper Amazon in Southeastern Peru, Montgomery and Johnson (1977) have recommended a technique using randomly selected observations of all members of a population. Basically, this method utilizes randomized spot visits made during one year and the observations of activity are gathered by sex and age groups to characterize the use of time at each period of the year. This new type of time-allocation is meant to represent more satisfactorily the composite activity profile of free-ranging groups of individuals. Its use with the classical respirometer technique allows determination of the energy cost of each separate type of activity.

Ancey (1974) and Inserm (Brun et al. 1979; Delegation Generale 1980; Geissler et al. 1981) have used a similar technique on a large sample in Upper Volta. Departing from the method of Montgomery and Johnson (1977), farmers and their families were visited at regular intervals 32 times a year, and the record of activity for each member was recorded for the entire day. A total of 28,160 days was recorded of which 21,388 days represented 657 adolescents and adults, aged 15 to 59 years old. Results were processed by region, sex, and age categories. Monthly variations of energy expenditure were computed from measured metabolic rates for each important activity. A summary of the results is given later in this chapter.

The discrepancies observed between average energy intake and expenditure has led several authors to suggest that the diary-respirometer technique might lead to a systematic overestimation of energy expenditure. Durnin (1981) notes that validation is lacking for the extrapolation of short measurements made with a portable respirometer.

Webb et al. (1980) and Webb and Troutman (1970) have presented puzzling results showing a large unmeasured energy gap between direct and indirect calorimetry. The calorimeter used by WEBB and his co-workers is made of a thermo regulated garment. This portable, water-cooled calorimeter presents many advantages over classical calorimeters but its use is, unfortunately, restricted to laboratory measurements. A continuous recording of both metabolic rate (from oxygen uptake and CO_2 output) and heat output (from the water-cooled garment) enables a precise and almost immediate comparison of both direct and indirect calorimetry.

Webb and the Inserm research group are presently comparing the extrapolation of short measurements (9' to 15') over 36 hours to both continuous oxygen uptake and heat output measurements.

For 8 Asian subjects studied for 36 hour periods in a metabolic unit, the mean daily energy output was found to be 1912 ± 72 kcal by direct calorimetry, 1998 ± 88 kcal from the ventilated hood, and 1745 ± 120 kcal from the diary-respirometer technique. Reasons for the discrepancies were investigated. At rest, either lying or sitting, the portable respirometer technique underestimated energy output by 20% in comparison to reference methods. Comparisons between respirometer results per minute for subjects wearing the water-cooled garment and subjects without the garment, suggest that the thermo-regulated garment induces relaxation and reduces thermal losses in these subjects by 15%. In contrast, during work periods, the weight of the water-cooled suit (7 kg) increased energy output by 11%. The mean dietary intake measured for 10 days was closer to the diary-respirometer technique results. Final computations are in progress, but it is already apparent that the more accurately energy expenditure is measured, the greater the modification of the behavior of the subject. In the case of the thermo-regulated water-cooled suit used as a direct calorimeter, an additional effect seems to be lowering the resting metabolic rate and raising energy expenditure during work on an ergocycle.

Several laboratories are presently experimenting with doubly labeled water (Deuterium and ^{18}O) to determine CO_2 output over periods of more than 2 weeks. Westerterp and DeBoer (1983) have presented a preliminary validation of the method in humans:

...using doubly labeled water allows observations of energy expenditure while daily routines are maintained without interference.

The oxygen of expired CO_2 is in isotopic equilibrium with the oxygen of body water. When a subject is loaded with $^2H^{18}O$ (by oral administration), the decrease in ^{18}O in the body water (determined in blood or urine) is a measure for H_2O output plus CO_2 output and the decrease in ^2H is a measure for H_2O output alone. Hence the CO_2 output can be obtained by difference. The method, as used in small animals, has been validated with respirometry in giving errors less than 10%, usually less than 5%.

The applicability of the method in humans has long been limited by the cost to enrich the body water with the stable isotopes, especially with ^{18}O as ^2H is not expensive. Now, with high resolution mass-spectrometers, we can afford these experiments by working at very low concentrations. Using this method, energy expenditure in man has been measured over two week intervals and differed from dietary intake plus change in body composition by an average of 2% (Schoeller and Van Santen 1982). Westerterp and de Boer compared the method with direct measurements of CO_2 production over 24 hour intervals.

CO_2 production in two subjects was measured simultaneously with doubly labeled water and respirometry, in the respiration chambers of the department of Animal Physiology in Wageningen. Both subjects were observed over three consecutive days including one or two days on a high activity level (19 MJ·day^{-1}) and the remaining day(s) on a low activity level (11 MJ·day^{-1}).

Results suggest that this technique could be useful for studies of two weeks duration or more when no detailed daily breakdown of energy expenditure is needed. However, the cost of the ^{18}O labeled water is a limiting factor for large-scale use in developing countries.

Garby (personal communication) has stressed the need for a light economical instrument which gives a reliable index of activity. He has initiated research on an improved pedometer which would measure acceleration as well as the number of movements. This instrument, once developed, could be worn as a watch or attached to the leg, and would be calibrated against the standard method of calorimetry.

The traditional Kofranyi-Michaelis respirometer, which has not been significantly improved since World War II, could be replaced in the near future by the P.R.A.M., the Portable Respiratory Air Monitor. The latter instrument was designed by Harvard Appartatus, Ltd. and is still in the testing stage. Presently, the flow rate measure is dependent upon the respiratory rate, which makes calibration awkward, but this limitation should be solved by further improvements to the components of this light respirometer.

Although all physiologists agree that the law of conservation of energy holds true for the human body, there is continued disagreement over how to account for external work. All energy supplied in food is either stored or recovered sooner or later in the form of heat and mechanical energy. It has been shown that to do a given amount of work, approximately five times as much body fuel must be oxidized as would be represented by the work alone; the rest appears as heat as measured by direct calorimetry. Unpublished results by Webb and co-workers suggest that external work may be a cause of error in energy balance studies. Significant external work may be present even in those situations in which it appears to be absent, such as walking on the level, but this awaits experimental proof.

The renewed interest in human calorimetry, and the existence of various excellent calorimeters in Europe and North America, should permit us, in the near future, to overcome the various obstacles presented here in the validation of appropriate field techniques.

ASSESSMENT OF SEASONAL VARIATIONS IN ACTIVITY

It may seem futile or irrelevant to measure the activity of poor, rural populations exposed to malnutrition, parasite infestations, and infections as it can be argued that priority should be given to intervention programs in agriculture and public health, and that the assessment of activity is an academic exercise of little or no value in alleviating malnutrition. Although there is some truth in that statement, it can be demonstrated, for example, that a better knowledge of the activity of traditional farmers, can be a useful tool in the formulation and evaluation of agricultural development projects. The data presented here illustrates the potential justification for measuring activity of free living individuals in the context of rural development schemes.

The tragic famine which occurred in the Sahel region in 1972-74 and the frequent episodes of seasonal hunger have demonstrated the incapacity of agricultural systems of this area to resist prolonged period of drought (Brun 1975; Brun and Bleiberg 1980). Production is in bare equilibrium with basic food needs and minor changes in environmental parameters can produce disproportionate effects on productivity. The agricultural sector is dominated by dry-land farming and pastoralism and, therefore, it is highly dependent on annual rainfall. Irrigation is seldom feasible, mechanical ploughing and fertilizers are often too expensive for local producers, and precipitation is unpredictable and subject to wide monthly and annual variation. The only practical way in which traditional farmers can increase staple food production is by extending hand cultivated areas with intensive hoeing and weeding during the rainy season. The entire available work force, men, women, and children, must be mobilized to protect the crop against invasion by weed or destruction by wandering animals. Most agricultural tasks are performed by hand with rudimentary tools, and human energy devoted to production is, after rainfall, the major parameter which determines the volume of cereal production in the Sahel. For this reason, the study described here undertook the documentation of farmers' activities in the Sahel country in terms of agricultural and non-agricultural tasks.

Methods

Essentially three methodological approaches have been used in this attempt to assess the time and energy utilization of Mossi farmers. In the first approach a sociologist (Ancey 1974) and his team of interviewers conducted a time allocation study for a period of one year on approximately 900 individuals from 5 test villages. This portion of the study was followed by one in which researchers from three complementary fields - agronomy, nutrition, and public health - undertook an accurate recording of activity and measured the rate of energy expenditure for the major activities in five control villages of the same region. Finally, this second portion of the study was repeated at three different periods of the year as part of a more general survey of the disequilibrium between food availability and food requirements (Delegation General 1980).

Most subjects were of Mossi origin and families were selected randomly from five villages: Zorgho, Koudougou, Yako, Dedougou, and Tougan. During a quarter, each of the study families was visited every three days. When the next quarter began the interviewer would move to another family of the same village. This process allowed the investigators to sample a large number of subjects and to represent more adequately the pattern of village activity throughout the year. During a visit the investigator obtained by interview, for all individuals over 12 years of age, the time spent on each activity in the previous 24 hours. Household occupation sheets were completed on the spot and later coded according to the list of selected major activities. Activities were recorded to the nearest ten minutes, and the monthly total was rounded to the nearest half hour. Since some of the subjects were absent on some occasions, it is more meaningful to express results in number of days of observation. Over one year in the five villages this amounted to 28,160 days, or an average of 77 adolescents and adult peasants, from 12 to over 60 years of age, interviewed per day (Ancey 1974).

In order to check the validity of the time allocation study, a second survey was designed using a small number of subjects from five control villages (Delegation General 1980). These subjects were under continuous 2 to 7 day observation during the dry season (December to March) when there is almost no agricultural activity, and during the rainy season (July to August), when heavy physical work is performed. Fifty-two subjects were followed by an observer throughout the waking day. The investigator, who was equipped with a chronometer and a watch, kept a diary and registered accurately the period of time spent in every activity, and described each task and the position of the body. Dietary intake was also measured accurately. The duration of each type of activity was totaled on a

24-hour basis for each participant and major activities were selected for measurements of their corresponding rates of energy expenditure (Bleiberg et al. 1980; 1981; Brun et al. 1981).

The energy cost of both agricultural and non-agricultural activities was calculated by the technique described by Durnin and Passmore (1967). This method, based on indirect calorimetry, uses Kofranyi-Michaelis respirometers for measurement of the pulmonary ventilation and a Servomex paramagnetic oxygen analyser for the determination of the O_2 content of the expired air. Each measurement period lasted approximately fifteen minutes.

Type of Work and Distribution of Activity

Most agricultural activities are concentrated in the wet season as water pumping is not used for gardening during the dry season, except in very limited areas not included in the study villages. Harvests are from October to December. At that time, food resources are abundant and some cash is obtained from groundnut, tobacco, cotton, sesame, or tubers sold on the markets. However, granary and monetary resources are usually exhausted before May or June when fields have to be cleared for the next crop.

Cultivated areas, the concession fields or "champs de case," typically include three circles of cultivation. The first circle consists of a limited area around the mud huts which is constantly and regularly cultivated. It receives most of the manure from the small ruminants, horses, and cows kept in the concessions as well as the wastes from food preparation. Corn, red sorghum, beans, tubers, tobacco, okra, garden-sorrel and spices are cultivated in those fields, but the amount is generally insufficient for most families and a semi-permanent circle of plots, the second circle, is cultivated in the vicinity with similar crops in addition to peas and groundnuts. The third circle is made up of additional fields which are normally cultivated in the bush. This land is left fallow for periods of from two to six years, depending on family needs and the distance of the land from the village. Since walking between those plots and the village is rather time-consuming, some family members usually settle in the bush from the period of cultivation through the completion of the harvest. Crops cultivated in those fields include millet, white or red sorghum, groundnuts, peas, and beans.

Animal husbandry is practiced throughout the year in the village, but to avoid devastating the crops the cattle is led outside cultivated areas during the cereal growing season. Although there are often conflicts between the agriculturalists and the pastoralists, the Fulani herders often settle near cultivated areas in order to trade their milk and butter with villages. They sometimes take charge of the Mossi cattle in exchange for cash or kind and they may be allowed to pasture the harvested plots in December.

Both men and women participate in agricultural tasks; however, the men do most of the heavy physical work such as clearing the land of bushes, burning the stubs, sowing, weeding, and harvesting. Women contribute a fair amount of time to sowing and weeding, activities performed from May to September. If all forms of rest are excluded, either lying, sitting, or standing, the mean annual time spent daily in various activities is 6 hours 20 minutes for women and 5 hours 30 minutes for men (Table 1). Sleeping, measured accurately on the sub-sample, was similar for both men and women and is equal to ten hours in the dry season and 8½ hours in the rainy season.

Large seasonal variations are observed for each category of activity. For men the range for land farming varies from less than ¼ hour per day in February (dry season) to more than 6 hours per day in the middle of the rainy season, mostly for hand hoeing, tillage, and weeding sorghum and millet plots. By contrast, animal maintenance takes up to one hour a day in the dry season (mostly January to April) and only ¼ hour in the middle of the rainy season (Table 2). On the average, adult women dedicate more than two hours per day to household tasks and up to three hours per day or more during the month preceding the rainy season (April, 3½ hours) and following major harvests (November and December, 3 hours). Their contribution to agricultural activities amounts to 4 hours daily in June, 5 hours in July, more than 4 hours in August, and less thereafter. Walking to and from the fields is not included in those "agricultural activities," and it represents an additional half-hour for men and an hour for women as the latter must collect wood, wild fruits, and leaves for the preparation of the evening meal. Resting

TABLE 1

Average time (in minutes) spent daily by women in selected
types of activities per month (Upper Volta)

ACTIVITIES	MONTHS												MEAN
	Jan.	Feb.	Mar.	Apr.	May.	Jun.	Jul.	Aug.	Sep.	Oct.	Nov.	Dec.	
Land farming from clearing to harvest	5	0	1	1	84	246	317	259	165	216	212	20	127
Animal husbandry, gathering from bush, and hunting...	16	27	16	27	31	11	5	14	24	16	11	26	19
Crafts	96	133	145	111	31	1	0	2	10	4	2	57	49
Households tasks	125	156	188	226	169	138	123	130	124	145	172	185	157
At the market	15	26	12	15	15	20	3	6	17	5	14	34	15
Social activities	21	19	7	13	22	4	9	1	3	5	6	9	10
Resting (lying, sitting, standing)	1162	1079	1071	1047	1088	1020	983	1028	1097	1049	1023	1109	1063

TABLE 2

Average time (in minutes) spent daily by men in selected
types of activities per month (Upper Volta)

ACTIVITIES	MONTHS												MEAN
	Jan.	Feb.	Mar.	Apr.	May.	Jun.	Jul.	Aug.	Sep.	Oct.	Nov.	Dec.	
Land farming from clearing to harvest	41	13	36	65	162	318	377	312	239	255	221	37	173
Animals husbandry, gathering from bush, and hunting...	79	76	67	74	44	18	14	12	15	20	47	51	43
Crafts	49	41	44	67	58	9	1	3	7	17	43	37	31
Households tasks	10	3	3	8	2	0	0	0	0	1	0	1	2
At the market	20	70	86	50	49	42	25	33	48	33	40	69	47
Social activities	45	44	46	51	27	19	26	18	23	29	22	51	33
Resting (lying, sitting, standing)	1196	1193	1158	1125	1098	1034	997	1062	1108	1085	1067	1194	1110

time spent in the field, measured on a subsample, was
nearly 25% of the working time. Therefore, in July, women
spent more than seven hours daily either in the field or on
their way back and forth. Little time was left for handi-
crafts or for other commercial or social activities from May
to November. On the average, women devoted only 10
minutes daily to social, non-productive activities and spent
an average of 15 minutes in the market.

The energy expenditure corresponding to each type of
activity has been measured in most cases (Bleiberg et al.
1980; 1981; Brun et al. 1981). When actual measurements
were not performed, estimates from similar activities or from
the literature were used (Table 3). On that basis, the
daily energy expenditure was computed for both men and
women (Table 4).

TABLE 3

Estimated energy expenditure in various activities, for a
60 kg standard weight for men and 55 kg for women

	Men	Women
	Kcal/min	Kcal/min
1. Agricultural activities		
land clearing	6.9	6.4
clearing after burning the bush	3.5	3.2
protecting crops and scaring birds	2.1	1.9
irrigations	4.2	3.9
sowing	3.9	3.8
hoeing-transplanting	4.7	4.2
earthing up crops	5.0	4.6
land clearing and weeding of fields	4.6	4.2
manure spreading	3.8	3.5
ploughing	4.8	4.4
pesticides spraying	4.0	3.7
planting	2.5	2.3
tending rice field	4.0	3.7
shelling groundnuts for seeds	1.5	1.4
collecting millet straw	3.0	2.8
miscellaneous agricultural activities	4.0	3.7
2. Harvest	3.3	3.0
3. Tending animals	3.0	2.8
4. Gathering miscellaneous products from		
the bush		
wood	3.8	3.0
leaves and wild fruits	3.3	2.8
clay	3.2	2.8
miscellaneous other	3.6	3.0
5. Collecting termites and hunting	3.6	3.0

TABLE 3 (cont'd)

	Men Kcal/min	Women Kcal/min
6. Craft		
building and cementing a well	3.0	2.6
threshing, winnowing dehulling, grinding, sieving	2.7	1.9
tool and granary repair	2.8	1.8
basket work	2.3	2.0
ginning and spinning cotton	-	1.4
weaving and sewing	2.5	1.4
miscellaneous crafts	2.5	2.3
other crafts	2.3	1.4
making "soumbala"[a] or "karite"[b] butter	-	2.8
pottery	3.0	2.7
house and granary repair	3.0	2.6
7. Household tasks		
making fermented sorghum beer[c]	2.5	2.3
fetching water	4.1	4.0
washing clothes	3.5	3.2
food preparation	3.2	3.1
other home activities	3.2	2.0
8. Market activities	2.5	2.0
9. Social activities		
ceremonies: baptism, funerals	2.0	1.7
chatting	1.4	1.6
school	2.0	1.8
visiting friends	2.4	1.9
other social activities	2.7	1.4
religious practices	1.5	2.0
10. Daily activities		
miscellaneous: lying resting, sitting or standing at the market or during small journeys	1.44	1.29

a. fermented seeds from Parkia biglobosa

b. from cooked seeds of Butyrospermum parkii

c. "Dolo"

TABLE 4

Mean daily energy expenditure of farmers
and wives in Upper Volta

Month	Men		Women	
	Per 60 kg standard weight Kcal/24 h	Per actual body mass Kcal/24 h	Per 55 kg standard weight Kcal/24 h	Per actual body mass Kcal/24 h
J	2,470	2,430	2,180	2,020
F	2,420	2,390	2,230	2,070
M	2,500	2,480	2,280	2,120
A	2,590	2,560	2,430	2,260
M	2,700	2,650	2,490	2,310
J	3,040	2,960	2,810	2,580
J	3,320	3,180	3,000	2,710
A	3,160	2,980	2,890	2,590
S	2,950	2,730	2,620	2,330
O	2,700	2,500	2,570	2,300
N	2,700	2,560	2,600	2,360
D	2,410	2,340	2,330	2,160
Mean	2,750	2,650	2,540	2,320

Impact of Rural Intervention Programs on Activity of Men
and Women

The observations made during this study raised a
number of questions related to activity, among them:

1. Is food energy availability, during the "hungry sea-
    son," a limiting factor for work capacity?
2. Does the apparently excessive work-load of women
    during most periods of the year have detrimental
    effects on pregnancy and lactation?
3. What is the contribution of hand and foot pumps to the
    reduction of the work-load of women?
4. What are the contributions of grain processing innova-
    tions such as mechanical threshing, dehulling, and
    grinding?

5.   What could be the benefits of animal traction in terms of human energy savings as well as increased productivity?

No definitive answers were obtained for any of those questions, but information was collected on each problem.

During the rainy season, the average weight loss of 1 to 3 kg for adult males and ½ to 1 kg for women engaged in agriculture suggests that the mobilization of fat stores is necessary during the "hungry season." Considering the high level of energy expenditure required during the rainy season, it may be that the long resting period observed for men in the dry season is necessary in order to reconstitute their physical fitness after a period of strenuous work (Brun et al. 1981).

At this point in the study no data has been collected on work productivity, but other authors have shown a direct relationship between low intake and poor work performance (Keys et al. 1950). Similarly, an excessive work load for women during pregnancy is suspected of being responsible for a high rate of premature births and low birth weights. According to Briend (1980):

> The need for rest at the end of pregnancy was first suggested in 1895 by the French obstetrician A. Pinard (42). He noticed that there was a difference in mean birth weight of 280g between infants born to mothers who had spent at least ten days at rest in a Parisian Council refuge for the indigent and those whose mothers came directly to the maternity hospital for delivery. His samples consisted of 500 consecutive births in each group.... Early this century, social measures were taken in all industrialized countries to allow pregnant women to stop their industrial work and this possible contibution to perinatal mortality is considered to have progressively disappeared although it is well known that domestic work is sometimes more physically demanding than occupational work, especially in low income groups.

The study described in this chapter indicated that, on the average, rural women dedicate one hour a day during the rainy season to threshing, washing, dehulling, and grinding grains, and 1¼ hours a day to the same activities during the dry season. Those tasks are among the most exhausting activities performed by women at home and are similar in difficulty to fetching water or hoeing in the fields. Pounding requires 4.5 Kcal/minute and grinding 4.1 Kcal/minute for a woman of 55 kg of body weight. Mechanical grain processing equipment, therefore, could be a significant benefit to rural women but, if the equipment is to save time and physical energy, it must not be not too distant from their residence nor too expensive. On several occasions, it was observed that the time required to walk to the village mill and back was greater than the time needed to grind the required quantity of grain at home. In addition, the cost of this service, for those who used paid, mechanical grinding, imposed additional handicraft work or commercial activity on the women. In another study, conducted in the village of Koumbidia (Senegal), the benefits derived by women from home vegetable gardening in the dry season were assessed (Unpublished document). It appeared that watering the vegetable plots by hand represented a heavy, additional work load on women. A minimal improvement of the diet was observed and the largest fraction of the additional income was used to buy clothes, jewelry, and miscellaneous non-food items at Kounghel, the local market.

The introduction of animal draft power to improve farm productivity and alleviate labor constraints has been studied by Barett et al. (1982) in Upper Volta. Field trials compared control plots which were scarified manually with a hoe to experimental plots which were plowed using animal traction. The latter produced an average increase of 17% in sorghum and millet yields and of 18% in groundnut yields. The study could not control for many factors that could obscure results and, therefore, the effect of animal traction could not be demonstrated clearly by the average yield differences between hoe and traction farmers. The impact of animal traction on household labor allocation was striking: on the average, the animal traction households devoted 174 fewer worker-equivalent hours to labor per hectare than did hoe households (Table 5). This represents a reduction of 25% in the average labor time per hectare. The reduction in labor time was greater in oxen zones (31%) than in donkey zones (20%). The savings in field labor associated with animal traction are somewhat offset by the

TABLE 5

Average worker equivalent hours of
family labor use per hectare for
major field activities on all
crops in animal traction
zones[a] (Upper Volta)
(Barrett et al. 1982)

Field Activity	Cultivation by	
	Hoe	Animal Traction
Seeding[b]	60	43
Tillage [c]	418	299
Harvest	148	134
Other[d]	60	36
Total	685	511

[a]Labor time was evaluated for 36 hoe
and 41 traction households.

[b]Includes planting, transplanting, and
thinning,

[c]Includes hand hoeing, weeding and
ridging; and plowing, weeding and
ridging with traction.

[d]Includes transport, threshing, fence
building, and off-season land clearing.

additional labor required to feed and maintain draft animals.
When this labor requirement is taken into account, the net
labor saving effect for oxen vs hoe farming is 11% and for
donkey vs hoe farming 15%.

Another effect outside the peak periods of June and
July, was the replacement of activities such as hoeing by
less intensive tasks related to animal care. The impact of
animal traction on the allocation of potential labor time to
actual work and leisure is shown in Table 6. Apparently

TABLE 6

Allocation of potential labor time to leisure,
farm and non-farm activities (Upper Volta)
(Barrett et al. 1982)

| | Households Using: | |
	Hoe	Animal Traction
Number of Households	36	41
Hours Worked:		
Men	5.5	5.4
Women	7.4	5.8
Household mean	6.5	5.6
Hours Resting, Walking, III:		
Men	6.5	6.4
Women	4.6	6.2
Household mean	5.5	6.4

[a]Potential labor time is defined as a 12-hour day; the
daylight hours in the Eastern Region. Leisure is derived as a residual time not accounted for by work
activities.

the hours worked were unchanged for men but were reduced by 22% for women. Similarly, leisure time (resting,
walking, attending the market, or illness) increased by 35%
for the same women. Contrary to expectations, however,
women from traction households spent less time daily in
household chores (2 vs. 3.4 hours for hoe household wom-
en), but the same amount of time (2 hours daily) for agricultural work. According to the authors of the study
(Barett et al. 1982), the apparent effect of the introduction
of draft animals can be attributed to the differing demographic structures of sample households: traction households are larger and have more women to share household
chores. It could also be argued that traction households
have more women as a result of the wealth of the head of
the household, but is it because of animal traction that
wealthier farmers could afford additional wives, or is it
because of wealth that they could afford draft animals?
The study does not provide the answer, nor does it suggest other relationships between the observations reported
here.

CONCLUSION

It is usually easier to measure the amount of primary good incorporated in a manufactured product than to estimate the quantity of work it has required. In addition, work is usually evaluated in terms of duration rather than physical intensity. In developing countries, where many tasks are still very strenuous, efforts should be made by national and international agencies to alleviate exploitive work conditions which often are imposed on the weakest and most vulnerable socio-economic groups. Men benefit first from technological .innovations, while women and children are left with the numerous time-consuming and poorly paid traditional chores of domestic and productive activities. The International Labour Organization (ILD) of the United Nations estimates that more than 50 million children under 15 years of age work in environments that are dangerous and detrimental to their mental and physical development. Similarly, millions of mothers are left in charge of all agricultural activities in their home villages by their husbands who have migrated to urban centers in search of employment. While men labor for wages that are largely consumed by urban necessities and taxation, the production responsibilities and, therefore, the workloads, of women and children increase. It is imperative that strategies designed to increase the availability of food at the village level take into account these parameters. The exploitive relationship that has developed between the modern sector and the traditional domestic economy tends to exclude the most vulnerable members from the benefits of labor-saving technologies. The estimation of human activity, not only in terms of time but also of fatigue and physical suffering, should be introduced as a tool in the evaluation of the impact of development projects. This objective emphasizes the need for improved field measurement techniques and also for a genuine commitment to alleviating the workload of the most deprived segments of impoverished populations.

REFERENCES

1. Ancey G (1974). Facteurs et systémes de production dans la sociéte Mossi d'aujour d'hui. ORSTOM, Centre de Ougadougou.
2. Barett V, Lassiter G, Wilcock D, Baker D and Crawford E. (1982). Animal traction in Eastern Upper

Volta - A technical, economic and institutional analysis. Michigan State Univ. Development Paper, No. 4. East Lansing, Michigan: Dept. of Economics, Michigan State University.

3. Basta S, Soekirhan S, Kariadi D and Scrimshaw N (1979). Iron deficiency anemia and the productivity of adult males in Indonesia. Am J Clin Nutr 32:916-925.

4. Bleiberg FM, Brun TA and Goihman S (1980). Duration of activities and energy expenditure of female farmers in dry and rainy seasons in Upper Volta. Brit J Nutr 43: 71-82.

5. Bleiberg FM, Brun TA, Goihman S and Lippman D (1981). Food intake and energy expenditure of male and female farmers from Upper Volta. Brit J Nutr 45: 505-515.

6. Bradfield RB, Huntzicker P and Fruehan G (1969). Simultaneous comparison of respirometry and heart-rate telemetry techniques as measures of human energy expenditure. Am Clin Nutr 22: 696-700.

7. Briend A (1980). Maternal physical activity, birth weight, and perinatal mortality. Med Hypotheses 6: 1157-1170.

8. Brun TA (1975). Manifestations nutritionnelles et medicales de la Famine. Auge, M. et J. Copans, Secheresse et Famine au Sahel. Paris: Maspero.

9. Brun TA and Bleiberg F (1980). Cereal shortage and adjustment in the Sahel. Food Policy 5:3.

10. Brun TA, Bleiberg F, Bonny S et Ancey G (1980). Alimentation et dépense énergétique du paysan Mossi. Environ Afric 14-15-16, IV, 2-3-4.

11. Brun T, Bleiberg F and Goihman S (1981). Energy expenditure of male farmers in dry and rainy seasons in Upper Volta. Brit J Nutr 45:67-75.

12. Brun T, Geissler CA, Mirabagheri I, Hormozdiary H, Bastani J and Hedayat H (1979). The energy expenditure of Iranian agricultural workers. Am J Clin Nutr 32: 2154-2161.

13. Bureau pour le Développement de la Production Agricole (BDPA) (1965). Techniques rurales en Afrique. Les temps de travaux. V. 21 et annexes 1 and 2.

14. Collins KJ, Brother-Hood RJ and Davies CTM (1976). Physiological performances and work capacity of Sudanese cane cutters with Shistosoma mansoni infection. Am J Trop Med Hyg 25(3):410-421.

15. Consolazio CF, Johnson RE and Pecora LE (1963). "Physiological Measurements of Metabolic Functions in Man. New York: McGraw Hill, pp 40-54 and 72-83.
16. Délégation Générale á la Recherche Scientifique et Technique (1980). "Conditions et limites de l'adjustement alimentaire et nutritionnel en milieu aride." (Action concertée: "Lutte contre l'aridite" en milieu tropical. Compte rendu de fin d'étude, Octobre.
17. Durnin JVGA (1979). Energy balance in man, with particular reference to low intakes. Biblio Nutr Dieta 27: 1-10.
18. Durnin JVGA (1981). Basal Metabolic Rate. A Critical Review of the Literature. Joint FAO/WHO/UNU Expert Consultation on Energy and Protein Requirement. Rome 5-17, October 1981. ESN.FAO/QHO/UNU.
19. Durnin JVGA and Passmore R (1967). Energy, work and leisure. London: Heinemann Educational Books.
20. Edmundson W (1977). Individual variations in work output per unit energy intake in East Java. Ecol Food Nutr 6: 147-151.
21. Edmundson W (1979). Individual variations in basal metabolic rate of mechanical work efficiency in East Java. Ecol Food Nutr 8: 189-195.
22. Edmundson W (1980). Adaptation to undernutrition. How much food does man need? Soc Sci Med Dec: 119-126, Pergamon Press, Ltd.
23. Ferro-Luzzi A and Durnin JVGA (1981). The assessment of human energy intake and expenditure. A critical review of literature. Joint FAO/WHO/UNU Expert Consultation on Energy and Protein Requirements. Rome 5-17 October 1981, ESN FAO/WHO/UNU.
24. Fox RH (1953). Energy expenditure of Africans engaged in various rural activities. Thesis for Ph.D., University of London.
25. Garby L. A Conceptual and Operational Definition of Energy Malnutrition. (Personal Communication).
26. Garrow JS (1974). "Energy Balance and Obesity in Man." London: North-Holland Publishing company.
27. Geissler CA, Brun TA, Mirbagheri I, Soheli A, Naghibi A and Hedayat H (1981). The energy expenditure of female carpet weavers and rural women in Iran. Am J Clin Nutr 34: 2776-2783.
28. Guzman de PE, Cabrera JP, Basconcillo RO, Gaurano AL, Yuchingtat GP, Tan RM, Kalaw JM and Recto RC (1978). A study of the energy expenditure, dietary intake and pattern of daily activity among various

occupational groups. V: Clerk-Typist. Philippine J Nutr 31: 147-156.

29. Guzman de PE, Dominguez SR, Kalaw JM, Bunung MN, Basconcillo RO and Santos VF (1974a). A study of the energy expenditure, dietary intake and pattern of daily activity among various occupational groups; II: Marikina Shoemakers and Housewives. Philippine J Sci 103: 53-65.

30. Guzman de PE, Dominguez SR, Kalaw JM, Basconcillo RO and Santos VF (1974b). A study of the energy expenditure, dietary intake, and pattern of daily activity among various occupational groups. I: Laguna rice farmers. Philippine J Sci 103: 53-65.

31. Guzman de PE, Kalaw JM, Tan RH, Recto RC, Basconcillo RO, Ferrer VT, Tombokon MS, Yuchingtat GP and Gaurano AL (1974c). A study of the energy expenditure, dietary intake and pattern of daily activity among various occupational groups; III: Urban Jeepney Drivers. Philippine J Nutr 27: 182-188.

32. Guzman de PE, Recto RC, Cabrera JP, Basconcillo RO, Gaurano AL, Yuchingtat GP, Ababto ZU and Math BS (1979). A study of the energy expenditure, dietary intake and pattern of daily activity among various occupational groups; VI: Textile Mill Workers. Philippine J Nutr 32: 134-148.

33. Keys A, Brozek A, Menchel J, Michelsen O and Taylor HL (1950). "The Biology of Human Starvation." Minneapolis: Univ. of Minnesota Press.

34. Maxfield ME (1971). The indirect measurement of energy expenditure in industrial situations. Am J Clin Nutr 24: 1126-1138.

35. Montgomery E and Johnson A (1977). Machiguenza energy expenditure. Ecol Food Nutr 6: 97-105.

36. Norgan NG (1981). Adaptation of energy metabolism to levels of energy intake. Joint FAO/WHO/UNU Expert Consultation on Energy and Protein Requirement. Rome, 5-17 October 1981. ESN. FAO/WHO/UNU.

37. Norgan N, Ferro-Luzzi A and Durnin JVGA (1974). The energy and nutrient intake and the energy expenditure of 204 New Guinean adults. Phil Trans Roy Soc London 268: 309-348.

38. Passmore R and Durnin JVGA (1955). Human Energy Expenditure. Physiol Rev 35: 801-840.

39. Phillips PG. The metabolic cost of common west African agricultural activities. J Trop Med 57:12.

40. Pinard A (1895). Note pour servir à l'histoire de la puériculture intrautérine. Ann de Gyn et d'Obstet 44:417-422.
41. Satyanarayana K, Naidu AN, Chatterjee B and RAO BSN (1977). Body size and work output. Am J Clin Nutr 30:322-325.
42. Schoeller DA and Van Santen E (1982). Measurement of energy expenditure in humans by doubly labeled water method. J Appl Phys 53:955-959.
43. Spurr GB, Barac-Nieto M and Maksud MG (1975). Energy expenditure cutting sugar cane. J App Phys 39(6):990-996.
44. Szalai A (1972). "The Use of Time: Daily Activities of Urban and Suburban Populations in 12 Countries." The Hague and Paris: Mouton.
45. Viteri FE, Torun B, Galcia JC and Herrera E (1971). Determining energy costs in agricultural activities by respirometer and energy balance techniques. Am J Clin Nutr 24:1418-1430.
46. Webb P, Annis JF and Troutman SJ Jr (1980). Energy balance in man measured by direct and indirect calorimetry. Am J Clin Nutr 33:1287.
47. Webb P and Troutman SJ Jr (1970). An instrument for continuous measurement of oxygen consumption. J Appl Phys 28:867-871.
48. Weir JB de V (1949). New methods for calculating metabolic rate with special reference to protein metabolism. J Phys 109:1-9.
49. Westerterp K and de Boer J (1983). Energy expenditure in humans using doubly labeled water. Fourth European Nutrition Conference, abstracts. Amsterdam, 24-27 May, W F-3, 66.

METHODOLOGY–CHILDREN

Energy Intake and Activity, pages 159–184
© *1984 Alan R. Liss, Inc., 150 Fifth Avenue, New York, NY 10011*

PHYSIOLOGICAL MEASUREMENTS OF PHYSICAL ACTIVITY
AMONG CHILDREN UNDER FREE-LIVING CONDITIONS

Benjamin Torún

Institute of Nutrition of Central America and Panama
Apartado Postal 1188, Guatemala, Guatemala

INTRODUCTION

The measurement of physical activity among children is necessary in order to assess energy expenditure, a prerequisite for establishing dietary energy requirements and recommendations (FAO/WHO/UNU 1984). These measurements are also necessary for evaluating energy-demanding behavior, an important functional indicator of health and nutritional status (Viteri and Torún 1981). The evaluation of energy requirements implies quantitative assessments of energy expenditure. In contrast, physical activity as a functional indicator of nutritional adequacy can be assessed quantitatively (e.g., in terms of energy expenditure), qualitatively (e.g., determining the types of activities spontaneously performed) or semi-quantitatively (e.g., assessing the relative amounts of time allocated to various types of activities).

Measurements should be done under free-living conditions that do not limit the spontaneous, natural activities of children. To do otherwise is to risk that values obtained for energy expenditure might be artifacts and that behavioral determinants might be masked by conditions that impair some activities and stimulate others. Physiological techniques used to measure physical activity fall within three general categories: (1) recording of activities and assessment of their energy costs; these are the so-called factorial or time-and-motion studies (Passmore and Durnin 1955; Wolff 1959); (2) evaluation of physiological phenomena that are quantitatively associated with energy expenditure; these include heart rate monitoring (Berggren and Christensen 1950; Bradfield 1971; Goldsmith et. al 1966) and estimates of total CO_2 production using doubly labeled water (Lifson et al. 1949; Lifson and McClinton 1966; Schoeller and Van Santen 1982); and, (3) quantification of body movements and displacement using motion sensors, such as pedometers, accelerometers and actometers (La Porte et al. 1979; Morris 1973; Schulman and Reisman 1959). The main advantages and limitations of these techniques are discussed below.

TIME AND MOTION TECHNIQUES

These consist of: (a) a time component, whereby an observer or the experimental subject himself records the duration of his various activities; and (b) an energy cost component, whereby the energy used to perform the activities is measured or obtained from published data. The time spent in each activity is then multiplied by the corresponding energy cost and the total energy expenditure is calculated by summation.

Several investigators have pointed out advantages and limitations of these techniques (Acheson et al. 1980; Bradfield 1971; Consolazio et al. 1963; Curtis and Bradfield 1971; Durnin and Brockway 1959; Durnin and Namyslowski 1958; Mundel 1970) The main advantages can be summarized as follows: (1) the time component gives qualitative or semi-quantitative behavioral information about the subject's life pattern, the types of activities or tasks performed, the frequency of their performance, and the time allocated to each activity; (2) the combination of the time component with the energy cost component provides quantitative information about energy expenditure over a period of time; and (3) the average energy cost of most activities per unit of body weight can be reproduced within acceptable limits in many populations of the same age group and physical training. The main pitfalls and limitations are: (1) direct observations are cumbersome and require one observer per subject; (2) observers must be familiar to the subjects in order to minimize the possibility of inducing behavioral changes by their presence; and (3) keeping personal activity records is tedious and reliability decreases as time between performance and recording is lengthened.

Time-and-motion studies have additional advantages and limitations when applied to children of different ages. The main pitfall is that the energy cost of work per unit of body weight is not constant throughout childhood, and adjustments must be made in order to use data from persons of an age that differs from that of the children observed (Torún 1983; Torún et al. 1983). In infants, the energy cost of activities may be quite variable (Morgan 1981). This may be due to the frequency of eating and the subsequent thermogenic effect of food (specific dynamic action), and to the relatively large energy cost of growth, which does not occur in a regular, uninterrupted manner throughout a day's 24 hours.

Preschool children cannot log their own activities and their parents or trained external observers must record them (Ku et al. 1981). Such activities can be quite varied: in a recent study (Torún et al., unpublished) with free-living preschool children, more than 40 different activities were recorded, with many children performing 10-15 activities in one day. The recording and analysis of such a large number of activities and tasks can be simplified by classifying them within a relatively small number of categories based on the predominant activity (lying down, standing, walking, etc.) or their relative energy cost (resting, walking, grooming, playing alone or with others, working, etc.). The observer must record the duration of each activity by writing down the exact time of its beginning and end. This cumbersome procedure can also be simplified by dividing the observation periods into short time intervals (e.g., 5-15 minutes); the observer records the number of times an activity is performed in each time interval, estimates the time spent in each activity, and divides the duration of the time interval by the number of recordings. Table 1 shows an example of such simplified recording. It should be noted, however, that this simplified method can overestimate the time spent in heavy energy-demanding activities that are usually done for very brief periods, such as running or hopping (Rutishauser and Whitehead 1972). This error may be of little importance when the same method is used to compare two groups of children with similar life patterns or to study a group of children repeatedly.

Time-and-motion observations have shown that the time allocated by preschool children to activities divided into specific categories can be related to their nutritional status: Table 2 shows that free-living children who had a

TABLE 1
SIMPLIFIED FORM TO RECORD ACTIVITIES OF CHILDREN IN TIME AND MOTION STUDIES

TIME	LYING DOWN		SITTING		STANDING		WALKING		RUNNING		PLAYING		NUMBER OF OBSERVATIONS
	asleep	awake	still	active	still	active	slowly	rapidly	slowly	rapidly	quietly	actively	
8:00 8:10		✓✓ 6.7*									✓ 3.3		3 (3.3'each)
8:10 8:20						✓ 2.5	✓✓ 5		✓ 2.5				4 (2.5'each)
8:20 8:30				✓ 10									1 (10')
8:30 8:40			✓ 2	✓ 2		✓✓ 4				✓ 2			5 (2' each)
.. ..													
.. ..													
.. ..													

*Minutes spent in each activity = (10 minutes/total number of observations) × number of times the activity was observed.

TABLE 2

TIME ALLOCATED TO LIGHT, MODERATE AND HEAVY
ACTIVITIES PERFORMED BY PRESCHOOL-AGED
CHILDREN, WITH OR WITHOUT WEIGHT
DEFICIT, IN A LOW-INCOME
MARGINAL NEIGHBORHOOD
OF GUATEMALA[a]

	Children with weight deficit (n = 19)	Children with adequate weight (n = 51)
Age, months	41 ± 15	43 ± 12
Weight-for-height, % of standard[b]	87 ± 2**	102 ± 6**
Proportion of daytime spent in:		
- sedentary and light activities	75 ± 9*	68 ± 12*
- moderate activities	22 ± 8	25 ± 10
- heavy activities	3 ± 2**	7 ± 5**

[a]Torún et al., unpublished observations.

[b]Relative to 50th percentile of World Health Organization
--U.S. National Center of Health Statistics Standards.

* Groups differ, p<0.05
**Groups differ, p<0.01

weight-for-height deficit of 10-19%, spent more time in
sedentary and light activities and less time in heavy activities than their counterparts with an adequate
weight-for-height (Torún et al., unpublished). Similar
findings were reported in rural Ugandan preschoolers,
compared to a small number of British children living in
Kampala (Rutishauser and Whitehead 1972). Time and motion
techniques are now being used by Torun and colleagues to
study the effect of nutritional supplementation on activity.

The use of this method has also shown that a short-
term (one week) decrease in energy intake changed the
physical activity of preschool children (Figure 1): energy-
demanding games and activities that implied standing,
walking, or running were reduced, whereas more time was
spent resting or playing while lying down (Viteri and Torún
1981). In addition, with weighting factors applied to
activities classified as inactive, light or active, it
has been used to explore the relationship of fatness in

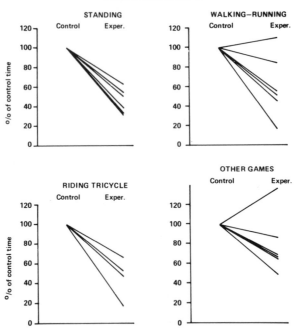

FIGURE 1
RELATIVE CHANGES IN TIME SPENT IN ACTIVITIES REQUIRING
INCREASED ENERGY EXPENDITURE
(0/o OF CONTROL TIME)

infants and preschool children to current and past patterns of physical activity (Ku et al. 1981). That study suggested that fatness may be more closely related to the child's previous activity than to present activity.

The assessment of energy expenditure of preschool children from time-and-motion records must take into account the energy cost of activities performed by children of this age group. The information available is scanty but indicates that the energy expended per unit of body weight is not the same in a child as in an adult doing the same task or activity (Table 3) (Torún et al. 1983). Consequently, the energy cost component in time-and-motion studies of preschool children must be derived from measurements obtained directly from children of that age group. Based on the figures shown in Table 3, Torún et al. (1983) have suggested that when such information is not available, it is possible to use the average basal metabolic expenditure for the child's age

TABLE 3

COMPARISON OF ENERGY COST OF ACTIVITIES OF PRESCHOOL CHILDREN (1.5-4 YEARS) AND ADULTS[a]

	Energy Cost, cal/kg/min			Basal Metabolic Energy Times[b]		
	child	adult[c]	child/adult	child	adult[c]	child/adult
Basal metabolism	38	18	2.1	-	-	-
Lying down, awake	44	20	2.2	1.2	1.2	1.0
Sitting quietly, playing, or in sedentary work	47	22	2.1	1.2	1.2	1.0
Walking leisurely on level ground	71	58	1.2	1.9	3.4	0.6
Walking up- and downhill	87	80	1.1	2.3	4.6	0.5
Walking rapidly at a grade	98	85	1.2	2.6	4.7	0.6
Leisure ride on tricycle (children) or bicycle (adults)	75	58	1.3	1.9	3.3	0.6
Climbing stairs slowly	94	85	1.1	2.5	4.7	0.5

[a] Adapted from Torún et al. (1983). Data for adults are from various sources.

[b] Ratio of energy cost of the activity/basal energy expenditure.

[c] Combining data for men and women.

group, multiplying it by 1.2, 2 and 2.5, respectively, to calculate the energy cost of sedentary, light and moderate activities. Another option is using values for adults, expressed per unit of body weight, but multiplied by 2 for sedentary activities and by 1.2 for other activities.

The logging of activities by school-age children and adolescents, or "diary technique," has been used in studies which showed that British adolescents of an upper social group engaged in less active exercise than those of poorer groups (Durnin 1967), that "plump" girls spent less time in activity than thin and "normal" girls (Durnin 1967), that there was usually no correlation between the activity pattern of North American 8-year-old children with their activity at a younger age (Ku et al. 1981), and that total energy expenditure correlated with some assessments of physical working capacity (Bouchard et al. 1983). The latter pointed out, however, that the validity of the diary technique has not been determined.

As in the case of preschool children, the use of the energy cost of activities performed by adults can lead to errors in the estimate of total energy expenditure (Torún 1983). Table 4 illustrates this problem and indicates that the younger the child, the greater the error. Although energy expenditures were not measured by the same investigators in all age groups, the rates of workloads or the tasks were not identical, and the indirect calorimetry methods used were not always the same, the data in Table 4 shows a trend of decreasing energy expenditure per unit of body weight as age increases. The existence of such a trend is supported by Astrand's report (1952) that the net oxygen uptake per kilogram of body weight during treadmill work at a given speed fell progressively as age increased from 5 to 15 years. It appears that the use of adult energy cost data may be valid during the later adolescent years, but more experimental information is required before a definitive statement can be made in this regard.

HEART RATE MONITORING

This method is based on the fact that heart rate increases with physical activity and that the increment is associated with a proportional linear rise in oxygen consumption. Hence, measurements of heart rate (HR) allow the estimation of oxygen uptake (VO_2), and energy expenditure can then be calculated using standard indirect calorimetry equations (Consolazio et al. 1963; Weir 1949). The evolution of these physiological inter-relations and the use of heart rate as an indirect indicator of energy expenditure, beginning with F.G. Benedict's reports in 1907, have been summarized by Booyens and Hervey (1960). The method has two components: (a) establishment of the subject's heart rate-energy expenditure regression equation; and, (b) cumulative counting or continuous monitoring of heart beats. Its use to assess the daily energy expenditure of free-living persons became widespread in the late 1960's with the development of lightweight, portable, unobtrusive heart-beat counters and electrocardiographic recorders (Baker et al. 1967; Bradfield 1971; Cunningham et al. 1981; Kennedy et al. 1976; Masironi and Mansourian 1974; Saris and Binkhorst 1977).

The advantages and limitations of the this method have been discussed by several investigators (Acheson et al. 1980; Andrews 1971; Bradfield 1971; Christensen et al. 1983; Dauncey and James 1979; Durnin 1978; Lange-Andersen 1978).

TABLE 4
COMPARISON OF THE ENERGY COST OF SELECTED ACTIVITIES AT DIFFERENT AGES, PER UNIT OF BODY WEIGHT (CAL/KG/MIN)[a]

Age in Years	BMR[b]	Sitting[c]	Standing Still[d]	Light Activities Standing[e]	Light-to-Moderate Activities[f]	Dressing and Undressing	Walking Leisurely[g]	Carpentry	Bicycle Ergometer[h]	References[i]
2-4	38	47			73		79			73
6-8	31	52							110	68
8-9	28	37								66
9-11	26	35	38	47	62	69			85	7,23,67 68-70
12-14	21	32	31	44	56		70	75	75(96)[j]	7,23,43 64,65,68
14-16	20	27	26	47					(82)[j]	28,64,65
19		24								65
Adult	18	23	23	38	52	49	62	63	55	4,17,20 22,42,74, 79

[a] No major differences between boys and girls until 12 years of age. After that, add a 5-10% for males and subtract 5-10% for females from the figures shown.
[b] Basal metabolic rate calculated from references 20,22,42,73 and standard BMR tables.
[c] Sitting quietly, reading, doing schoolwork, listening to a lecture or to the radio, doing puzzles, playing cards or singing.
[d] Standing casually or singing without doing many body movements.
[e] With light-to-moderate body movements or displacement in tasks such as playing musical instruments, cooking and light house-cleaning chores.
[f] Playing in schoolgrounds, doing light or moderately heavy domestic work, performing light or moderate agricultural tasks.
[g] Walking indoors or outdoors at a slow or moderately fast pace.
[h] Pedalling against a moderately heavy load at a constant rhythm.
[i] Average of values obtained, adapted or calculated from various sources. The number of observations were not always available.
[j] Different workload than the load used in the preceding column.

The main advantages are that: (1) it does not require direct observation of the subject, and has little or no influence on his behavior; (2) the small, lightweight, heart rate monitors do not burden the subject or interfere with his usual activities; (3) energy expended during leisure time activities can be measured without intruding in the subject's privacy; and (4) fewer personnel are needed than in time-and-motion studies that require external observers. The main shortcomings and limitations are: (1) the relationship between heart rate and energy expenditure varies from one individual to another and it is affected by factors related to the subject, the environment, and the circumstances under which the relationship is assessed; (2) there is a poor correlation between heart rate and oxygen consumption at low levels of energy expenditure; (3) the method does not give information about activity patterns nor about the time allocated to different activities; and (4) technical problems can lead to loss of lengthy information, although this can be ameliorated by the use of electrocardiographic recordings and adequate electrode placement (Hanish et al. 1971).

The individual nature of the HR-VO$_2$ relationship and the factors that may affect it, such as the child's age, physical fitness and health, environmental temperature, type of work, body position and muscle groups involved, make it necessary to establish the regression equation of oxygen consumption on heart rate for each child whose energy expenditure will be assessed. This equation is the so-called "calibration curve" for an individual. If changes in physical fitness or health are taking place, the calibration curves must be determined close to the time when heart rate will be monitored, and must be repeated as necessary. This is illustrated by the weekly increase in slope or regression coefficient observed in preschool children being treated for severe protein-energy malnutrition (Torún et al. 1979, Figure 2). It should be noted, however, that as Christensen et al. (1983) have reported in adults and Torún and Viteri (unpublished) have observed in preschool children, there is a random day-to-day variation in HR-VO$_2$ relationships which may lead to over or underestimation of energy expenditure in an individual when his heart rate is measured. At a group level and in population studies these random errors tend to cancel out, and some investigators (Andrews 1967; Bradfield et al. 1970) calculated that the heart rate prediction method applied to adults with individual calibration curves resulted in errors of the same order as those of other indirect measures of energy expenditure.

It is not always feasible to obtain individual calibration curves. An alternative is the use of the average regression equations of persons of the same sex and similar age and physical fitness; however, the coefficient of variation of the energy expenditure, predicted from heart rate, increases 1.5 to 3 times as compared with the use of individual regression equations (Bradfield et al. 1970; Payne et al. 1971). Another alternative is based on observations that individual regression lines of school-age children with cerebral palsy (Berg 1971; Berg and Bjure 1970) and of malnourished preschoolers (Torún et al. 1979) tended to converge near a common point (Figure 2). Berg (1971) reported that for two children the use of that group cross-over point, plus one or

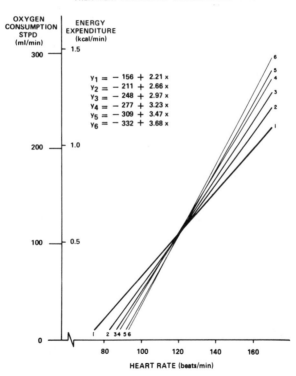

FIGURE 2
MEAN WEEKLY REGRESSION LINES OF OXYGEN CONSUMPTION
ON HEART RATE OF 19 CHILDREN DURING SIX WEEKS OF
TREATMENT FOR PROTEIN–ENERGY MALNUTRITION

OXYGEN CONSUMPTION STPD (ml/min)

ENERGY EXPENDITURE (kcal/min)

$y_1 = -156 + 2.21\,x$
$y_2 = -211 + 2.66\,x$
$y_3 = -248 + 2.97\,x$
$y_4 = -277 + 3.23\,x$
$y_5 = -309 + 3.47\,x$
$y_6 = -332 + 3.68\,x$

HEART RATE (beats/min)

two individual calibrations points to obtain each child's $HR-\dot{V}O_2$ regression equation, gave the same energy expenditure results as those with individual calibration curves, but that the results differed by 20% in two other children.

Another pitfall related to the $HR-VO_2$ relationship of children is that the exercise done to begin establishing the calibration curve of a young child frequently results in a relatively large increase in energy expenditure in relation to resting values, whereas subsequent workloads produce smaller changes. This may produce a clustering of the data points and requires a resting value of HR and $\dot{V}O_2$ in order to calculate an adequate regression equation, especially, as is often the case, when only 3 or 4 exercising measurements can be done. At least in 2- to 4-year-old children the resting $HR-\dot{V}O_2$ point should be obtained while lying down, since measurements in the sitting and standing positions give highly variable results compared to the supine position, either at rest or under basal metabolic conditions (Torún and Viteri, unpublished).

A major shortcoming is the poor correlation between heart rate and oxygen consumption at low levels of energy expenditure, when factors such as shifts in body position, emotions, and smoking can modify heart rate with little or no influence on oxygen consumption. This makes heart rate an unsuitable predictor of energy expenditure in persons who engage in sedentary or light daily activities because their average 24-hour heart rate is only slightly above their resting pulse (Christensen et al. 1983; Dauncey and James 1979). Using heart-rate monitoring and direct calorimetry simultaneously, Dauncey and James (1979) showed that the errors in the prediction of heat production from heart rate were particularly large when the experimental subjects were resting at night and that the reliability of the prediction was much better during daytime. Their best estimates of energy expenditure based on HR were obtained by calibrating the subjects' HR over a 24-hour period within the whole-body calorimeter; the second best estimate was obtained using various resting and exercising points and fitting a logistic curve constrained to pass through the lower calibration points. Comparing the heart-rate monitoring method with time-and-motion studies, Acheson et al. (1980) found that heart rate was a better predictor of energy expenditure when a linear regression equation was calculated from heart rate and the logarithm of energy expenditure.

A practical approach to calculating daily energy expenditure for heart rate in partially sedentary persons is the use of multichannel heart-beat accumulators and continuous electrocardiographic recorders. This equipment discriminates between periods of low and high physical activity defined in terms of heart rate thresholds; energy expenditures during periods of activity may be calculated from heart rate by regression equations, and estimates of resting energy expenditure can be used to calculate the energy expended during the remaining time. A similar approach with single-channel heartbeat accumulators has been used in preschool (Torún et al. 1984; Torún and Viteri 1981a; 1981b) and school-aged (Spady 1980) children. It consists of the combination of energy expenditure estimated from heart rate during the active hours of the day, and from basal metabolic rate during the night or daytime naps. The accuracy of these measurements, however, has not been validated.

In the absence of calibration curves, heart rate can be used to determine whether two groups of children of the same age, sex, health and physical fitness have similar levels of physical activity. The use of multi-channel heart-beat accumulators and continuous electrocardiographic recordings may also provide some information about activity patterns based on changes in HR that may indicate the intensity and relative duration of peak activities. Although strong emotions can raise heart rate markedly, with only a small increase in oxygen consumption, it can be assumed that prolonged, strong emotions are usually absent in everyday performance of routine activities; in many circumstances, therefore, heart rate may be an acceptable indicator of the intensity of physical activity. Nevertheless, heart rate monitoring does not give information about the type of activities performed or about behavioral changes in activity patterns.

In spite of its limitations, heart-rate monitoring is a useful technique for studying habitual physical activity and energy expenditure in individuals and population groups. If its limitations are taken into consideration, and the pitfalls discussed above are avoided or solved, the social acceptability of the method, its relatively low influence on behavior, the objectivity of the information, and the amount and ease of retrieval, all favor its use. It has been successfully used in infants, preschool-age children, school-age children, and adolescents for purposes such as assessing energy expenditure and physical activity of normal, obese, malnourished, anemic and mentally retarded children (Berg 1971; Berg and Bjure 1970; Bradfield 1971; Bradfield et al. 1971; Gandra and Bradfield 1971; Griffiths and Payne 1976; Heywood and Latham 1971; Saris et al. 1977; Spady 1980; Torún et al. 1984; Torún and Viteri 1981a; 1981b), calculating the energy cost of growth (Spady et al. 1976), evaluating the relationship between daily energy expenditure and physical fitness (Cunningham et al. 1981), investigating functional aspects of protein-energy malnutrition (Torún et al. 1979; Viteri and Torún 1981) and studying the effect of environmental and social influences on behavior (Wade and Ellis 1971).

DOUBLY LABELED WATER METHOD

This method, developed by Lifson and co-workers (Lifson et al. 1949; Lifson et al. 1955; Lifson and McClintock 1966; Lifson et al. 1975), is based on the observation that through the action of carbonic anhydrase (Lifson et al. 1949) the oxygen of expired CO_2 is in isotopic equilibrium with the oxygen of body water. Consequently, when a known dose of water labeled with both deuterium (or tritium) and heavy oxygen (^{18}O) is given, there is a rapid exchange of the isotopes with the hydrogen and oxygen of body water and with the oxygen of CO_2. After equilibrium is reached, the decrease in concentration of the hydrogen isotope indicates body water output, and the decrease in concentration of the oxygen isotope indicates body water plus CO_2 outputs. The outpout of CO_2 can be obtained by difference, using the formula:

$$r_{CO_2} = (W/(2 \times 1.04)) (K_O - K_H) - 0.015 \, WK_H$$

where r_{CO_2} is the rate of CO_2 output, W is the total body water, and K_O and K_H are the fractional turnover rates of the labeled oxygen and hydrogen of the body water. The factor of 2 is used because CO_2 has the oxygen equivalent of 2 molecules of water, and 1.04 and 0.015 are correction factors for isotopic fractionation of water lost as vapor. Lifson and McClintock (1966) have discussed in detail the assumptions and mathematical derivation of the formula.

Measurements done in the water of urine or blood samples collected shortly after isotopic equilibration with endogenous hydrogen and oxygen (about 12 hours after administration of the doubly labeled water) and several days later, allow calculation of total CO_2 excretion during that time interval. Total respiratory oxygen uptake during those days can be calculated from estimates of the average respiratory quotient (RQ), since:

$$RQ = CO_2 \text{ production}/O_2 \text{ consumption}.$$

Energy expenditure can then be calculated from oxygen consumption using standard indirect calorimetry equations (Consolazio et al. 1963; Weir 1949).

Measurements of CO_2 production with accuracy within ± 8% have been made in several laboratory animals, but errors may be larger in field studies (Nagy 1980). However, a 14-day study (Shoeller and Van Santen 1982) in three men and one woman gave measurements of energy expenditure that differed within ± 7% from calculations derived from dietary intakes plus changes in body composition.

The method seems highly promising for studies in free-living children, although it must still be validated under those conditions. Its main advantages are that: (1) it is noninvasive (using urine samples for the isotopic measurements); (2) it does not interfere with the subject's activities or behavior; (3) it does not require field personnel or complex data collection; and (4) it can be carried out over a period of several days, either continuously or serially, to assess changes in energy expenditure with different activity patterns. Its major limitations are: (1) the need for a mass spectrometer to measure stable isotopes; (2) the high cost of the heavy-oxygen labeled water and the spectrometric analyses; (3) that it does not provide information about the nature of the activities performed or about the subject's activity pattern; (4) and that it is necessary to measure the subject's average respiratory quotient. The latter can be estimated from the composition of ingested food and/or by measurements of exhaled oxygen and CO_2 repeated several times throughout the experimental period. An alternative for individuals consuming a mixed diet is to assume that their average RQ is 0.85. Table 5 shows that if the actual RQ was either 0.80 or 0.90, the error in the energy expenditure assessment would be within ± 5%. This error range is

TABLE 5
ERRORS IN THE CALCULATION OF ENERGY EXPENDITURE USING
DIFFERENT RESPIRATORY QUOTIENTS (RQ) WITH THE
DOUBLY LABELED WATER METHOD. EXAMPLE BASED
ON A DAILY CO_2 PRODUCTION OF
340 LITERS, STPD[a]

Non-Protein RQ	Oxygen Consumption, l/day, STPD		Energy Equivalent of Oxygen, Kcal/l		Energy Expenditure, Kcal/day	Energy Deviations from RQ of 0.85
0.80	425	x	4.801	=	2,040	+4.9%
0.85	400	x	4.862	=	1,945	--
0.90	378	x	4.924	=	1,861	-4.3%

[a]Standard conditions of temperature (0°C) and pressure (760 mm Hg), dry gas.

within, and usually lower than, those for energy expenditure estimates obtained by other methods. The method has potential pitfalls associated with theoretical assumptions that must be made, but some of these assumptions can be controlled experimentally and others lead to negligible errors or do not apply in humans (Nagy and Costa 1980).

BODY MOTION SENSORS

These techniques involve the use of small, portable, lightweight instruments that provide semi-quantitative information on physical activity by registering distance traveled or the number or speed of movements performed. In some instances, statistically significant correlations have been reported between activity recorded by these instruments and the energy expenditure of children and adults walking on a treadmill (Saris and Binkhorst 1977; Schulman et al. 1961), performing specific exercises (Rose and Mayer 1968), or the ratio of work metabolic rate/basal metabolic rate estimated from activity questionnaires (La Porte et al. 1982; 1979; Rieff et al. 1967). However, the existence of such correlations has not been consistently shown and their accuracy and validity have not been demonstrated.

The main advantages of these devices are that: (1) they do not interfere with the subject's usual activities and behavior; (2) many of the instruments are relatively inexpensive; and (3) they determine whether one group of persons is more or less active than another. Their main limitations are that: (1) the sensitivity and specificity of the recordings has not been consistently demonstrated; (2) their accuracy in estimating daily energy expenditure has not been tested with measurements of direct or indirect calorimetry; (3) they do not provide information about the type of activities performed or the subject's activity pattern; and (4) they do not record adequately certain body movements.

The following are among the instruments used as body motion and displacement sensors:

Actometers are modified automatically winding calendar watches from which the escape mechanism has been removed in order to connect the rotor directly to the hands (Schulman and Reisman 1959). They measure movements in horizontal and vertical planes. Actometers have been used to assess activity of 4- to 6-month-old infants, indicating that obese babies tended to be hypoactive in comparison to their leaner counterparts (Rose and Mayer 1968). A more sophisticated motion sensor, the Large-Scale Integrated Activity Monitor, or LSI, was developed by La Porte, et al. (1979). It is a small cylinder with a ball of mercury that rolls and makes contact with a mercury switch when the instrument deviates 3% from the horizontal plane; the number of body movements are registered by the closures of the mercury switch. It was used with twenty-two free-living boys, aged 12 to 14 (La Porte et al. 1982); although activity measures during school hours were correlated with those after school hours (r=0.43), they did not correlate consistently with estimates of food energy intake or with the results of leisure time activity questionnaires. Their developers, however, believe that the instrument has an excellent potential as an objective measure of physical activity in large population studies.

Pedometers or step counters are either watch-like devices with a moveable inner part that swings with each step and drives a counter connected to a digital dial (Chirico and Stunkard 1960; Lange-Andersen et al. 1978), or pressure-sensitive electrical resistors placed in the shoe sole that send an electrical signal to either a digital counter or a magnetic tape every time the shoe touches the ground (Lange-Andersen et al. 1978). Pedometers only count steps and do not provide information about movements of the upper part of the body. Furthermore, many pedometers tend to overestimate the number of steps during fast walking and running since they are sensitive to both horizontal and vertical movements. In contrast, they underestimate the actual step rate during slow walking (Saris et al. 1977).

Accelerometers placed on various parts of the body can measure the increase in speed of movements (Morris 1973). The output from the accelerometers are electrical signals that may be stored on magnetic tape or transmitted by telemetry to a receiver. Retrieval and computing of the signals are very complex and the validity of accelerometers to measure habitual physical activity has not been proven.

CONCLUSIONS

The assessment of physical activity and energy expenditure of children are of great importance because of their functional and practical implications. They are of special interest in the field of nutrition since it has been recognized that

> ...the energy requirement of an individual is that level of energy intake from food which will balance energy expenditure when the individual has a body size and composition, and level of physical activity consistent with long-term good health, which will allow for the maintenance of economically necessary and socially desirable physical activity, and which will satisfy the energy needs associated with the deposition of tissues in growing children (FAO/WHO/UNU 1984).

Furthermore, the level and pattern of physical activity are important functional indicators of nutritional status, especially in relation to energy intake, but probably also in relation to other nutrients.

Although there are many studies of the physical fitness of children and its relationship to body composition or anthropometry, there is little information about the usual physical activity and energy expenditure of free-living children. Most of the information available is from children, particularly those of school age, who live in the urban areas of industrialized countries. The principal constraints to obtaining more information about age, cultural, social, ethnic and geographic groups are related to the complexity and high cost of the methods that currently exist. Time-and-motion investigations by direct observation require that a fairly large number of children be observed within a relatively short period of time without inducing major behavioral changes. Costs increase when observations must be repeated at different times of the year in children who have important seasonal activity changes. The diary or questionnaire techniques would reduce costs, but the reliability of the information obtained from most low-income groups with a high rate of illiteracy is questionable. Even if the practical problems related to the time component could be solved, more information on the energy cost of activities performed by children is needed to convert the timed activity observations into assessments of energy expenditure. Heart rate monitoring requires an investment in equipment to perform the oxygen uptake measurements that are necessary for the $HR-VO_2$ calibrations, and to monitor the children's heart rate. Although the cost of this equipment has decreased somewhat in the last decade, the instruments needed to obtain better quality information, such as multi-channel heart rate discriminators and portable electrocardiographic recorders, are more expensive than single-channel heart-beat accumulators. This method must be combined with other assessments of energy expenditure during periods of low physical activity. Actometers, including the Large-Scale Integrated Activity Monitor, are cheaper than heart rate monitors but, because the estimations of activity patterns and energy expenditure using these instruments are questionable, their use may be limited to assessing changes in activity. Pedometers, in particular, seem to be very unreliable indicators of activity. Doubly labeled water is the most expensive method at the present time and its use to calculate total energy expenditure must still be validated in children and under field conditions. If valid, the simplicity of the field work and the objectivity of the information make it the most attractive method to assess total energy expenditure in free-living children, specially if the economic limitations can be overcome. It does not, however, give information about the types and patterns of activity.

Some general recommendations to overcome these and other constraints in view of the important applications of physical activity and energy expenditure assessments, are:

1) Organization of a coordinated international effort using comparable standardized techniques to obtain more information on activity and energy expenditure of children from different social and geographic environments. Physiologists, nutritionists and behavioral scientists should interact in this effort.

2) Stimulation of the improvement of current methodology and development of new techniques to measure activity accurately. This includes validation of methods such as the use of doubly labeled water, which may become an accurate standard of comparison for simpler or cheaper techniques.

3) Provision of technical and financial support to investigators who may obtain new and reliable information on physical activity and energy expenditure of children, especially in the context of their nutritional applications and consequences.

REFERENCES

1. Acheson KJ, Campbell IT, Edholm OG, Miller DS and Stock MJ (1980). The measurement of daily energy expenditure - an evaluation of some techniques. Am J Clin Nutr 33:1155-1164.
2. Andrews RB (1967). Estimation of values of energy expenditure rate from observed values of heart rate. Human Factors 9: 581-586.
3. Andrews RB (1971). Net heart rate as a substitute for respiratory calorimetry. Am J Clin Nutr 24:1139-1147.
4. Apfelbaum M, Bostsarron J and Lacatis D (1971). Effect of caloric restriction and excessive caloric intake on energy expenditure. Am J Clin Nutr 24:1405-1409.
5. Astrand PO (1952). "Experimental Studies on Physical Working Capacity in Relation to Sex and Age," Munksgaard, Copenhagen. Cited in: Astrand PO and Rodahl K (1970). "Textbook of Work Physiology," New York: McGraw-Hill.
6. Baker JA, Humphrey SJE and Wolff HS (1967). Socially acceptable monitoring instruments (SAMI). J Physiol 188:4-5P.
7. Bedale EM (1923). Energy expenditure and food requirements of children at school. Proc Roy Soc (London), 94B:368-404. Cited by Bradfield RB, Chan H,

Bradfield NE and Payne PR (1971). Am J Clin Nutr 24:1461-1466.

8. Berg K (1971). Heart-rate telemetry for evaluation of the energy expenditure of children with cerebral palsy. Am J Clin Nutr 24: 1438-1445.

9. Berg K and Bjure G (1970). Methods for evaluation of the physical working capacity of school children with cerebral palsy. Acta Pediat Scand Suppl 204:15-26.

10. Berggren G and Christensen EH (1950). Heart rate and body temperature as indices of metabolic rate during work. Arbeitsphysiologie 14:255-260.

11. Booyens J and Hervey GR (1960). The pulse rate as a means of measuring metabolic rate in man. Can J Biochem Physiol 38:1301-1311.

12. Bouchard C, Tremblay A, Leblanc C, Lortie G, Savard R and Thériault G (1983). A method to assess energy expenditure in children and adults. Am J Clin Nutr 37:461-467.

13. Bradfield RB (1971). A technique for determination of usual daily energy expenditure in the field. Am J Clin Nutr 24:1148-1154.

14. Bradfield RB, Chan N, Bradfield NE and Payne PR (1971): Energy expenditures and heart rates of Cambridge boys at school. Am J Clin Nutr 24:1461-1466.

15. Bradfield RB, Huntzicker PB and Freuhan GJ (1970). Errors of group regressions for prediction of individual energy expenditure. Am J Clin Nutr 23:1015-1016.

16. Bradfield RB, Paulos J and Grossman L (1971). Energy expenditure and heart rate of obese high school girls. Am J Clin Nutr 24:1482-1488.

17. Chen H-C (1981). Studies of energy intakes, expenditures and requirements in China. In Torún B, Young VR and Rand WM (eds): "Protein-Energy Requirements of Developing Countries: Evaluation of New Data," Tokyo: United Nations Univ., Food Nutr Bull Suppl 5:150-158.

18. Chirico AM and Stunkard AJ (1960). Physical activity and human obesity. N Engl J Med 263:935-940.

19. Christensen CC, Frey HMM, Foenstelien E, Aadland E and Refsum HE (1983). A critical evaluation of energy expenditure estimates based on individual O_2 consumption/heart rate curves and average daily heart rate. Am J Clin Nutr 37:468-472.

20. Consolazio CF (1971). Energy expenditure studies in military populations using Kofranyi-Michaelis respirometers. Am J Clin Nutr 24: 1431-1437.

21. Consolazio CF, Johnson RE and Pecora LJ (1963). "Physiological Measurements of Metabolic Functions in Man." New York: McGraw-Hill.

22. Consolazio CF, Pollack H, Crowley LV and Goldstein DR (1956). Calorie cost of work and energy balance studies. Metab Clin Exptl 5:259-271.

23. Cullumbine H (1950). Heat production and energy requirements of tropical people. J Appl Physiol 2:640-653.

24. Cunningham DA, Stapleton JJ, MacDonald IC and Paterson, DH (1981). Daily energy expenditure of young boys as related to maximal aerobic power. Can J Appl Sport Sci 6:207-211.

25. Curtis DE and Bradfield RB (1971). Long-term energy intake and expenditure of obese housewives. Am J Clin Nutr 24:1410-1417.

26. Dauncey MJ and James WPT (1979). Assessment of the heart-rate method for determining energy expenditure in man, using a whole-body calorimeter. Br J Nutr 42:1-13.

27. Durnin JVGA (1967). Activity patterns in the community. Can Med Ass J 96:882-888.

28. Durnin JVGA (1971). Physical activity by adolescents. Acta Pediatr Scand Suppl 217:133-135.

29. Durnin JVGA (1978). Indirect calorimetry in man: a critique of practical problems. Proc Nutr Soc 37:5-12.

30. Durnin JVGA and Brockway JM (1959). Determination of the total daily energy expenditure in man by direct calorimetry: assessment of the accuracy of a modern technique. Brit J Nutr 13:41-53.

31. Durnin JVGA and Namyslowski L (1958). Individual variations in the energy expenditure of standardized activities. J Physiol 143:573-578.

32. FAO/WHO/UNU (1984): Report of Joint Expert Consultation on Energy and Protein Requirements, Rome, 1981. Geneva: WHO, In press.

33. Gandra YR and Bradfield RB (1971). Energy expenditure and oxygen handling efficiency of anemic school children. Am J Clin Nutr 24: 1451-1456.

34. Goldsmith R, Miller DS, Mumford P and Stock MJ (1966). The use of long-term heart rate to assess energy expenditure. J Physiol 189: 35-36P.

35. Griffiths M and Payne PR (1976). Energy expenditure in small children of obese and non-obese parents. Nature 260:698-700.

36. Hanish HM, Neustein RA, Van Cott CC and Sanders RT (1971). Technical aspects of monitoring the heart rate of active persons. Am J Clin Nutr 24:1155-1163.

37. Heywood PF and Latham MC (1971). Use of the SAMI heart-rate integrator in malnourished children. Am J Clin Nutr 24:1446-1450.

38. Kennedy HL, Underhill SJ and Warbasse JR (1976). Practical advantages of two-channel electrocardiographic Holter recordings. Am Heart J 91:822-823.

39. Ku LC, Shapiro LR, Crawford PB and Huenemann RL (1981). Body composition and physical activity in 8-year-old children. Am J Clin Nutr 34:2770-2775.

40. La Porte RE, Cauley JA, Kinsey CM, Corbett W, Robertson R, Black-Sandler R, Kuller LH and Falkel J (1982): The epidemiology of physical activity in children, college students, middle-aged men, menopausal females and monkeys. J Chron Dis 35:787-795.

41. La Porte RE, Kuller LH, Kupfer DJ, McPartland RJ, Matthews G and Caspersen C (1979). An objective measure of physical activity for epidemiologic research. Am J Epid 109:158-168.

42. Lange-Andersen K, Masironi R, Rutenfranz J and Seliger V (1978). "Habitual Physical Activity and Health." Copenhagen: WHO Reg Publ Ser No. 6.

43. Legun AF and Moltschanowa OP (1935) Uber den 24 Stundigen Energiever brauch von Kindern in Schulpflchtigen Alter 8-14 Jahre. "Problems of Nutrition, Moscow," 4: 43-60. Cited by Passmore R and Durnin JVGA (1955). Physiol Rev 35: 801-840.

44. Lifson N, Gordon GB, Visscher MB and Nier AOC (1949). The fate of utilized molecular oxygen and the source of the oxygen of respiratory carbon dioxide, studied with the aid of heavy oxygen. J Biol Chem 180: 803-811.

45. Lifson N, Gordon GB and McClintock R (1955). Measurement of total carbon dioxide production by means of D_2O^{18}. J Appl Physiol 7: 704-710.

46. Lifson N and McClintock R (1966). Theory of use of the turnover rates of body water for measuring energy and material balance. J Theoret Biol 12:46-74.

47. Lifson N, Little WS, Levitt DG and Henderson RM (1975). $D_2^{18}O$ method for CO_2 output in small mammals and economic feasibility in man. J Appl Physiol 39:657-664.

48. Masironi R and Mansourian P (1974). Determination of habitual physical activity by means of a portable R-R

interval distribution recorder. Bull Wld Hlth Org 51:291-298.

49. Morgan J and Mumford P (1981). Preliminary studies of energy expenditure in infants under six months of age. Acta Pediatr Scand 70: 15-19.

50. Morris JRW (1973). Accelerometry: A technique for the measurement of human body movements. J Biomech 6:729-736.

51. Mundel ME (1970). "Motion and Time Study." Englewood Cliffs, NJ: Prentice-Hall.

52. Nagy KA (1980). CO_2 production in animals: analysis of potential errors in the doubly labeled water method. Am J Physiol 238: R466-R473.

53. Nagy KA and Costa DP (1980). Water flux in animals: analysis of potential errors in the tritiated water method. Am J Physiol 238: R454-R465.

54. Passmore R and Durnin JVGA (1955). Human energy expenditure. Physiol Rev 35:801-840.

55. Payne PR, Wheeler EF and Salvosa CB (1971). Prediction of daily energy expenditure from average pulse rate. Am J Clin Nutr 24: 1164-1170.

56. Rieff GG, Montoye HJ, Remington RD, et al. (1967). Assessment of physical activity by questionnaire and interview. J Sports Med Phys Fitness 7:135-142.

57. Rose HE and Mayer J (1968). Activity, calorie intake, fat storage, and the energy balance of infants. Pediatrics 41:18-29.

58. Rutishauser IHE and Whitehead RG (1972). Energy intake and expenditure in 1-3-year-old Ugandan children living in a rural environment. Br J Nutr 28:145-152.

59. Saris WHM and Binkhorst RA (1977). The use of pedometer and actometer in studying the daily physical activity in man. Part I: Reliability of pedometer and actometer. Eur J Appl Physiol 37:219-228.

60. Saris WH, Snel P and Binkhorst RA (1977). A portable heart rate distribution recorder for studying daily physical activity. Eur J Appl Physiol 37:17-25.

61. Schoeller DA and van Santen E (1982). Measurement of energy expenditure in man by the doubly labeled water method. J Appl Physiol 53(4):955-959.

62. Schulman JL and Reisman JM (1959). An objective measure of hyperactivity. Amer J Ment Defic 64:455.

63. Schulman JL et al. (1961). Studies on activity levels of children. Presented to the American Psychiatric Asso-

ciation and cited by Rose HE and Mayer J (1968). Pediatrics 41:18-29.

64. Seliger V, Cermak V, Handzo P, Horak J, Jirka Z, Macek M, Pribil M, Rous J, Skranc O, Ulbrich J and Uranek J (1971). Physical fitness of the Czechoslovak 12- and 15-year-old population. Acta Pediatr Scand Suppl 217:37-41.

65. Sobolova V, Seliger V, Grussova D, Machovcova J and Zelenka, V (1971). The influence of age and sports training in swimming on physical fitness. Acta Pediatr Scand Suppl 217:63-67.

66. Spady DW (1980). Total daily energy expenditure of healthy, free ranging school children. Am J Clin Nutr 33:766-775.

67. Spady DW, Payne PR, Picou D and Waterlow JC (1976). Energy balance during recovery from malnutrition. Am J Clin Nutr 29:1073-1078.

68. Taylor CM, Lamb MW, Robertson ME and MacLeod G (1948). The energy expenditure for quiet play and cycling of boys seven to fourteen years of age. J Nutr 35:511-521.

69. Taylor CM, Pye OF and Caldwell AB (1948). The energy expenditure of 9- to 11-year-old boys and girls (1) standing drawing and (2) dressing and undressing. J Nutr 36:123-131.

70. Taylor CM, Pye OF, Caldwell AB and Sostman ER (1949). The energy expenditure of boys and girls 9 to 11 years of age (1) sitting listening to the radio (phonograph), (2) sitting singing, and (3) standing singing. J Nutr 38:1-10.

71. Torún B (1983). Inaccuracy of applying energy expenditure rates of adults to children. Am J Clin Nutr 38: 813-814.

72. Torún B, Caballero B, Flores-Huerta S and Viteri F (1984). Habitual Guatemalan diets and catch-up growth of children with mild-to-moderate malnutrition. In Rand WM, Uauy R and Scrimshaw NW (eds.): "Protein Energy requirements in Developing Countries: Results of International Research," United Nations Univ Food Nutr Bull Suppl 8 (In press).

73. Torún B, Chew F and Mendoza RD (1983). Energy cost of activities of preschool children. Nutr Res 3:401-406.

74. Torún B, McGuire JS and Mendoza RD (1982). Energy cost of activities and tasks of women from a rural region of Guatemala. Nutr Res 2: 127-136.

75. Torún B, Schutz Y, Viteri F and Bradfield RB (1979). Growth, body composition and heart rate/VO₂ relationship changes during the nutritional recovery of children with two different physical activity levels. Bibl Nutr Dieta 27:55-56.

76. Torún B and Viteri FE (1981a). Capacity of habitual Guatemalan diets to satisy protein requirements of pre-school children with adequate dietary energy intakes. In Torún B, Young VR and Rand WM (eds): "Protein-Energy Requirements of Developing Countries: Evaluation of New Data," Tokyo: United Nations Univ Food Nutr Bull Suppl 5:210-228.

77. Torún B and Viteri FE (1981b). Energy requirements of pre-school children and effects of varying energy intakes on protein metabolism. In Torún B, Young VR and Rand WM (eds): "Protein-Energy Requirements of Developing Countries: Evaluation of New Data," Tokyo United Nations Univ Food Nutr Bull Suppl 5:229-241.

78. Viteri FE and Torún B (1981). Nutrition, physical activity and growth. In Ritźen M, Aperia A, Hall K, Larsson A, Zetterberg A and Zetterström R (eds): "The Biology of Normal Human Growth," New York: Raven Press.

79. Viteri FE, Torún B, Galicia JC and Herrera E (1971). Determining energy costs of agricultural activities by respirometer and energy balance techniques. Am J Clin Nutr 24:1418-1430.

80. Wade MG and Ellis MJ (1971). Measurement of free-range activity in children as modified by social and environmental complexity. Am J Clin Nutr 24:1457-1460.

81. Weir JB de V (1949). New methods for calculating metabolic rate with specific reference to protein metabolism. J Physiol 109:1-9.

82. Wolf HS (1959). Modern techniques for time and motion study in physiological research. Ergonomics 2:354-362.

Energy Intake and Activity, pages 185–203
© 1984 Alan R. Liss, Inc., 150 Fifth Avenue, New York, NY 10011

MEASUREMENT OF OPEN-FIELD ACTIVITY IN YOUNG
CHILDREN: A CRITICAL ANALYSIS

Charles F. Halverson, Jr.
Joan C. Post-Gorden

Department of Child and Family Development,
University of Georgia, Athens, Georgia   30602,
and Department of Psychology, University of
Southern Colorado, Pueblo, Colorado   81001.

INTRODUCTION

The study of activity level has long been of interest to
developmental researchers.   Childrens' motor activity has
probably been one of the more frequently studied constructs
in the area of personality and social development.   Some of
the early studies of children's social and personality development included thorough and extensive analyses of
open-field activity (Fales 1938; Goodenough 1930).   In later
years theorists focused on the importance for personality
development of individual differences in activity level
(Escalona 1968; Fries 1944; Shaffer 1966).   Recently the
concept of activity level has been incorporated as a fundamental individual difference dimension in the burgeoning
research area of infant and childhood temperament (Buss and
Plomin 1975; Goldsmith and Gottesman 1981; Routh et al.
1974).   Finally, it is the central construct in the area of
childhood hyperactivity (Barkley and Cunningham 1979; Klein
and Gittelman-Klein 1975).

Many investigators, however, have become either disillusioned or suspicious about the use of activity level because
of the limitations of measurement and its apparent instability
over time.   Campbell and Fiske (1959) stated that a meaningful construct should be shown to be more than the measure
of it.   It is necessary to collect data across methods, situations, behaviors and, hopefully, across time before it is
possible to assess whether activity level in open field

settings is a robust variable that can function in a predictive way. Little data is available on the convergent validity of activity measures and most of it is fairly disappointing.

For example, Rapoport and Benoit (1975) used multiple activity level measures to study 20 boys, 6 to 12 years of age, in both home and laboratory settings. They found only modest convergence; significant correlations ranged from .46 for observations of activity level and a parental diary, to .59 for a global rating of free play behavior and the parental diary. The data tend to show that there is limited generality, and that different ways of measuring the same construct are not necessarily comparable simply because the categories have the same names. The parental diary, however, proved to be a relatively good source of activity data. Parents kept an objective, low inference record of the number of activities the child engaged in over time. In a very similar study Rapoport et al. (1971) found that intercorrelations for grid crossings, pedometers, and global activity ratings by observers were about .50 for 19 boys. The data were based on 20 minute observations for 5 days conducted over an eleven-week period.

Barkley and Ullman (1975) also present extensive data on the comparability of measures of activity level. Based on 15 minutes of free play, 32 boys were assessed for differences in activity level. The subjects wore wrist and ankle actometers and wrist and ankle pedometers adjacent to one another (the authors do not indicate what effects wearing the numerous devices may have had on the criterion measures). The boys also were coded for quadrant changes and toy changes, and the parents filled out the Werry-Weiss-Peters Home Activity Rating Scale (HARS). The data show modest convergence for actometers and quadrant changes (r's = .44 and .67) but little for toy changes or wrist pedometers (no r's were significant--presumably a sensitivity problem). More importantly, there was no convergence with the HARS. None of the categories shared any variance with activity level as rated at home. In a similar vein Routh et al. (1974) found no convergence between the HARS, a factored version of the HARS, the number of toy changes in a play session, or the number of quadrant entries.

Grunewald-Zuberbier et al. (1972), in a telemetric study of activity level in 21 high and low-activity

12-year-old boys, found within setting convergence between both telemetered body movement and a time sampled observation of the same movement (r = .89), and global ratings of activity level with telemetered activity (r's ranging from .44 to .45). The boys were observed in two sessions totaling approximately 16 minutes.

Willoughby (unpublished manuscript, no date) studied 40 children aged 4 to 7 for 2 one-hour periods, using free play codes and the HARS, and found no convergence among play measures and no convergence with the HARS. Eaton and Keats (1982) compared actometers and teacher rankings based on solitary play and play in triads. Teacher actometer correlations for 69 children were: alone, r = .33, in triads, r = .32. Similarly, for 11 children Loo and Wenar (1971) found no correlation between an in-class actometer worn from ½ to 2 hours and teacher ratings of activity level (r = .12). McConnell et al. (1964) showed no relationship between a 10-item activity checklist for young children and a mechanical measure of activity (r = .20). Walker (1967), using a 16-item energy scale checklist, found reasonable internal consistencies(.61) and modest test-retest correlations over one year (boys = .58, girls = .44), but found little convergence between data sources using the same instrument, e.g., peer-teacher, r =.48; peer-self, r = .29; teacher-self, r = .16.

Data such as those summarized above have disillusioned many researchers. Sandoval (1977) writes, "Because of the possibility of instrument unreliability, the expense of the equipment, the obtrusive nature of some of the instruments, and problems of controlling the context of measurement in a field study, direct measures of physical activity are less attractive than the other diagnostic instruments" (p. 307). Maccoby and Jacklin, in their influential review of sex differences, write,

> We have repeatedly encountered the problem that so-called 'objective' measures of behavior yield different results than ratings.... Ratings are notoriously subject to shifting anchor points... in one study teachers rated each child in their class on activity level; the boys received higher average ratings; but 'actometer' recordings for the same groups of children did not show boys to be engaging in more body movement. Obviously, the

possibility exists that teachers are noticing and remembering primarily behavior that fits their stereotypes. There is another possibility, however, that teachers are analyzing clusters or patterns of behavior that simple single attribute measurement such as the actometer score does not capture (1974, p. 356).

In fact, the variability in the results of activity level studies led Maccoby to conclude that there may be no general sex difference in activity level; that activity level seems to depend on aspects of the situation in which the measurements are taken.

Maccoby and Jacklin (1974) cited Loo and Wenar's 1971 study as an example of the lack of convergence among measures. In the cited study, teacher global ratings were compared to actometers. The ratings of activity level were based on months of observing and comparing the children in a number of situations. The "objective" measure was an actometer worn in class one time for about 1½ hours. No data are available on stability or on whether the time sampled was typical of larger samples. Yet Maccoby and Jacklin (1974) believe it reasonable to rely on the objective measure.

Brooks and Lewis (1973, 1974) measured activity level in twins for 15 minutes of play. The activity of the 13 month old subjects was measured by the number of grids traversed. As usual, interrater reliabilities are excellent because the measurements require only counting. No data is provided, however, on whether this sample of activity level demonstrates stability. On the basis of this very short sample of behavior, Brooks and Lewis (1973) make a number of rather startling generalizations.

We found no activity level differences between the boy and girl twins. Rheingold and Eckerman (1969) and Goldberg and Lewis (1969) also find no sex differences in activity level. In a working class sample Messer and Lewis (1972) found that girl infants tended to be more active in terms of number of squares traversed than did boys; mobility, however, was not related to proximal attachment. It seems that boys do not exhibit more activity than do girls. Therefore, the girls' tendency to seek proximity to their mothers cannot be attributed to a low activity level. That is, girls do not spend more time near their mothers than do boys because they move about the room less. Reviews of sex differences often state that there are innate activity differences, despite the fact that there is little evidence to substantiate this hypothesis (Maccoby and Jacklin 1973). For example, Bell, Weller and Waldrop (1971) found no activity level differences in neonates when birth trauma is controlled and, in a longitudinal study, report that two-and-a-half-year-old boys and girls do not differ in restless movement or high vigor behavior. In addition, activity level does not seem to be a stable characteristic, and it has been found to vary across repeated measures (Brooks and Lewis, 1973; p. 9, emphasis added).

There is yet another possibility from those outlined by Maccoby and Jacklin (1974). If measurements of activity level have been poorly collected and poorly analyzed, for the most part, then we are plagued with measures that are generally unreliable and situation bound. Reviewing the literature allows us to illustrate the utility of data aggregation and the problem of reliability of individual difference measures.

DATA AGGREGATION

It will be helpful, in defining data aggregation, to review some recent work by Seymour Epstein (1979, 1980) on the stability of behavior. Epstein concurs with many others that a crisis in behavioral research is approaching because findings resist empirical generalization. He cites Mischel (1968) as one of the leading proponents of the antitraits position:

he observed that when objectively measured behavior in one situation is correlated with objectively measured behavior in another situation or with scores on a personality inventory, the correlations are almost invariably below .30. This led him to dub such correlations 'personality coefficients' and to conclude that "with the possible exception of intelligence, highly generalized behavioral consistencies have not been demonstrated, and the

concept of personality traits as broad predisposi-
tions is thus untenable" (Epstein, 1980,
pp. 790-791) (Mischel 1968, p. 146).

Epstein entertains the idea that, instead of critiquing
trait theory, Mischel could have examined measurement
strategies. He also suggests that the failure of objective
data to intercorrelate and to relate to more global measures
often may be the result of inadequate event sampling and
consequent "measurement noise." He states,

> In most cases the objective data consisted of single
> behavioral observations, usually obtained in the
> laboratory. Single items of behavior, <u>no matter</u>
> <u>how</u> <u>objectively</u> <u>measured</u>, can be expected, like
> single items on a test, to be low in reliability and
> lack generality and therefore be inadequate to the
> task of demonstrating stability in behavior and of
> measuring personality traits.... Stability can be
> demonstrated over a wide range of variables <u>so</u>
> <u>long</u> <u>as</u> <u>the behavior</u> <u>in</u> <u>question</u> <u>is</u> <u>averaged</u> <u>over</u>
> <u>a</u> <u>sufficient</u> <u>number</u> <u>of</u> <u>occurrences</u>.... Reliable
> relationships can be demonstrated... so long as
> the objective behavior is sampled over an appro-
> priate level of generality and averaged over a
> sufficient number of occurrences" (1980, p. 791,
> emphasis in original).

The studies reviewed here are striking confirmation of
one aspect of Epstein's thesis: most of the studies that
used low inference measures of activity level collected data
on only one or two occasions, and then proceeded to draw
far-reaching conclusions about activity level as a personality
variable in young children. In fact, there is really no basis
on which to evaluate the strong conclusions. None of the
studies cited by Brooks and Lewis (1973, 1974) aggregated
data. Rheingold and Eckerman (1969) used one-time grid
crossings, as did Goldberg and Lewis (1969), and Messer
and Lewis (1972). Bell, Weller and Waldrop (1971) did
aggregate data on actometers, and did find a sex difference
(reported in Pederson and Bell 1970), but the data cited
were global ratings. The conclusions may not be war-
ranted because the data is potentially very unreliable.

Maccoby <u>et</u> <u>al</u>. (1965) also used actometers on a single
occasion for 2 hours and found low reliabilities. One

occasion may not be sufficient. Other examples of one-time observations abound in the literature, e.g., Schwarz (1972) used grid crossings during a 5-minute observation session; Maccoby and Feldman (1972) brief episodes (e.g., 3 minutes) of grid crossings on one occasion; Maccoby and Jacklin (1973) 9 minutes of grid crossings on one occasion; Routh et al. (1974; 1978) grid crossings for 15 minutes, once or twice; Schwarz and Wynn (1971) footsteps in three 2-minute samples; Zern and Taylor (1973) a 5 minute observation setting, etc., etc. This list could be extended, but the point is made: most of the data which purport to measure a generalized temperamental trait were measured only on one or two brief occasions and usually within one setting.

Most of the above studies are the legacy of experimental research with its implicit values of control and the explora- tion of efficient causes. When open-field activity level has been assessed, it has been done most often in the very restricted paradigm of the psychological experiment. Anoth- er legacy of the psychological experiment is that data are not usually replicated or collected over a number of occa- sions (aggregated). Epstein (1980) suggests several reasons why most behavioral scientists have accepted such a ques- tionable paradigm. Some are mundane, such as journals tending to reject replications, or the short-term experiment fitting conveniently into professors' and students' schedules. Other reasons, however, are more important. Epstein be- lieves that most researchers fail to distinguish between concurrent and temporal reliability: many investigators think that it is enough to establish satisfactory interrater reliabil- ity and to obtain a statistically significant effect...

> After all, a statistically significant finding at the .01 level indicates that if the experiment were identically reproduced a hundred times, in no more than one case would a difference as large as that obtained be expected by chance. A critical as- sumption here is that the experiment would have to be reproduced identically in all its minor relevant details, including subtle contextual ones. The .01 reliability estimate would not hold if all factors that could affect the outcome were not held con- stant... the reliability estimate refers to a theoret- ical condition that connot be met with respect to actual replication... (Epstein 1980, pp. 796-797).

Temporal reliability, however, is more akin to predictive validity as used in tests and measurement theory. A test can show good concurrent validity (same-day correlations, interrater reliability), but poor predictive validity (correlations over time). Most studies of activity level reviewed here have failed to take into account the idea of temporal stability even while making generalizations which imply that such stability had been demonstrated by short, one-shot assessments. For the most part, behavioral scientists simply do not have the data on activity level to decide many of the issues relating to sex differences, age differences, relations to social interaction with caregivers and peers, etc.

In the opinion of the authors, then, the basic issue in the measurement of activity level is cross-occasion stability. A priority must be to establish whether activity level differences have such cross-occasion stability and then, if such stability exists, the relationships of such a variable should be investigated. The authors do not wish to deny that situations may have dramatic effects on activity level or that such effects are unimportant. In fact, as Epstein so aptly put it:

> The conclusion that there are relatively broad, stable response dispositions, or traits, does not conflict with the assumption that situations often exert a strong influence on behavior. By the same token, demonstrations that behavior varies with situations cannot be taken as evidence against traits. The fact that people read in a library and swim in a swimming pool does not establish that there is no generality, or cross-situational stability, in either swimming or in reading behavior. More to the point is that some people are more prone to swim than others when there is a reasonable opportunity to do so, and this may include swimming in pools, in lakes, and in oceans. Further, one cannot test such a cross-situational proclivity to swim by observing a person once in the vicinity of a lake, as there may be many reasons for that person to forego swimming on that particular occasion. Behavior is obviously determined by more than response dispositions. Given an adequate sample of occasions, however, response dispositions will out (1975, pp. 1122-1123).

The authors believe that Epsteins' position has merit and have reviewed the literature both to identify studies which do aggregate activity level over occasions, and to determine whether aggregation improves the quality of the data as Epstein predicts. A brief review follows of the studies in which data were aggregated, either through global ratings of multiple data sources or through repeated observations. Subsequently, the viability of the position will be demonstrated on the basis of the data the authors have collected.

STUDIES OF ACTIVITY WITH AGGREGATE DATA

One of the early studies (Fales 1938) of the vigorousness of play activities in preschool children aggregated data. Fales made 2 forty-minute observations on two different days and reported that activity showed low short-term stability (r for boys = .38, for girls = .15), a typical finding for data collected on only one or two occasions. Fales went on, however, to make Epstein's point some 40 years before his position was stated. She took the 80 minutes of observations done on one day and divided it into 16 5-minute intervals, compared odd scores with even scores, and discovered that the stability was impressive: r = .79 for boys, .87 for girls and .85 for the total sample. She commented that data within the session were stable even if between session data showed almost no stability. Unfortunately, she did not extrapolate to multiple days and the issue ended there.

Bell, Weller and Waldrop (1971) used actometers in an outdoor setting and composited data collected on six days spread over five weeks. They report an odd vs. even-day stability of .68, and in another publication (Pederson and Bell 1970) report significant sex differences on this measure based on the same sample. Halverson and Waldrop (1973), in a sample of 58 preschool children, collected actometer data on 6 days of outdoor play over a period of 5 weeks. For this sample the odd-day vs. even-day stability correlations for males were r = .81, and for females, r = .92. When aggregated the actometers showed excellent stability. Furthermore, when aggregated activity scores were compared with independent observer scores, that were also aggregated over days (6 days, odd vs. even stabilities averaged .82), the correlations of activity recorders with a count of "runs" was .80 and .82 for boys and girls respectively. Objective data on activity level were also compared to teacher ratings of the same children. Of 27 daily ratings, 25 were significantly related to mechanically recorded activity level for boys; for girls the figure was 21 of 27. The average correlations were .51 for boys and .44 for girls. Examples were: vigor in play .72, seeking help -.53, excitability, .55. Finally, these aggregated activity scores showed substantial sex differences with boys being much more active than girls. In fact, 31% of the variance in activity level was accounted for by gender. (Contrast these findings to most of those reviewed in the 1974 Maccoby and Jacklin volume). In addition, reasonably good stability was found for these measures over 5 years; early activity level was related to vigor and excitability and later activity level (r's from .31 to .57) (Halverson and Waldrop 1976).

Similarly, in the Block's longitudinal study (Block 1976; Buss et al. 1980) aggregated data were collected on 129 children, 65 boys and 64 girls. Two hours a day of wrist activity was measured and the 3 data collection days for 3 year olds, and 4 days for 4 year olds were separated by a period of one week. The composite activity data were then compared to the 100 items on the California Child Q set (CCQ) done by 3 teachers at age 3, 9 new teachers at age 4, and 67 teachers at age 7 years. The aggregated actometers showed reliabilities of .86 and .62 for ages 3 and 4 respectively. Teacher rated activity and actometers correlated .61 and .50 for boys and girls respectively at age 3 years. Most impressive, however, was the finding that activity level (when aggregated) makes a considerable contribution to teacher-rated personality variables. As Buss et al. (1980) stated "... these core correlations... provide striking evidence for the independent construct validity of the actometer... preschool-identified active children try to stretch the limits, try to take advantage of others, try to be the center of attention, like to compete, are self-assertive, and are not obedient, shy or reserved" (1980, pp. 405-406). The authors contend that it would have been impossible to obtain these data with short samples of behavior, not because activity level is inherently unstable, as many have implied, but because of the unreliability of measurement.

Other studies using aggregated activity recorder data provide evidence for the validity of activity level: Victor et al. (1973) had 6-day composite actometer scores correlated

.77 with a hyperactivity rating and found that reliable actometers also distinguish between hyperactive and normal boys in a free play setting. In a similar study, Victor and Halverson (1975) found that actometers related to behavior problem-checklist data for both boys and girls when the activity data were composited over 5 days of in-class activity.

Eaton (1983) provides even further validity data for aggregated activity level in his one facet generalizability study of 27 children (13 males and 14 females) with mean age of 50 months. Children wore wrist actometers between 13 and 14 days in a free play setting during the one month period in which data were collected. In addition, Eaton's staff made global ratings of activity, and the parents made ratings on the Colorado Childhood Temperament Inventory (CCTI).

As Epstein (1979, 1980) would predict, Eaton's actometer data showed increases in reliability as the number of actometers (days) increased. Reliability for one day of activity recording was low (.33), but rose to nearly .90 with 14 days of recorded activity. Clearly the one or two days of recording which is typical of most studies provides unreliable data. In addition, when Eaton compared his aggregated actometer scores with staff ratings (.69) and the parental CCTI (.75) he found excellent convergent validity for the three measures. These correlations are further confirmation that activity level can be measured very reliably if the investigator aggregates data over a sufficient number of occasions. When this is done, parent and staff ratings indicate that there is strong cross-method and cross-setting generality of activity level.

Data collected by the authors will illustrate some of the issues concerned with measuring activity (Halverson CF Jr, 1983, manuscript in preparation). As part of a larger longitudinal study of development, data was collected on 132 children (65 boys, 67 girls). Ages ranged from 30 to 42 months and children were from predominantly white middle class homes. Over a four week period activity level was measured daily in a variety of open field settings. For the first several days actometers were worn in a free play setting, first in solitary free play and then with one or two same-or-other-sex peers. During the subsequent 3 weeks, activity level was assessed in mixed-sex groups of 5

children, in free-play indoors, a "rough and tumble" session, and a free-play setting outdoors. Actometers which
measured activity level in two dimensions were sewn in
pockets on the backs of shirts the children wore. Each
child wore a different actometer in each setting each day
(132 children X 3 daily settings X 20 days = 7920 observations). In addition, their activity level was coded independently on a daily basis by 2 independent observers in each
setting. Daily ratings were also done on each child by 2
teachers.

This paper will explore aspects of the data on activity
level in order to highlight certain issues. The first concerns the relationship between increases in reliability and
the number of actometers worn. The actometer measure of
activity level in the freeplay indoor setting for 40 of the
children shows the negatively accelerated pattern of reliabilities found in many aggregations studies (Epstein 1979;
1980). Reliability for one day of actometers was .18 but
rose to .96 for 10 days of aggregated data[1]. Similar patterns held for other settings and between genders. The
message is clear: it is likely that studies based on short
samples of behavior have been dealing with very unreliable
data on activity level. If actometer data is considered, both
Eaton's work (1983) and the authors' work indicate that
reliable data require at least 6-7 observations to achieve
reasonable stability. This point can be made another way.
Recall that both daily ratings and observations of activities
were obtained for these same children. The correlation
between the rating of activity level by the teachers
(inter-rater r = .88) for 1 day of activity level and that
day's actometer scores was r = .17. When actometer data
was aggregated over an increasing number of days the r
rose to .46 for 6 days of activity, to .67 for 10 days, and
to .88 for 20 days.

Teacher daily rating data can also be assessed for
reliability increases associated with aggregation. The increases for ratings of activity level are modest, however,

---

[1]The larger sample has been divided into 3 replication
samples for analysis to be reported elsewhere. Unless
noted, the data from only one of the samples is used for the
analyses reported here. Minor variations across samples do
not compromise the conclusions noted.

because reliability for this sample was high on day 1 (e.g., one day = .86, two days = .89, 4 days = .92). Teachers apparently "mentally aggregate" data in a fairly efficient manner. The lack of correlation between "objective" actometers and "subjective" rating data based on small samples (Maccoby and Jacklin 1974) may be more closely related to the unreliability of the "objective measure" than to the rating.

Similar results were found on a daily variable of "runs" coded by observers: 1-day correlations of "runs" and corresponding actometer data tended to be in the low 20's (range .15 to .44 for 10 individual-day correlations) but rose to .77 ($\underline{n}$ = 132) for data composited across days for both actometers and observation code (which also increased in stability as data were aggregated). Again, the message is clear. Had the study been based on 1 or 2 days of observations and rating, it would have been logical to con-clude that there was little convergence among activity level measures and, therefore, little reason to pursue the con-struct further. Or the result may have been to puzzle over the lack of replications of earlier studies. If the data were considered as 20 studies of 132 children the correlations, mean levels, etc. would demonstrate that the data vary considerably. This is confirmed in the literature, and is the result of failing to aggregate data over occasions long enough to achieve stability.

A second issue is cross-setting stability. These data can be examined correlationally and/or by mean level differ-ences by setting. When correlations are calculated between the aggregated scores for each setting (4-week totals), activity level is fairly predictable in across setting: Free play vs. Rest $\underline{r}$ (130) = .50; Free Play vs. Outside, $\underline{r}$ (130) = .54 and Rest vs. Outside $\underline{r}$ (130) = .69.

An examination of the mean levels reveals situation effects as well. Children were much more active in the "rest" period and outdoors than they were in free play. These setting effects are highly significant (repeated mea-sures ANOVA, $\underline{F}$'s all < .001), but a comment about the settings may clarify the differences. The free play room was large and furnished with many toys; consequently activity level was attenuated. The "rest" room had only 5 children, 2 teachers, and some pillows, and "rest" time was a misnomer. Without toys children, especially boys, turned to high levels of peer interaction and rough and tumble play. Outdoor play took place in a large, grassy area furnished with swings, wagons, tricycles and other gross-motor toys. Activity level was also high in this setting. Consequently, even though children tended to be moderately stable in their rank orders across settings, the actual amount of activity differed greatly. Another consistency was maintained throughout: in every setting where actometer data was gathered girls were significantly less active than boys, even in solitary play and when playing with one or two peers (Halverson, in preparation).

The issue of cross-setting generality is at the heart of Epstein's (1979; 1980) argument about personality traits. Using actometers, data can be collected and aggregated over occasions within a setting (i.e. free play) and the same can be done for another setting (i.e. outdoor play) if we wish to assess the amount of situational variance present. Depending on research needs, data could be aggregated over occasions and settings to get a stable estimate of activity averaged across many different settings. Using the actometer, or a similar low inference observational technique, allows us to assess setting variance directly. In fact, there may be a subtle irony here. If children wore the actometers across settings where high and low activity typically occurred, and if the children spent comparable times together in each setting, the between subject variance would tend to reflect setting differences rather than individual differences. For example, Plomin and Foch (1980) had twins wear actometers each day, all day, for a week. When they examined the intra-class correlations for both MZ and DZ pairs, they found the rs to be .99 and .94 respectively. If the twins went through the day's activities together the measure was, ironically, one of situation more than trait. In this special case, the concern is with yolking of activity scores - and the unit is then the pair. Preliminary investigation has been done on the authors' actometer data and some modest yolking of actometer scores was found for a subsample of 25 children. (intra-class r = .40), but the bias for larger groups of children does not appear to be serious. In situations where all subjects perform the same activities the result may be literally a group score. These problems, by and large, are assessed by aggregating data over many occasions and situations and checking the relationships.

One other issue bears mentioning. What is lacking in the literature is come concept of norms of activity for different ages. This is perfectly understandable given the welter of methods and situations of questionable reliability that have been used in the past. No generalizable or generalized activity score has been available to assess issues of over-or under-activity, certainly an important diagnostic issue. If aggregate data were available, however, it would be possible to begin to assess activity level by age. Norms would aid tremendously in diagnosing activity disturbance in children and these norms are most valuable when constructed with data aggregated across setting and time.

CONCLUSIONS AND IMPLICATIONS

Where does this leave the investigator with regard to assessing open-field activity level? While not simple, the answer may not be as complex as many had previously thought. When the authors began to survey the extant literature on open-field activity level in children, they were convinced that, for research purposes, low-inference observations, actometers, grid crossings, etc. were, almost exclusively, the way to arrive at useful descriptors. While they still believe this to be true, they also feel that "global ratings," parent ratings, and clinician ratings may have been unduly maligned. For many applications, well-constructed and well-applied ratings of motor activity do a remarkably good job of distinguishing different levels of activity. In those studies where data have been aggregated over occasions, the convergence among both low and high inference measures is quite high. It must be remembered that the goal in measurement is first to achieve concurrent and predictive validity of measures of activity, and then to relate these stable, reliable measures of open-field activity to other measures of interest. Understanding of the role of activity differences in children will be enhanced when our measures are perfected as much as possible. The authors believe that activity level differences are extremely important in the social development of young children, and that these differences and their impact on peers and caregivers has been under-estimated because of the measurement problems inherent in much of the research.

ACKNOWLEDGMENTS

The preparation of this chapter was supported by funds from the College of Home Economics, University of Georgia.

REFERENCES

1. Barkley RA and Cunningham CE (1979). The effects of methyphenidate on the mother-child interactions of hyperactive children. Arch Gen Psychiatry 36:201-208.
2. Barkley RA and Ullman DG (1975). A comparison of objective measures of activity and distractibility in hyperactive and nonhyperactive children. J Abnorm Child Psychol 3:231-244.
3. Bell RQ, Weller GM and Waldrop MF (1971). Newborn and preschooler: Organization of behavior and relations between periods. Monogr Soc Res Child Dev 36:1-145.
4. Block J (1976). Issues, problems, and pitfalls in assessing sex differences: A critical review of the psychology of sex differences. Merrill-Palmer Q 22:283-308.
5. Brooks J and Lewis M (1973). Attachment behavior in thirteen-month-old, opposite sex twins. Paper presented Soc Res Child Dev, Philadelphia.
6. Brooks J and Lewis M (1974). Attachment behavior in thirteen-month-old opposite sex twins. Child Dev 45:243-247.
7. Buss AH and Plomin R (1975). "A Temperament Theory of Personality Development." New York: John Wiley.
8. Buss DM, Block JH and Block J (1980). Preschool activity level: Personality correlates and developmental implications. Child Dev 51:401-408.
9. Campbell DT and Fiske DW (1959). Convergent and discriminant validation by the multitrait multimethod matrix. Psychol Bull 56:81-105.
10. Eaton WO (1983). Measuring activity level with actometers: reliability, validity, and arm length. Child Dev 54:720-726.
11. Eaton WO and Keats JG (1982). Peer presence, stress, and sex differences in the motor activity levels of preschoolers. Dev Psychol 198:534-540.
12. Epstein S (1979). The stability of behavior: I. On predicting most of the people much of the time. J Pers Soc Psychol 37:1097-1126.

13. Epstein S (1980). The stability of behavior. II. Implications for psychological research. Am Psychol 35:790-806.
14. Escalona SK (1968). "The Roots of Individuality: Normal Patterns of Development in Infancy." Chicago: Aldine.
15. Fales E (1938). A rating scale of the vigorousness of play activities of preschool children. Child Dev 8:15-46.
16. Fries ME (1944). Psychosomatic relations between mother and infant. Psychosom Med 6:159-162.
17. Goldberg S and Lewis M (1969). Play behavior in the year-old infant: Early sex differences. Child Dev 40:21-31.
18. Goldsmith HH and Gottesman I. (1981). Origins of variation in behavioral style: A longitudinal study of temperament in young twins. Child Dev 52:91-103.
19. Goodenough FL (1930). Inter-relationships in the behavior of young children. Child Dev 1:29-47.
20. Gruenwald-Zuberbier E, Grunewald G and Rashe A (1972). Telemetric measurement of motor activity in maladjusted children under different experimental conditions. Psychiat Neurol Neurochir 75:371-378.
21. Halverson CF Jr and Waldrop MF (1973). The relations of mechanically recorded activity level to varieties of preschool play behavior. Child Dev 44:678-681.
22. Halverson CF Jr and Waldrop MF (1976). Relations between preschool activity and aspects of intellectual and social behavior at age 7½. J Dev Psychol 12:107-112.
23. Klein DF and Gittelman-Klein R (1975). Problems in the diagnosis of minimal brain dysfunction and the hyperkinetic syndrome. Int J Ment Health 4:45-60.
24. Loo C and Wenar C (1971). Activity level and motor inhibition: Their relationship to intelligence-test performance in normal children. Child Dev 42:967-971.
25. Maccoby EE, Dowley EM, Hagen JW, and Degern R (1965). Activity level and intellectual functioning in normal preschool children. Child Dev 36:761-770.
26. Maccoby EE and Feldman SS (1972). Mother attachment and stranger-reactions in the third year of life. Monogr Soc Res Child Dev 37:1-85.
27. Maccoby EE and Jacklin CN (1973). Stress, activity, and proximity seeking: Sex differences in the year-old child. Child Dev 44:34-42.

28. Maccoby EE and Jacklin CN (1974). "The Psychology of Sex Differences." Stanford University Press, California.

29. McConnell TR, Cromwell R, Biale I and Son C (1964). Studies in activity level: VII. Effects of amphetamine drug administration on the activity level. Am J Ment Defic 68:647-651.

30. Messer SB and Lewis M (1972). Social class and sex differences in the attachment and play behavior of the one-year-old infant. Merrill Palmer Q 18:295-306.

31. Mischel W (1968). "Personality and Assessment." New York: John Wiley.

32. Pederson FA and Bell RQ (1970). Sex differences in preschool children without histories of complications of pregnancy and delivery. Dev Psychol 3:10-15.

33. Plomin R and Foch TT (1980). A twin study of objectively assessed personality in childhood. J Pers Soc Psychol 39:680-688.

34. Rapoport JL, Abramson A, Alexander D and Lott J (1971). Play-room observations of hyperactive children on medication. J Child Psychiatry 10:524-534.

35. Rapoport JL and Benoit M (1975). The relation of direct home observations to the clinic evaluations of hyperactive school age boys. J Child Psychol Psychiatry 17:141-147.

36. Rheingold HL and Eckerman CO (1969). The infant's free entry into a new environment. J Exp Child Psychol 8:271-283.

37. Routh D, Schroeder C and O'Tuama L (1974). Development of activity level in children. Dev Psychol 10:163-168.

38. Routh DK, Walton MD and Padan-Belkin E (1978): Development of activity level in children revisited. Effects of mother presence. Dev Psychol 14:571-581.

39. Sandoval J (1977). The measurement of the hyperactive syndrome in children. Rev Educ Res 47:293-318.

40. Schaffer HR (1966). Activity level as a constitutional determinant of infantile reaction to deprivation. Child Dev 37:595-602.

41. Schwarz JC (1972). Effects of peer familiarity on the behavior of preschoolers in a novel situation. J Pers Soc Psychol 24:276-284.

42. Schwarz JC and Wynn R (1971). The effects of mothers' presence and previsits on children's emotional reactions to starting nursery school. Child Dev 42:871-881.

43. Victor JB and Halverson CF Jr (1975). Distractibility and hypersensitivity: Two behavior factors in elementary school children. J Abnorm Child Psychol 3:83-94.
44. Victor JB, Halverson CF Jr, Inoff G and Buczkowski HJ (1973). Objective behavior measures of first and second grade boys' free play and teachers' ratings on a behavior problem checklist. Psychol Schools 10:439-443.
45. Walker RN (1967). Some temperament traits in children as reviewed by their peers, their teachers, and themselves. Monogr Soc Res Child Dev 32:6,1-36.
46. Zern D and Taylor AL (1973). Rhythmic behavior in the hierarchy of responses of preschool children. Merrill-Palmer Q 19:137-145.

FIELD STUDIES–ACTIVITY, PRODUCTIVITY, METABOLISM

Energy Intake and Activity, pages 207–261
© 1984 Alan R. Liss, Inc., 150 Fifth Avenue, New York, NY 10011

PHYSICAL ACTIVITY, NUTRITIONAL STATUS, AND
PHYSICAL WORK CAPACITY IN RELATION TO
AGRICULTURAL PRODUCTIVITY

G.B. SPURR

Department of Physiology
Medical College of Wisconsin
Milwaukee, Wisconsin 53226

The condition of exercise is not a mere variant of
the condition of rest. It is the essence of the
machine.
J. Barcroft

INTRODUCTION

In the developing countries of the world, where mechanization of industry, including agriculture, is at a minimum, it is human labor which provides much of the power
to fuel economic productivity (Smil 1979). From data published by the United Nations (1980) it is possible to estimate that in Africa (6 countries) 38% of the economically
active males are engaged in work classified as agriculture,
hunting, forestry, and fishing. In Latin America (8 countries) the figure is 47%, but in the U.S. and Canada combined, the proportion is only 6%. While figures are not
readily available, it is likely that the larger portion of
these groups is engaged in some type of farming as their
principal activity. The energy costs of agricultural activities have been reported by a number of investigators
(Durnin and Passmore 1967; Phillips 1954; Ramana Murthy
and Belavady 1966; Viteri et al. 1971) and, in general,
levels of energy expenditure range from moderate to heavy
physical work. Unmechanized farming is one of the more
labor intensive occupations and has mean values just under
those for coal mining and forestry (Durnin and Passmore
1967). The value of 3550 Cal·24 Hr^{-1} reported by Durnin
and Passmore (1967) is very similar to the 3694 Cal·24 Hr^{-1}
which Viteri et al. (1975, 1971) found for Guatemalan

agricultural workers. It is also similar to the crude estimate of energy expenditure of 3426 Cal·24 Hr-¹ in Colombian sugar cane cutters (Spurr et al. 1975), although the
latter value may be too low. Brun et al. (1979) have
reported daily energy expenditures of 3400 Cal·24 Hr-¹ for
Iranian agricultural workers during seasons of high
activity.

In the discussion which follows, agricultural productivity refers to man's ability to accomplish successfully
those physical labors usually associated with farming, and
not to the economic productivity resulting from the operation of mechanized and highly technical agriculture involved
in food production in the developed countries of the world.
In this sense, agricultural productivity is similar to the
productivity of any human endeavor which requires moderate to heavy physical work.

In discussing physical work in developing countries
there are two separate problems which must be considered
(Arteaga 1976). First is the malnutrition which occurs
during the period of growth and leads to the small adult
stature characteristic of populations from developing countries (Habicht et al. 1974; Martorell et al. 1978; Spurr et
al. 1978). Figure 1 presents the average adult heights of

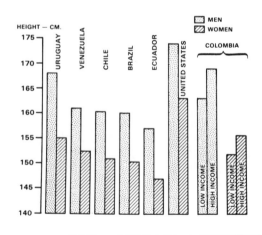

FIGURE 1: Average heights of adult men and women
from several Latin-American countries and the United
States. (Spurr et al. 1978)

men and women in Latin America (ICNND 1963a) and in the United States (Stuart et al. 1964). In all of the Latin American countries represented in Figure 1 adult heights for both men and women are considerably below those for the U.S. population.

The second problem which needs to be addressed is the nutritional deficiencies in the diet of the adult population. Arteaga (1976) analyzed the average daily caloric intake of 5 Latin American countries during the years 1960-1970 in relation to the percentage of the population engaged in heavy, moderate, and light activities, and the occurrence of undernutrition and obesity (Figure 2). It is evident that the populations with the lowest caloric intake and the highest incidence of undernutrition are precisely those engaged in the hardest work. On the other hand, as would be expected, the more sedentary populations, with the highest available calories in the diet, have the highest incidence of obesity.

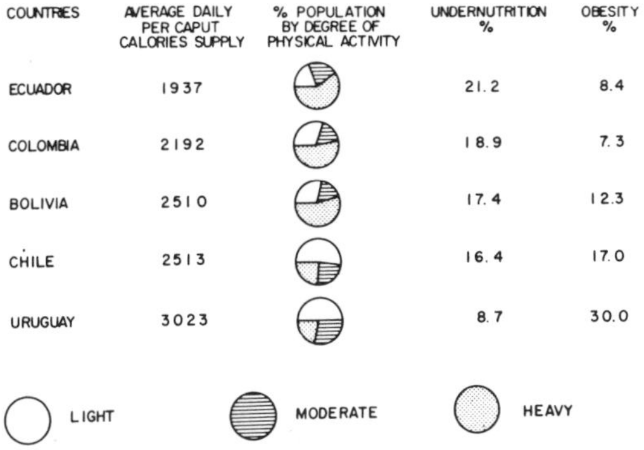

COUNTRIES	AVERAGE DAILY PER CAPUT CALORIES SUPPLY	% POPULATION BY DEGREE OF PHYSICAL ACTIVITY	UNDERNUTRITION %	OBESITY %
ECUADOR	1937		21.2	8.4
COLOMBIA	2192		18.9	7.3
BOLIVIA	2510		17.4	12.3
CHILE	2513		16.4	17.0
URUGUAY	3023		8.7	30.0

◯ LIGHT   ⬤ MODERATE   ◯ HEAVY

FIGURE 2: Average daily per capita calorie supply, degree of physical activity, and obesity in five Latin American countries, 1960-70. (Arteaga 1976).

Figure 3 is a somewhat simplistic diagram of the inter-relations which exist among physical activity, nutritional status, physical work capacity, and productivity, and is an attempt to organize the present discussion into four major sections. Productivity in the present context refers to that

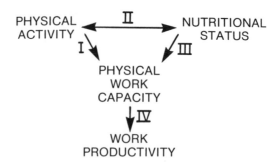

FIGURE 3: Relations among physical activity, nutritional status, physical work capacity and productivity.

which is accomplished by moderate to heavy physical work, in contrast to sedentary occupations where the intellectual component may be of greater importance. In addition to the biologic component, work, and therefore productivity, involves psychological (motivational), type of work, and work setting components (Viteri et al. 1981).

The present discussion will deal with only the biologic component. It is clear from Figure 3 that, with the exception of possible direct effects of nutritional intake, the final common pathway of the biologic component is the physical work capacity (PWC) as measured by the maximum oxygen consumption ($\dot{V}O_2$ max), or as estimated by a variety of sub-maximal work tests (Astrand and Rodahl 1977; Shephard 1978). Physical work capacity may be affected, in turn, by the level of physical activity and the nutritional status of the individual. Nutritional status influences activity and, conversely, physical activity influences nutritional status, or at least nutritional requirements. Nutritional status reflects nutritional intake, although other factors may contribute (disease, intestinal parasitism, etc.) In addition to its direct effect on physical work capacity, nutritional status may have an indirect effect; smaller adult size may be the result of poor nutrition during the growth period. Because of the prevalence of undernutrition in large segments of the world's population and the usual necessity for these people to participate in heavy physical work (Figure 2), the present discussion will concentrate on this aspect of nutritional status.

PHYSICAL ACTIVITY AND PHYSICAL WORK CAPACITY

There is general agreement that increased habitual physical activity leads to an increase in physical work capacity as measured by $\dot{V}O_2$ max (Astrand and Rodahl 1977). The vast majority of the evidence for this improvement comes from the extensive literature on physical training for various sporting events (Astrand and Rodahl 1977) or for the improvement of health through physical activity (Pollock et al. 1978). The relationship of occupation to $\dot{V}O_2$ max is less clear. Some authors state that there is a definite trend for mean values for $\dot{V}O_2$ max to vary to some degree with the nature of the occupation. They also point out that this may be related to subject selection since those with a naturally strong constitution may be over-represented in physically demanding work (Astrand and Rodahl 1977). Irma Astrand (1967a) related $\dot{V}O_2$ max ($1 \cdot min^{-1}$) to both the occupation of the subjects and their ages and found that, in general, the more strenuous professions were associated with a higher $\dot{V}O_2$ max throughout the age range studied. Kozlowski et al. (1969) also found that men doing heavy manual labor had higher values for $\dot{V}O_2$ max ($1 \cdot min^{-1}$) than those engaged in clerical or light manual work; the latter two groups were not significantly different from each other. All three groups had the same rate of decrease with age; however, no data on weights or heights of the subjects were given in either study, so the contribution of body size cannot be determined.

Others have reported that occupations which demand relatively heavy physical work do little to improve endurance fitness (Allen 1966; Anderson 1964). This led Shephard (1978) to speculate that leisure activities may have more influence on physical work capacity than occupational effort. In mechanized societies, where sedentary life styles are more common, one usually encounters lower physical work capacities (Shephard 1978). Cumming and Bailey (1974) found that Canadian men engaged in grain farming, a highly mechanized form of agriculture, had $\dot{V}O_2$ max values (~ 40 ml$\cdot$kg$^{-1}\cdot$min^{-1}) more nearly representative of sedentary individuals. Miller et al. (1972) measured the $\dot{V}O_2$ max of Jamaican farmers and suburbanites, Trinidadian shopkeepers and clerks, and English factory workers who were doing fairly heavy work, and related it to the lean body mass (LBM) of the subjects. $\dot{V}O_2$ max was higher in subjects with higher values for LBM and the sedentary shopkeepers and clerks of Trinidad had lower values than the more active Jamaican and English subjects. The investigators concluded that $\dot{V}O_2$ max was determined mainly by body muscle (LBM) and the level of habitual activity.

Aghemo et al. (1971) compared the maximal aerobic powers of two groups of Tarahumara Indians: one group followed their ancient custom of long distance running while the other had become adapted to modern ways and had lost the habit of running. The average aerobic power of the runners was 63 ml·kg^{-1}·min^{-1} while that of the non-runners was only 39 ml·kg^{-1}·min^{-1}. Rode and Shephard (1973) have observed similar results in predicted aerobic power of Eskimos in the process of' acculturation. Indeed, Shephard (1978) reports the development of an empirical acculturation index of Eskimos based on such variables as time in school, English vocabulary, type of housing and domestic equipment, wage income, etc. The index was significantly correlated with skinfold thickness in both men and women and, in men at least, negatively correlated with maximal aerobic power. On the other hand, Awad el Karim et al. (1981) estimated $\dot{V}O_2$ max from submaximal exercise tests in urban and rural populations in the Sudan. Rural dwellers who were engaged in manual labor which demanded a high energy output during working hours had higher mean values for estimated $\dot{V}O_2$ max (ml·kg^{-1}·min^{-1}) than townspeople, but the differences were not statistically significant. These results are in accord with the findings of others concerning Africans (Ojikutu et al. 1972; Van Graan et al. 1972).

There would seem, therefore, to be a consensus, if not universal agreement, that daily levels of habitual activity, whether of a recreational (training) or occupational nature have a positive effect on physical work capacity. The effects of physical training programs on maximum aerobic power, where intensity and duration are controlled, are relatively easy to demonstrate. However, the relationship between intensity of occupational activity (i.e., Cal·Kg^{-1}·24 Hr^{-1} expended) and PWC seems not to have been quantitated, and indeed may be very difficult to quantify. In this regard, some very brief comments about the principles of physical training, as distinct from physical activity, may be pertinent. For the ordinary person beginning a training program, a work or exercise load in excess of about 50% of his/her maximum capacity will probably produce a significant training effect (Astrand and Rodahl 1977). However, not only the intensity of work but also its duration, and the age of the subject, must be considered. Furthermore, in more physically fit individuals, higher work loads must be undertaken than for sedentary persons and, as physical fitness improves, more intense training schedules must be followed if additional improvement is to occur (Astrand and Rodahl 1977).

In laboratory experiments on the treadmill (Michael et al. 1961), and in occupational activities (Astrand 1967b; Spurr et al. 1975), it has been shown that the level which can be sustained for an 8 hr work day is about 40% or less of maximum capacity. This does not preclude the possibility that spurts of activity in excess of this value may produce training effects if sustained long enough. Most of the studies in which an attempt is made to show the relationship between occupation and physical work capacity are based on the changes from active to more sedentary life styles alluded to previously. It is well known that enforced idleness results in reduced $\dot{V}O_2$ max (Saltin et al. 1968). Wyndham et al. (1962; 1966) did find that Bantu tribesmen who entered the mines to perform a moderate level of work 6 days a week, after a previously sedentary existence, showed an improvement in work capacity ($\dot{V}O_2$ max) during their first month of work, even when expressed in terms of body weight, and showed a further slight increase after 4 months (Wyndham et al. 1962). However, at least a part of this change was probably related to their markedly improved diet (4000 Cal. and 136 g. of protein per day) (Wyndham 1966; Wyndham et al. 1966). In any event, physical training is different from habitual physical activity in terms of its effects on physical work capacity.

The improvement in physical work capacity of untrained individuals following endurance training programs is unquestioned, but the effects of occupational activity on maximum work capacity are somewhat more tenuous. It is possible that chronically high daily energy expenditures, even when they do not include significant periods of activity which could be considered to have training effects ($> 50\%$ $\dot{V}O_2$ max), do indeed have positive results on physical work capacity. Systematic studies of the relationship between habitual physical activity and physical work capacity are needed. They should take into account not only body size and composition, but also should distinguish between work related and recreational activities. Ideally these studies should include longitudinal measurements of physical work capacity when there is a change from lighter to heavier work, and when nutrition is not a factor. In reality, such studies may be more difficult to carry out than they are to suggest.

NUTRITIONAL STATUS AND PHYSICAL ACTIVITY

The influence of undernutrition on the physical activity of children is discussed elsewhere in this publication (Reina and Spurr 1984; Torun 1984). In considering the effects of chronic undernutrition in adults, a distinction should be made between daily energy expenditure and habitual physical activity. The contribution of basal metabolism (BMR) to the maintenance of life makes up a large component of daily energy expenditure. The reduction of BMR in adults, associated with below normal calorie intake, has been a consistent feature of all studies during this century (Apfelbaum 1978). The data of Keys et al. (1950) show that 24 weeks of semi-starvation (~ 1600 Cal$\cdot$24-1) resulted in a 39% decrease in basal $\dot{V}O_2$, a 31% reduction in terms of body surface area, and a 19% reduction when expressed per Kg of body weight. The other component of daily energy expenditure which is of specific concern is the physical activity which makes up the rest of daily energy expenditure.

Graham Lusk's statement that "walking gives no pleasure to a seamstress nor golf to a half-starved professor" (1921, p. 538) illustrates the largely anecdotal nature of observations on the relation between reduced caloric intake and physical activity. Lusk (1921) describes 3 subjects of Jansen (1917) on a low calorie intake (1628 Cal$\cdot$24 Hr-1) who developed excessive fatigue and exhaustion after completing walks which ordinarily would have been easily undertaken. The results for Benedict et al. (1919) are somewhat equivocal because the subjects were encouraged to increase physical activity to compensate for weight gains during the period of semi-starvation. They reported a decreased endurance in chin-up exercise and a tendency toward reduced walking distances. In general there were fairly common complaints of fatigue and weakness, and observers noted reductions in endurance, alertness and performance in their athletic activities. In the Minnesota Experiment, most of the subjects felt weak and tired easily during semi-starvation, but daily energy expenditure was not measured (Keys et al. 1950). Consequently, most of the earlier work which is sometimes quoted as evidence for decreased daily energy expenditure in malnutrition is based on impressions rather than measurements.

The classic studies of Viteri (1971) and Viteri and Torún (1975) in nutritionally supplemented and unsupplemented Guatemalan agricultural workers are an outstanding exception. These investigators employed time-motion studies and measures of the energy costs of various types of activity common to agricultural work in order to determine daily energy expenditure (Viteri 1971) and the energy cost of assigned work tasks (Viteri and Torún 1975). They also made detailed studies of dietary intake during a 3-day period by weighing the food ingested (Viteri and Torún 1975) and measured body composition and physical work capacity (Viteri 1971) as well. Two groups of agricultural workers are of primary concern for the present discussion. One group consisted of 18 men employed on a farm which paid higher than usual wages and which, for the 3 years preceding the study, had been receiving dietary supplementation in the form of 5.5g of high quality protein and 250 calories, 6 days per week. These men also had ready access to milk for themselves and their families. The second group, also composed of 18 workers, was not so fortunate. These men had no access to dietary supplementation and did not enjoy the higher wages of the supplemented farmers. Both groups were from poor regions of Guatemala and were engaged in similar agricultural activities. All the subjects were healthy, had blood hemoglobins above $13g \cdot dl^{-1}$ and plasma protein levels within the normal range. In Figure 4, physical characteristics of the two groups are compared with a group of military cadets from middle to upper socioeconomic level and good nutritional backgrounds. It can be seen that the supplemented group was older than the other two groups. Both groups of agricultural workers were significantly shorter than the cadets but not different from each other. The latter is probably a reflection of similarly poor nutritional backgrounds during childhood. The weights of the

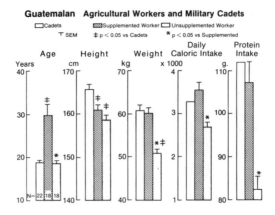

FIGURE 4: Physical characteristics and dietary
intakes of Guatemalan military cadets, supplemented
and unsupplemented agricultural workers. (Viteri 1971;
Viteri and Torún 1975)

unsupplemented workers were significantly less than either
the cadets or supplemented workers, which were not different from each other. When these data are expressed as
weight/height ratios, the two groups with good nutritional
intake have average values of 36.6 and 35.8 Kg·m^{-1} respectively, compared to the significantly lower value of 32
Kg·m^{-1} for the unsupplemented farm workers. Also, the
latter group had significantly lower body fat than the
others. Finally, estimates of muscle mass from measurements of daily creatinine excretion showed significant differences between all groups, with the cadets having a mean
value of 167 g·cm^{-1} of height and the supplemented and
unsupplemented groups 145 and 119 g·cm^{-1}, respectively.
Consequently, the poorer farmers probably were in a state
of at least marginal malnutrition when these studies were
conducted. The calorie and protein intakes of the 3 groups
are also shown in Figure 4. The cadets and supplemented
workers were ingesting 3279 and 3555 calories, respectively,
and protein well in excess of 100 g per day, while the
unsupplemented worker ingested 2695 calories and 82g of
protein per day. The percentages of protein intake with
high biologic value were 44, 26 and 8%, respectively.

The results obtained by Viteri and Torún (1975) from
their time-motion studies and caloric balance measurements

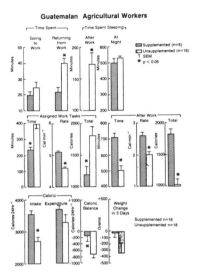

FIGURE 5: Time studies, energy expenditure and caloric balance of supplemented and unsupplemented Guatemalan agricultural workers. (Viteri and Torún 1975)

of agricultural workers are summarized in Figure 5. The time required to get to work each morning was approximately the same in each group, but the unsupplemented workers took significantly longer to return, with more rest stops and a slower pace. The two groups slept about the same amount of time at night, but the unsupplemented group used the siesta period to sleep or rest almost 3 additional hours during the day, while the supplemented group did not rest, taking advantage of their leisure time to work at home, walk around town, or even play football. In the work studies, each group was assigned a series of work tasks to be accomplished. The supplemented workers completed their work in a shorter period of time by working at a higher rate for a total energy expenditure which was considerably less than that expended by the unsupplemented group performing the same work tasks. This allowed them more time and higher energy expenditure for leisure activities than the unsupplemented workers who spent most of their non-working hours resting. The caloric intake, expenditure, caloric balance, and changes in body weight of the two groups are shown at the bottom of

Figure 5. The large caloric imbalance of the unsupplemented group is evident and, during the 3-day study,
led to an average weight loss of 346g compared to a
weight loss of only 29g in the supplemented workers. The
authors point out that the negative balances were the result
of the subjects' desire to please the investigators
(Hawthorne effect) (Hanson 1967) by expending energy
clearly in excess of their intakes, and was not a situation
that could be maintained for any significant period of time.
By assuming that the daily energy expenditures of the unsupplemented workers outside the context of the scientific
study would be more nearly equal to their intake (2700
Cal·24 Hr^{-1}) and subtracting the 24 Hr BMR, the investigators calculated that the supplemented group would have
1852 Cal available for physical work or other activities,
while the lower intake group would have only 1167 Cal
(Viteri 1971). No direct measurements of productivity were
made in these studies, but the implications of lower productivity for the unsupplemented workers and the improved
working ability of those receiving dietary supplementation
are clear. Furthermore, as these authors (Viteri and
Torún 1975) emphasize, the provision of adequate nutritional intake for these (agricultural) workers would allow
them to provide more adequately for their families, to
participate in community activities and, in general, to
improve the quality of their lives. Presumably the same
would be true of any group involved in moderate to heavy
physical labor.

In addition to the impact of nutritional intake and
status on physical activity, it is well known that sustained
high levels of activity are associated with higher caloric
intake (Mayer et al. 1956). The effects of physical activity
on protein requirements are less certain, but recent work
summarized by Young (1981) and Young and Torún (1981)
bring into question the prevalent view that physical exercise per se does not result in an increased requirement for
dietary protein. They have presented evidence from their
own work and that of others which seems to indicate that
moderate and heavy exercise in adult subjects does, indeed,
result in an increase in the need for specific amino acids
and/or total protein. Accordingly, they have called for a
careful and extensive exploration of the affects of various
types, intensities, and durations of physical activity on the
amino acid and protein requirements of human subjects

(Young and Torún 1981). The reader is referred to these reviews for specific details.

NUTRITIONAL STATUS AND PHYSICAL WORK CAPACITY

Nutritional status, although influenced by disease and sanitary conditions, is the result of nutrient intake, and its assessment is based on anthropometric, biochemical and/or body composition measurements, and physical examination, used either separately or in combination. The determination of nutritional status of communities and of individuals has been the subject of a number of reviews (Brozek 1963; ICNND 1963b; Jelliffe 1966; Keys and Brozek 1953; Malina 1980; Moore et al. 1963; Simopoulos 1982), and the topic of nutritional status and physical work capacity in a wide variety of subjects and conditions (not including malnutrition) has been reviewed extensively by Parizkova (1977). In this discussion, the effects of nutritional intake and status on physical work capacity will be limited to the results of acute starvation or reduced caloric intake (semi-starvation) and chronic malnutrition as evidenced by changes in body composition. This chapter will not consider the influence on work capacity of either obesity or anemia, the latter a consistent feature of protein-calorie malnutrition (Viteri et al. 1968). There is general agreement that both acute and chronic reduction in levels of blood hemoglobin (low O_2 carrying capacity) reduce work capacity and endurance in both animals (Edgerton et al. 1972; Koziol et al. 1982; Ohira et al. 1981) and adult humans (Davies et al. 1973; Gardner et al. 1975; Gardner et al. 1977; Viteri and Torún 1973). Edgerton et al. (1979) have measured significant increases in daily physical activity following treatment of anemic subjects with iron. The subject of nutritional status and physical work capacity, including obesity and anemia, has been reviewed recently (Spurr 1983).

Starvation

Two groups of workers have investigated the effects of acute starvation on $\dot{V}O_2$ max. Henschel et al. (1954) studied 12 men before and after a 4.5-day fast, before and during which they also performed heavy physical labor in order to maintain their levels of physical training. There was a significant 8% fall in $\dot{V}O_2$ max (1.min-1) associated with an 8% reduction in body weight at the end of the fast, and 34% and 44% reduction in fitness scores obtained on the Harvard Fitness Test (Johnson et al. 1942) on the 2nd and 4th days of the fast. There was no significant change in maximal aerobic power when expressed in terms of body weight (ml·kg-1·min-1). The investigators observed a marked increase in nitrogen excretion (protein catabolism) and only a part of the weight loss could be accounted for by reduced extracellular fluid volume (Taylor et al. 1954). This finding indicated that a decrease in muscle mass could account for the decreased aerobic power in absolute terms. Similar findings were obtained by Consolazio et al. (1967a; 1967b) except that their subjects demonstrated an increase in physical fitness score. This may have been a result of training effects (Consolazio et al. 1967a) since the men did not follow a routine of physical work during the experiments.

Semi-Starvation

Perhaps the most often quoted works on the effects of acute dietary restriction on normal men are those of Benedict et al. (1919) and Keys et al. (1950). Although a variety of functions were studied by Benedict et al. (1919), the primary goal was to determine the effects on the metabolic rate of a total weight loss of about 10%. The measurements of work were limited to the metabolic cost of level treadmill walking. The energy expenditure (Cal·min-1) for this task was slightly reduced (-6%), but the difference was not statistically significant (Keys et al. 1950).

Keys et al. (1950) made extensive measurements on the 32 men in their study at the University of Minnesota during World War II. Some of their results are summarized in Figure 6. Following several weeks of a control diet of 3500 Cal·24 Hr-1, the subjects underwent a 24-week period of semi-starvation on a diet of about 1600 Cal·24 Hr-1. During the recovery period, 4 groups of 8 subjects each (Groups Z,L,T and G) consumed increasing quantities of calories which averaged 2378, 2692, 2896 and 3123 Cal·24 Hr-1 respectively (Figure 6). During the period of semi-starvation average body weight was reduced 24%, body fat decreased from 14 to 6% of body weight, and performance on the Harvard Fitness Test declined to about 30% of

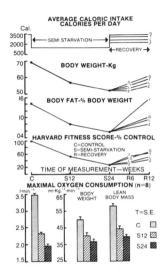

FIGURE 6: Constructed from data presented in "The Biology of Human Starvation" (Keys et al. 1950). Z, L, T and G at top refer to average recovery dietary intakes of 2378, 2692, 2896 and 3123 Cal·24 Hr^{-1} respectively. S12 and S24 are 12 and 24 weeks of semi-starvation; R6 and R12 are 6 and 12 weeks of recovery. (Spurr 1983)

control. The $\dot{V}O_2$ max expressed as $l \cdot min^{-1}$ or in terms of body weight or lean body mass (LBM = Body weight - fat weight) was also significantly ($p < 0.001$) depressed at both 12 and 24 weeks of reduced dietary intake (Figure 6). On the basis of nitrogen balance studies the authors estimated that there was a loss of 1990g of protein during the first 12 weeks of dietary restriction and another 690g during the last 12 weeks. Consequently, the reduced $\dot{V}O_2$ max during semi-starvation may have been due largely to a decline in muscle mass as protein was catabolized. Physical activity was maintained during this period by hiking 20 miles per week, walking to and from the mess hall, etc., but as already mentioned, voluntary movement was noticeably slower and, in general, energy output was markedly reduced. Some of the reduction in work capacity, therefore, may have been due to the detraining effects of a more sedentary life style, despite the programmed activities.

The recovery in the results of the Harvard Fitness Test was slow and roughly proportional to the caloric content of the recovery diets. It was not possible to recalculate the $\dot{V}O_2$ max values during the rehabilitation period, but from average data on 6 men at 12 weeks of rehabilitation, $\dot{V}O_2$ max was 74% of control and complete recovery did not occur until 20 weeks after the end of the period of dietary restriction (Keys et al. 1950). From estimates of the cross sectional area of the thigh, the authors concluded that in semi-starved subjects performing hard physical work, a unit of working muscle receives less O_2 than the same unit of muscle under normal conditions. They suggested that reduced O_2 carrying capacity of the blood (anemia), decreased cardiac output, and/or a poor capillary bed in the muscles themselves may have contributed to this low muscle O_2 supply. This last suggestion seems unlikely since, as muscle is lost during periods of undernutrition, there would have to be a disproportionate loss or closing of capillaries in order to have a detrimental effect on O_2 supply. While there is capillary growth in chronically stimulated skeletal muscle (Myrhage and Hudlicka 1978), there seem to be no studies of capillarization of skeletal muscle in malnourished humans or animals, or of cardiac output in undernourished subjects during sub-maximal or maximal work. The effects of anemia on work capacity have been alluded to earlier.

More intense caloric restriction of 580 Cal·24 Hr^{-1} for 12 days and 1010 Cal·24 Hr^{-1} for 24 days with average weight losses of 7.7% and 11% respectively has been studied by Brozek et al. (1957) and Taylor et al. (1957). Regular work tasks were performed by both groups of subjects before and during the studies to avoid detraining effects on $\dot{V}O_2$ max. Both groups showed slight reductions in $\dot{V}O_2$ max (5-10%) which were proportional to the fall in body weight. Taylor et al. (1957) suggested that the slow decline in $\dot{V}O_2$ max, down to a weight loss of 10% of body weight, was due primarily to a loss of muscle mass with the small change in blood hemoglobin contributing in a minor way. They also concluded that at weight losses greater than 10% (Keys et al. 1950) (Figure 6), cardiovascular inefficiency and increasing anemia are additional limiting factors. There is no question that $\dot{V}O_2$ max is closely related to muscle mass. Buskirk and Taylor (1957) reported a correlation coefficient of 0.91 between $\dot{V}O_2$ max and "active tissue," which is probably more closely related to muscle mass than to lean body mass. Also, it has been shown that over 80% of the difference in $\dot{V}O_2$ max between subjects with mild and severe malnutrition can be accounted for by differences in muscle mass. Perhaps much of the remainder may be accounted for by differences in blood hemoglobin (Barac-Nieto et al. 1978a). Even though a suggestion about "cardiovascular inefficiency" was made about 25 years ago (Taylor et al. 1957), we still do not have information about cardiac output, muscle blood flow, or aerobic enzymes of skeletal muscle in malnourished subjects during or immediately after physical exercise. The question about cardiac function is particularly pertinent since it has been shown that chronic malnutrition is associated with cardiac myopathies (Araujo et al. 1970; Correa et al. 1963; Gillanders 1951) which may affect function as described below.

In summary then, it would appear that acute malnutrition (starvation and semi-starvation) occurring under laboratory conditions results in a depression in physical working capacity ($\dot{V}O_2$ max) largely as a result of a loss in muscle mass.

Malnutrition

The malnutrition which occurs in the adults of developing countries, unlike that produced in the laboratory under controlled conditions, is chronic in nature and is usually the result of long exposure to a hostile environment and a losing battle for available energy intake. The nature of malnutrition is complex. It is most frequently characterized by a lack of calories, sometimes by a lack of protein, often by varying degrees of mineral and vitamin deficiencies, and by sanitary conditions which are not conducive to good health. These conditions apply particularly to children, but also to some agricultural and industrial societies (Buzina 1981). There appear to be some correlations between physical work capacity and mineral and vitamin status. Thus Buzina (1981) has shown that children with vitamin and mineral deficiencies have a slightly lower physical work capacity at a heart rate of $140 \cdot min-1$ (PWC_{140}). The estimated $\dot{V}O_2$ ($1 \cdot min-1$) of these children in submaximal exercise was significantly associated with vitamin A, riboflavin, and pyridoxin nutrition status and when expressed in terms of body weight ($ml \cdot kg-1 \cdot min-1$), was associated with serum iron, vitamin C, and riboflavin, although the correlations were not high. When treated with ascorbic acid, riboflavin, and pyridoxine for 12 weeks there was a significant improvement in PWC_{140} (Buzina 1981).

Lukaski et al. (1983) have recently shown that there is a significant difference in plasma copper levels between athletic (with higher $\dot{V}O_2$ max values) and non-athletic, nutritionally normal subjects, but that no difference existed between the two groups in plasma magnesium and zinc concentrations. In the trained subjects there was a significant correlation ($r = 0.46$; $p < 0.002$) between $\dot{V}O_2$ max ($ml \cdot kg^{-1} \cdot min^{-1}$) and plasma magnesium which was not seen in the untrained subjects. These results may reflect the fact that requirements differ for more active subjects. In general, the overall relationship between physical work capacity and mineral and vitamin nutritional status is somewhat tenuous. In animal studies it has been demonstrated that iron deficiency alone, without the associated anemia, results in a marked reduction in running ability (work performance) compared to controls (Finch et al. 1976; Ohira 1981). More information is necessary to determine the specific effects of mineral and vitamin deficiencies on physical work capacity in humans, but it is unlikely that studies of pure mineral or vitamin deficiency states in malnourished populations can be carried out.

In considering the relationship between nutritional status and physical work capacity the situation in adult agricultural workers and in rural children as future agricultural workers will be treated separately. The use of the term "working capacity" in reference to children is sometimes disturbing to the socially conscious, but physical work capacity is a widely accepted term to describe the physiological capability of individuals to perform exercise. In the case of children, an attempt will be made to relate their maximal exercise capacity to their work performance as adults, not as children.

Adults. Viteri (1971) compared the $\dot{V}O_2$ max of several groups of young Guatemalan adults. His unsupplemented agricultural workers, previously described, can probably be considered at least marginally malnourished on the basis of their adiposity, lean body mass (LBM), and muscle cell mass (MCM, calculated from daily creatinine excretion). This group, another group which consisted of recent inductees into the army who were from a similar rural socioeconomic background, and 10 of the supplemented agricultural workers discussed above had significantly lower $\dot{V}O_2$ max and maximal aerobic power (expressed as per Kg of body weight or LBM) than army cadets from middle or upper socioeconomic levels who had never been exposed to nutritional deprivation. When compared on the basis of "cell residue" (body weight less fat, water, and bone mineral), all differences in maximal aerobic power between groups disappeared. Viteri (1971) observed that the differences in maximal aerobic power were due to differences in body composition and not to differences in cell function.

Barac-Nieto et al. (1978b) studied three groups of chronically malnourished adult males who were selected for their existing degree of undernutrition. The most severely malnourished of these subjects were also studied during a 45-day basal period in the hospital and during 79 days of a dietary repletion regime (Barac-Nieto et al. 1979). Volunteer subjects from rural areas of Colombia were classified into those with mild (M), intermediate (I), and severe (S) malnutrition based on their weight/height (W/H) ratios, serum albumin (AL) concentrations, and daily creatinine excretion per meter of height (Cr/h.) as detailed in Table 1. Each group was significantly different ($p < 0.001$) from the other two with regard to each variable used in the classification. The W/H ratio of 107 nutritionally normal

Table 1
Selection criteria, means and standard deviations of mild (M),
intermediate (I) and severely (S) malnourished
adult males

Subject Groups	Weight/Height $kg \cdot m^{-1}$	Serum Albumin $g \cdot dl^{-1}$	Daily Creatinine/ Height $mg \cdot day^{-1} \cdot m^{-1}$
M (n=11)	>32	>3.5	>600
	33.3 ± 2.1	3.8 ± 0.5	660 ± 67
I (n=18)	29 - 32	2.5 - 3.5	450 - 600
	30.8 ± 2.0	3.0 ± 0.7	559 ± 75
S (n=18)	<29	<2.5	<450
	27.4 ± 2.1	2.1 ± 0.5	391 ± 76

agricultural workers was 36.3 ± 3.6 kg·m^{-1} (mean $\pm$ SD) and in 72 the serum albumin was 4.4 ± 0.3. Both values were significantly higher than those with mild malnutrition. Creatinine excretions in these control subjects were not obtained. Detailed body composition and biochemical measurements of the 3 undernourished groups were made shortly after admission to the hospital metabolic ward (Barac-Nieto et al. 1978b) and during the dietary repletion regime of Group S (Barac-Nieto et al. 1979). Upon entry into the hospital the subjects were placed on an energy intake (2240 Cal·day^{-1}) adequate for the sedentary conditions of the metabolic ward, but were maintained on the same protein intake (27g·day^{-1}) they were ingesting prior to entry. Studies of work capacity and endurance in the severely malnourished men were made at the beginning and end of the 45-day basal period on this diet (Barac-Nieto et al. 1980). The protein intake was then increased to 100 g·day^{-1} for the 79-day repletion regime; the increased caloric intake from proteins was balanced by reducing carbohydrate intake to maintain the diets isocaloric. Measurements of $\dot{V}O_2$ max and endurance were repeated at 90 and 124 hospital days (Barac-Nieto et al. 1980).

The results for the 3 groups, and the changes in the severely malnourished men during dietary repletion, are presented in Figures 7 and 8 and compared with data on 107 nutritionally normal control subjects (72 in the case of blood data) who were sugar cane cutters (Spurr et al. 1977b), loaders (Spurr et al. 1977a), or general agricultural workers (Maksud et al. 1976). There were progressive differences in body weight, W/H ratio, serum albumin and total proteins in the control (C), M, I and S groups (Figure 7). Groups C and M were not significantly different in regard to hematocrit and blood hemoglobin but I and S were significantly and progressively depressed in these measurements. There was a slight gain in body weight for Group S during the basal period, but otherwise the variables did not change. Weight, W/H ratio and the serum proteins showed progressive improvement during the repletion regime, but the hematological values did not show improvement until the final round of measurements (Figure 7).

Figure 8 presents the results for f_H max, maximal aerobic power and $\dot{V}O_2$ max (1/min) for the control and malnourished subjects. Average max f_H values did not

NUTRITIONAL STATUS

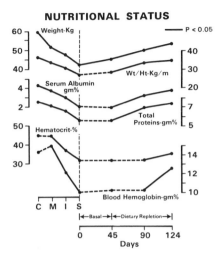

FIGURE 7: Average values of some anthropometric and blood variables in nutritionally normal (C) subjects and men with mild (M), intermediate (I) and severe (S) malnutrition. The severely undernourished were studied during a basal period on adequate calories and low protein followed by a dietary repletion period on an isocaloric but high protein diet. Solid lines connect points which are significantly different from each other and, in the case of the 4 groups to the left, have only this statistical meaning. (Spurr 1983)

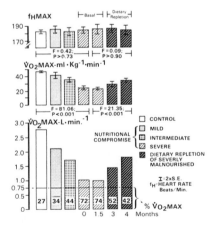

FIGURE 8: Maximum heart rates (f_H), aerobic power, and $\dot{V}O_2$ max in control, undernourished, and severely malnourished subjects and during dietary repletion of the latter. Lower panel shows a fixed sub-maximal work load (0.75 $1 \cdot min^{-1}$) in terms of % $\dot{V}O_2$ max. (From Spurr 1983)

differ in the various groups nor did they change during dietary repletion. However, $\dot{V}O_2$ max and maximal aerobic power were progressively less in C,M,I and S subjects, did not change in the latter during the basal period, and then progressively improved during dietary repletion, although they did not return to even the level of Group M during the period of study. Figure 8 also expresses a theoretical submaximal work load of 0.75 $1 \cdot min^{-1}$ $\dot{V}O_2$ in terms of % $\dot{V}O_2$ max for each of the groups. From Figure 8, it is clear that $\dot{V}O_2$ max and maximal aerobic power are markedly depressed in chronic malnutrition and that the degree of reduction is related to the severity of depression in nutritional status. Using the three groups of malnourished subjects, a stepwise multiple regression analysis (Barac-Nieto et al. 1978a) revealed that the W/H ratio ($Kg \cdot m^{-1}$), log of the sum of triceps and subscapular skinfolds in mm. (SK), total body Hb (TotHb) obtained as the product of blood Hb and blood volume ($g \cdot Kg^{-1}$ body weight), and daily creatinine (Cr) excretion ($g \cdot day^{-1}$ $\cdot kg^{-1}$) contributed signifiantly to the variation in $\dot{V}O_2$ max ($1 \cdot min^{-1}$). That is:

(1) $\dot{V}O_2$ max ($1 \cdot min^{-1}$) = 0.095 W/H - 0.152 SK +

0.087 TotHb + 0.031 Cr - 2.550

(r = 0.931; S.E.E. = 0.21)

All of the variables in the equation are, of course, related to nutritional status.

Figure 9 expresses the data for the 3 malnourished groups, and for Group S during recovery, in terms of various body compartments. It was not possible to do body composition studies on the control subjects. The salient feature of Figure 9 is that over 80% of the difference in $\dot{V}O_2$ max between M and S subjects is accounted for by difference in MCM. The remaining difference might be ascribed to reduced capacity for oxygen transport either because of low blood Hb (Figure 7) or reduced maximum cardiac output. A number of investigators have reported changes in cardiac muscle in nutritional deficiencies (Araujo et al. 1970; Correa et al. 1963; Gillander 1951), which could result in decreases in the force of contraction and perhaps, therefore, in maximal stroke volume. However,

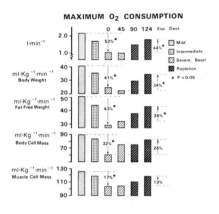

FIGURE 9: $\dot{V}O_2$ max expressed in terms of various body compartments for the undernourished and subjects and during dietary repletion of the most severely malnourished. (Spurr 1983)

there do not seem to be any reports of studies on maximum cardiac output in malnourished subjects.

Another possibility is that the skeletal muscle cells exhibit reduced maximal aerobic power because of reduced oxidative enzyme content. Tasker and Tulpule (1964) found a marked decrease in the activities of oxidative enzymes in the skeletal muscle of protein deficient rats, and Raju (1974) reported that after recovery from 13 weeks of re-duced protein intake, rat skeletal muscle had an increase in glycolytic and a decrease in oxydative enzymes and activi-ty. However, there are no studies which have measured similar biochemical changes in humans although Lopes et al. (1982) recently have shown that malnourished patients exhibited marked impairment in muscle function. Both an increased muscle fatigability in static muscular contraction and a changed pattern of muscle on traction and relaxation were reversed in patients undergoing nutritional supple-mentation. Their data would indicate the possibility of a decreased content of ATP and phosphocreatine in the skele-tal muscle tissue of malnourished subjects. The data of Heymsfield et al. (1982) indicate changes in the biochemical composition of skeletal muscle in both acute and chronic semistarvation, particularly with regard to glycogen and total energy contents.

In any event, it should be emphasized that the $\dot{V}O_2$ max not accounted for by differences in MCM is small (Figure 9). After 2-1/2 months of recovery the $\dot{V}O_2$ max increased significantly in $1 \cdot min^{-1}$ and when expressed in terms of body weight and LBM but, although mean values were elevated in terms of body cell mass and MCM, the increases were not statistically significant. At the termination of the experiment, however, physical work capacity had not returned to values comparable to those seen in mild malnutrition (Figures 8 and 9) which indicates that the recovery process is a long one, particularly when carried out under the sedentary conditions of the hospital metabolic ward. This slow recovery was also noted in the semi-starved subjects in the Minnesota Experiment (Keys et al. 1950). It is interesting to note that the $\dot{V}O_2$ max was increased 45 days after beginning the repletion diet (90 hospital days), when blood Hb concentration had not yet increased (Figure 7), but MCM was significantly increased over basal values (Barac-Nieto et al. 1980). This also points to a primary dependence of $\dot{V}O_2$ max on MCM (Figure 9). Furthermore, it appears that supplying adequate calories alone was not sufficient to bring about an increase in $\dot{V}O_2$ max or MCM and that only after increasing the protein intake to $100g \cdot day^{-1}$ was there improvement in these 2 variables.

The data in Figure 8 show that a fixed sub maximal $\dot{V}O_2$ (0.75 $1 \cdot min^{-1}$) represents differing relative work loads in terms of $\%\dot{V}O_2$ max. In these subjects the heart rate responses to submaximal work were examined using the linear relationship between f_H and $\dot{V}O_2$ which had been established by several measurements obtained during the max treadmill test on the way to $\dot{V}O_2$ max (Spurr et al. 1979). With the least squares regression line obtained it was possible to calculate the f_H at submaximal work levels of $\dot{V}O_2$, in terms of $1 \cdot min^{-1}$, Kg of body weight, or % of $\dot{V}O_2$ max. The results for the control subjects and the 3 groups of malnourished men are shown in Figure 10. At the same work load (250 $Kg \cdot m \cdot min^{-1}$), $\dot{V}O_2$ (0.75 $1 \cdot min^{-1}$), or $\dot{V}O_2$ per Kg body weight (30 $ml \cdot kg^{-1} \cdot min^{-1}$) there was a progressive increase in f_H from C to S subjects. Usually, when submaximal f_H is expressed in terms of the same % $\dot{V}O_2$ max, there are no differences (Saltin et al. 1968). This is the case for C, M, and I subjects, and indicates that it is the relative effort which determines f_H response. However, the S subjects show a significantly

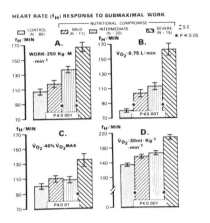

HEART RATE (f_H) RESPONSE TO SUBMAXIMAL WORK

FIGURE 10: Calculated heart rates at various submaximal work loads in control and undernourished adult male subjects. (Spurr et al. 1979)

higher f_H at 40% $\dot{V}O_2$ max than do the other groups (Figure 10). During the period of dietary repletion of Group S there was a progressive reversal of the f_H values toward control levels, but in the case of the f_H vs %$\dot{V}O_2$ max relationship the f_H was still significantly higher than control subjects at the end of the period of dietary repletion (Spurr et al. 1979).

Cotes et al. (1973) used bicycle exercise to relate submax f_H to body muscle as estimated from careful measurements of leg volume. They found it to be similar in men and women and also found that exercise f_H was correlated negatively with indices of body muscle. This is in general agreement with the results discussed here, i.e., the lower the MCM (Barac-Nieto et al. 1978a; Barac-Nieto et al. 1980), the higher the f_H at given submaximal work loads (Spurr et al. 1979). Thus when muscle mass is reduced, as in malnutrition, the work load relative to $\dot{V}O_2$ max is higher (Figure 8) and f_H is higher. But when f_H is expressed in terms of the same relative workload (%$\dot{V}O_2$ max), f_H is the same (Saltin et al. 1968) except in the case of severely malnourished subjects (Figure 10C). This indicates that Group S subjects may have undergone a physiologic change which is different from the less severely malnourished men. The nature of this change is unknown. The occurrence of cardiomyopathies associated with under-nutrition may be involved (Araujo et al. 1970; Correa et al. 1963). If these result in cardiac muscle weakening, they could contribute to the elevated heart rates observed. However, reduced stroke volume as a result of myocardial weakening from cardiac pathology (Correa et al. 1963) might not be as easily reversed as suggested by our data on the performance of Group S during dietary repletion (Spurr et al. 1979). This points to physiological rather than morpho-logical (pathological) alterations. It is clear that more detailed investigations of the cardiovascular responses to exercise in malnourished subjects are needed.

Endurance in Malnourished Subjects. An endurance test is carried out on a treadmill or bicycle ergometer at a work load ($\dot{V}O_2$) of 70-80% of the subject's maximum until exhaustion supervenes, usually with the f_H within about 5 beats of f_H max. Because of the difficulty in performing this test, few laboratories have attempted measurement of endurance times in normal individuals and, to the author's knowledge, only Spurr and colleagues have attempted it on malnourished subjects.

The relationship between relative work load (% $\dot{V}O_2$ max) and endurance time is a negative exponential one, having the form

$$(2) \quad \% \, \dot{V}O_2 \text{ max} = Ae^{-Kt}$$

where, in the linearized form, A = the intercept, K the slope and t the endurance time. Endurance times were measured in the three groups of malnourished subjects described above by two endurance tests carried out at 90-95% and 80-85% $\dot{V}O_2$ max (Barac-Nieto et al. 1978b; Barac-Nieto et al. 1980). Using the linearized form of equation 2 and substituting the actual values for %$\dot{V}O_2$ max and endurance times in the two tests, it was possible to calculate the endurance time at 80% $\dot{V}O_2$ max (T_{80}). No significant differences were demonstrated between the 3 groups (M, I and S) of malnourished men; T_{80} averaged 97 ± 12 min (mean ± S.E.) in all subjects.

In the case of Group S during dietary repletion, an interesting change in T_{80} was observed. Endurance times were significantly reduced from 113 min at the first measurement of the basal period to 42 min at the final determination at the end of the dietary repletion (Barac-Nieto et al. 1980). The explanation for this surprising reduction is still not clear. Hanson-Smith et al. (1977) reported decreased work endurance times in rats on high protein diets compared to animals ingesting an isocaloric carbohydrate diet, and Bergstrom et al. (1967) and Gollnick et al. (1972) have shown that diets in which the energy value of carbohydrate has been replaced with fat and/or protein, lead to reduced stores of muscle glycogen. Furthermore, Bergstrom et al. (1967) demonstrated that the maximum endurance time in humans is directly related to the initial glycogen content of skeletal muscle. During the dietary repletion period of the Group S subjects, carbohydrate intake was reduced from 64% to 50% of calories. In a normal individual this amount of carbohydrate should be sufficient to maintain muscle glycogen stores, but it appears that no definitive studies have been done (Durnin 1982). The rebuilt muscle tissue of Group S subjects may not store glycogen normally and, together with the lack of regular exercise in the protracted sedentary existence in the metabolic ward, may lead to reduced muscle glycogen and shorter endurance times.

The slowness of recovery from malnutrition under sedentary conditions (Barac-Nieto 1980; Keys 1950) makes one wonder what effects a regime of exercise training would have on the recovery process. Torún and Viteri (1981) have studied the effects of increased physical activity on the growth of 2-4 yr old children during recovery from protein-energy malnutrition, and found that more active children grew better in height and in lean body mass than children undergoing a traditional course of treatment without increased activity; that is, there was an increase in the efficiency of utilization of dietary energy and protein for growth. Regular exercise by adults during recovery from malnutrition may have similar effects, if not in growth at least in the rebuilding of muscle tissue. Other than those mentioned, there do not appear to be any studies of the effects, beneficial or otherwise, of exercise training in malnourished subjects. The subject of muscle nutritive supply and metabolism, and the endocrine responses which regulate them during both short term and prolonged exercise, has not been investigated in relation to malnourished individuals. Even though there is little reason, at the moment, to suspect abnormal muscle function in acute

exercise testing to maximum levels, the responses to prolonged exercise should be investigated.

In summary then, malnutrition is accompanied by a
reduced PWC as measured by $\dot{V}O_2$ max, and the degree of
depression is related to the severity of the depressed
nutritional status and to the loss of muscle mass. Dietary
repletion with protein ($100g \cdot day^{-1}$) is associated with a
rebuilding of MCM and a return of $\dot{V}O_2$ max towards normal
values, but 2.5 months of such a rehabilitation program
found severely undernourished subjects still in an intermediate to mild state of malnutrition. The reduction in endurance time during dietary repletion is not clearly understood
and indicates the need for further research to establish
mechanisms. The elevated f_H responses of severely
malnourished men to the same relative ($\%\dot{V}O_2$ max) work
load indicates some physiological change(s) as yet poorly
understood.

Children. When comparing the $\dot{V}O_2$ max of various
populations of children from different parts of the world,
race and socioeconomic status arise as possible confounding
variables. However, when studies were performed on
nutritionally normal Colombian children there were no differences in $\dot{V}O_2$ max in white, mestizo or black boys 6-16
years of age, nor did socioeconomic status influence their
maximum exercise response (Spurr et al. 1982).

There are few studies of exercise and work capacity in
malnourished children, and most of these have been carried
out using sub maximal exercise testing. Areskog et al.
(1969) determined the PWC_{170} in 10 and 13 year old
Ethiopian boys from public and private schools with the aim
of including both poorly nourished and well-nourished
subjects. The older public school boys were shorter,
weighed less, and had smaller skinfolds and mid-arm circumferences than their private school counterparts. The
height and weight differences in the younger children were
less clear-cut, although mid-arm circumference and
skinfolds were smaller in the public school boys, and the
average caloric and protein intakes lower, in both groups of
public school than private school children. The results on
PWC_{170} showed that the performance of the public school
boys (i.e., undernourished) was somewhat better than the
private school children. Davies (1973a) predicted $\dot{V}O_2$ max
from submaximal bicycle ergometry, demonstrating that

malnourished (underweight) children had low values for $\dot{V}O_2$ max, but that the maximal aerobic power in terms of body weight, LBM, or leg volume was well within the normal range. Satyanarayana et al. (1979) have also reported the results of measurements of PWC_{170} in boys 14-17 years of age categorized according to their nutritional status at age 5 years. They found that about 64% of the variation in PWC_{170} could be explained by the subjects' body weight at the time of the testing and another 10% by their habitual physical activity levels. But even severe malnutrition at age 5 had no effect on work performance when they expressed PWC_{170} in terms of body weight. However, the undernourished subjects had higher values for f_H at the same sub max work load, i.e., were working at a higher %$\dot{V}O_2$ max than normal children.

The results of work capacity studies in marginally malnourished and nutritionally normal, urban and rural Colombian boys 6-16 yrs. of age have been reported recently (Spurr et al. 1983a). Only the results obtained on the 327 rural boys will be presented here because it is presumably these children who will be the agricultural workers of the future in this region. The subjects were recruited from lower socioeconomic families living in 3 rural villages outside of the city of Cali. They were classified as nutritionally normal (N), low weight for age (W-A) but normal weight for height (past history of malnutrition but nutritionally normal at the time the studies were concluded), and low weight for age and height (W-H; presently malnourished). Classifications were based on the data of Rueda-Williamson et al. (1969) who used upper socioeconomic children as the reference population. The children ranged in age from 6 to 16 years and were divided into 5 age groups of 2-year intervals. The average height and weight values for the rural N boys varied between the 50th and 25th percentile of the U.S. National Center for Health Statistics reference population (Figure 11). In the W-A and W-H the children's height and weight fell at or below the 5th percentile. The W-H boys had significantly lower weights (F = 6.90; P =< 0.009) and were taller (F = 30.26; P<0.001) than the W-A groups. The average $\dot{V}O_2$ max for the 3 nutritional groups is plotted in Figure 12 as a function of the average age of each of the 5 groups. The n values for each group varied between 13 and 27. The W-A and W-H groups were both significantly lower in their values for $\dot{V}O_2$ max throughout the age range studied

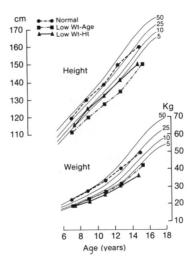

FIGURE 11: Average weights and heights of nutritionally normal, low weight for age, and low weight for height rural Colombian boys plotted as average group age on U.S. National Center for Health Statistics percentiles.

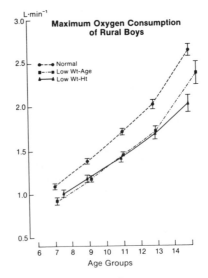

FIGURE 12: Average ± S.E. values of $\dot{V}O_2$ max ($1 \cdot min^{-1}$) of normal, low weight for age, and low weight for height Colombian boys.

(except in the case of the older W-A boys), but were not significantly different from each other. When expressed in terms of body weight (Figure 13), there were statistically significant age and nutritional group effects in a two-way analysis of variance, and the nutritionally deprived groups were slightly, though significantly, higher than the nutritionally normal boys.

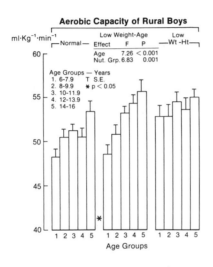

FIGURE 13: Maximum aerobic power ($ml \cdot kg^{-1} \cdot min^{-1}$) of normal, low weight for age, and low weight for height Colombian boys, with results of 2-way analysis of variance.

These results make it clear that the lower values of $\dot{V}O_2$ max for the nutritionally deprived children are due to their lower body weights. This is essentially the same conclusion reached by Davies (1973a) and Satyanarayana et al. (1979). Again, as mentioned earlier for adults, there does not appear to be any basic deficit in muscle function in marginally malnourished children, only in the quantity of muscle available for maximal work. The elevated values for maximal aerobic power in the undernourished boys (Figure 13) are no doubt a reflection of differences in body composition. The nutritionally deprived children had significantly lower summed skinfolds (triceps, subscapular, and abdominal) than N boys, and the values in W-H boys were significantly lower than W-A children (Spurr et al.

1983b), indicating corresponding differences in body fat. LBM was not calculated from skinfolds since it is improbable that the empirical equations in existence for European (Parizkova 1977) or North American (Lohman et al. 1975) children apply to the Colombian boys. This is particularly true in view of the finding that the correlation coefficients of skinfolds (triceps and subscapular) with body fat, calculated from measurements of total body water and extra-cellular fluid volume, decrease and finally disappear in moderately and severely malnourished adult males (Spurr et al. 1981). However, it is not difficult to envision that the nutritionally deprived children with presumably lower fat contents (reduced skinfold thickness) have a higher LBM, and therefore MCM, per unit of body weight than the N boys, and that this accounts for the higher values for maximal aerobic power in the former.

PHYSICAL WORK CAPACITY AND PRODUCTIVITY

In attempting to relate nutritional status to productivi-ty, one frequently finds that poor nutritional status results from lack of employment and that individuals in the poorest nutritional condition are too ill to work. Consequently, the direct relationship between nutritional status and produc-tivity has not been studied. Instead, the productivity of nutritionally normal workers has been determined and related to measurements of physical work capacity. Infer-ences about nutritional status and productivity can then be drawn from the results of studies described in the previous section.

In moderate and heavy piece work it has sometimes been possible to estimate productivity by measuring the quantity of product or amount of income produced. Sugar cane cutting and loading are heavy work tasks and the weight of cane cut or loaded is measured carefully because workers are usually paid by the tonnage cut or loaded. Because the pay scale in many sugar harvesting operations is very low, one might expect that the motivation factor would be fairly similar in different groups of workers and that they would work close to the limit of their physical capacities. Logging is also heavy physical work (Durnin and Passmore 1967) and has been used to relate productivi-ty to worker characteristics. Measuring the time required to accomplish standard work tasks is another method which has been utilized to estimate productivity.

Hansson (1965) measured submaximal work and estimated $\dot{V}O_2$ max in a group of "top" producing lumberjacks and a group of average producers. There were no differences between the two groups in measurements of height, weight, circumferences of lower and upper arms and chest, muscle strength in the hands and arms, or when vertically lifting with two hands. However, the top producers had a higher estimated $\dot{V}O_2$ max than the average group. Davies (1973b) studied sugar cane cutters in East Africa, dividing them into high, medium and low producers based on the daily tonnage cut. As in the case of Hansson's loggers (1965), he found no difference in the 3 groups in height, weight, summed skinfolds, LBM, leg volume, or circumferences of biceps and calf, but he did encounter a significant correlation between daily productivity and $\dot{V}O_2$ max ($r = 0.46$; $p<0.001$). Morrison and Blake (1974) observed that six Australian cutters, whose productivity was much higher than their Rhodesian counterparts, also had a higher estimated $\dot{V}O_2$ max, although the difference disappeared when the data were normalized for body weight. Davies et al. (1976) also measured productivity in Sudanese cane cutters during a 3-hr period of continuous cutting and reported a significant correlation between $\dot{V}O_2$ max and rate ($Kg \cdot min^{-1}$) of cane cutting ($r = 0.26$; $P < 0.01$).

Nutritionally normal sugar cane workers in Colombia have been studied (Spurr et al. 1975; Spurr et al. 1977a; Spurr et al. 1977c), where the the tasks of cutting and loading the cane are performed by separate gangs of men. Because of the warm climate harvesting is not seasonal in nature, but occurs throughout the year. Sugar cane cutting is a self-paced, continuous task, while the loading of cane is discontinuous and depends on the availability of wagons. The measurements of energy expenditure ($\dot{V}O_2$) while cutting cane were made for each subject with a Kofranyi-Michaelis Respirometer during two periods in the morning and two periods in the afternoon. During each period of measurement the cane cut was carefully collected and weighed, so that the energy cost of the work ($\dot{V}O_2$ per Kg of cane cut) could be determined. On a separate day the $\dot{V}O_2$ max of the workers was determined at the base laboratory (Spurr et al. 1975). During the measurements in the field it was estimated that the cutters were working at an average of 57% of their $\dot{V}O_2$ max. However, this value is considered to be higher than that which can be sustained during an 8 hr. work day. Michael et al. (1961) found in laboratory treadmill work that 8 hrs could be tolerated without undue fatigue when the relative load did not exceed 35% $\dot{V}O_2$ max. In the building industry, Astrand (1967b) reported that about 40% $\dot{V}O_2$ max was the upper limit that could be tolerated for an 8 hr work day. Knowing the rate of cane cutting ($kg \cdot min^{-1}$) during the periods of observation, it could be estimated that if cutters had sustained this rate for 8 hrs, their productivity would have been considerably higher than it actually was. With the O_2 cost of cutting cane ($1 \cdot kg^{-1}$) and the actual productivity of the workers, it was possible to estimate that, on the average, they worked at about 35% of their $\dot{V}O_2$ max during the 8 hr work day. This is in agreement with Michael et al. (1961) and Astrand (1967b) and is another clear example of the Hawthorne effect (Hanson 1967) and the eagerness of the subjects to please the observers during the periods of measurement (Spurr et al. 1975). A rough estimate of the activities of the 59 subjects during non-working hours was made by means of a questionnaire: 68% were classified as being almost completely inactive; 30% participated in some physical activity at least 4 hours per week; and only 2% (one subject) was involved

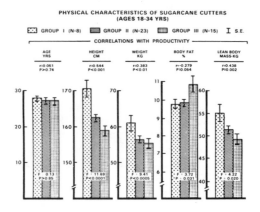

FIGURE 14: Physical characteristics of good (Group I), average (Group II), and poor (Group III) sugar cane cutters and their relationship to productivity. F-ratio values are from a one-way analysis of variance. (Spurr et al. 1977b)

in regular physical activity. In this respect at least, the majority of the sugar cane cutters studied by the author resemble the unsupplemented agricultural workers of Viteri and Torún (1975).

The cutters were divided into good (Group I), average (Group II), and poor (Group III) producers, depending on the daily tonnage cut. The correlations between productivity and various anthropometric measurements and age of the cutters are shown in Figure 14. There were statistically significant positive correlations of height, weight, and LBM with productivity. The correlations with age and body fat were not significant. Figure 15 summarizes the relation of $\dot{V}O_2$ max $(1 \cdot min^{-1})$ and maximal aerobic power $(ml \cdot Kg^{-1} \cdot min^{-1})$ with productivity, both of which were significantly correlated. A step-wise multiple regression analysis revealed that $\dot{V}O_2$ max $(1 \cdot min^{-1})$, % body fat (F), and height (H;cm) contributed significantly to the variation in productivity (tons·day^{-1}) so that

(3) Productivity = 0.81 $\dot{V}O_2$ max - 0.14 F + 0.03 H - 1.962

$$(r = 0.685; P < 0.001)$$

The $\dot{V}O_2$ max is influenced by physical condition and, together with body fat, by present nutritional status (Astrand and Rodahl 1977; Barac-Nieto et al. 1978a; Viteri 1971), and adult height is influenced by past nutritional status during the period of growth (Thomson 1968). Equation 3 simply states that those who are in poor physical condition, who are presently malnourished (low $\dot{V}O_2$ max), or whose height is stunted because of past undernutrition, are at a disadvantage in terms of ability to produce in cutting sugar cane. The negative coefficient for % body fat indicates that there is some advantage to low body fat contents. The relatively low correlation coefficients between productivity and $\dot{V}O_2$ max obtained in these studies and others (Davies 1973b; Davies et al. 1976) preclude the use of regression equations in the prediction of productivity and bring into question the homogeneity of motivation alluded to above. The results shown in Figure 15 indicate that the more physically fit subjects were better producers. This was also seen in the measurements made on these subjects in the field under their usual working conditions. The f_H during cutting was lowest in Group I, intermediate in Group II, and highest in Group III at the same $\dot{V}O_2$

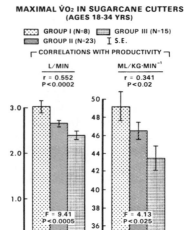

FIGURE 15: $\dot{V}O_2$ max and maximal aerobic power of good (Group I), average (Group II), and poor (Group III) sugar cane cutters. F-ratio values are from a one-way analysis of variance. (Spurr et al. 1977b)

(Spurr et al. 1975). Subjects in better physical condition have lower resting and work f_H than non-fit subjects (Astrand and Rodahl 1977). Even in the case of the sugar cane loaders, who do not work continuously, productivity was positively correlated with maximal aerobic power and negatively with resting and working f_H, demonstrating again the relationship of productivity to the physical condition of the worker (Spurr 1977a).

The results in Figure 14 show that in the case of sugar cane cutting, which at an average expenditure of 5 Cal·min-1 per 65 Kg of body weight during the 8-hr work day (Spurr et al. 1975) can be classified as moderate industrial work (Durnin and Passmore 1967), worker productivity is related to body size, height, weight and LBM. This has also been demonstrated by Satyanarayana et al. (1977; 1978) for industrial factory work which is presumably of less intensity than sugar cane cutting. Their subjects were nutritionally normal workers engaged in the production of detonator fuses, and productivity could be measured in terms of the number of fuses produced per day. They found that body weight, height, and LBM were significantly correlated with productivity and that, after partialing out the effect of height, weight, and LBM were still significantly correlated with productivity. That is, the total daily work output was significantly higher in those with higher body weight and LBM.

Martorell et al. (1978), in discussing the causes and implications of small stature in developing nations, quote several groups of investigators (Areskog et al. 1969; Banerjee and Saha 1970; Phillips 1954; Ramana Murthy and Dakshayani 1962; Wyndham 1966) as evidence that adults from developing countries are "mechanically more efficient than their taller counterparts from the developed nations; that is, that they require less oxygen per unit rate of work" (Martorell et al. 1978, p. 151). However, only two of the quoted groups purported to have measured efficiency. Banerjee and Saha (1970) and Ramana Murthy and Dakshayani (1962) measured the energy expenditure ($Cal \cdot min^{-1}$) of their subjects at specific activities (stone cutting, walking, running, etc.) and compared it with the energy expenditure in similar activities of subjects from Western nations. No energy expenditures per unit of work or activity done were made, so there were no measurements of efficiency. Areskog et al. (1969) found that the PWC_{170} was somewhat lower in their Ethiopian subjects than in Scandinavian subjects, which means that the former were in poorer physical condition, not more efficient. Phillips (1954) concluded that his results did not support the contention that the African is physiologically more efficient than the European. Finally, Wyndham (1966) did find that Bantu and Bushmen were mechanically more efficient than Caucasians in performing a stair-climbing procedure. However, he pointed out that the Bantu and Bushmen are more accustomed to walking and running than Caucasians in South Africa and that the latter had more body fat (greater skinfold thickness) than the other 2 groups. The greater O_2 cost of moving more body fat is well known (Buskirk and Taylor 1957). The author is unaware of any evidence that shorter, lighter people from developing countries are more efficient than their larger counterparts from the so-called developed world. Consequently, the contention of Martorell et al. (1978, p. 151) that "the ability of people with small body size to perform everyday tasks with less oxygen consumption (and hence, less energy) than larger ones is clearly advantageous" is true only because they do less in order to balance their lower energy intakes (Viteri and

Torún 1975). The advantages of smaller body size would derive from the smaller body mass that needs to be supplied with energy and there would be some advantage in moving body weight in work involving body translation. In view of the results presented in Figure 14 and the results of Satyanarayana et al. (1977; 1978), the statement of Martorell et al. (1978) that there is no clear advantage to being tall, would also seem to be incorrect.

The direct effects of caloric supplementation or of nutritional status on productivity have also been investigated. In World War II, during periods of caloric restriction, Kraut and Muller (1946) studied the influence of caloric deficiency or supplementation on the work output of workers in German industries. The productivity of one group of laborers, measured as tons of material moved per hr., improved 47% when caloric intake was increased 480 Cal·24 Hr^{-1}. Another group (coal miners) receiving 2800 Cal·24 Hr^{-1} and producing 7 tons per day per man increased their output to 9.6 tons when 400 extra Cal·24 Hr^{-1} were allowed for each man. Brooks et al. (1979) have shown that the nutritional status of Kenyan road workers was related to productivity. The time to complete 3 standard work tasks (wheelbarrow work, ditch digging, and earth excavation) was related to weight for height as the indicator of nutritional status. The lower the weight for height below the reference population, the longer the time (lower the productivity) for task completion. Also, Wolgemuth et al. (1982) have reported that successful dietary supplementation resulted in a statistically significant increase in worker productivity in road building, associated with increases in arm circumference and Hb levels.

In order to present more clearly the ideas discussed above and those to be discussed in relation to children, some theoretical conceptualization is necessary. Figure 16 shows imaginary data for normally nourished individuals with $\dot{V}O_2$ max values which differ for whatever reasons: genetic endowment, age, physical condition, etc. Also presented is the theoretical cost of some work task in terms of $\dot{V}O_2$. In the case of subject No. 1, this would represent 50% of his $\dot{V}O_2$ max, 60% of max in subject No. 2, and 75% of max in No. 3. An undernourished subject with severely reduced $\dot{V}O_2$ max (Barac-Nieto et al. 1978a) is also shown, in whom the work task might be 100% of his $\dot{V}O_2$ max. As already mentioned, up to 35-40% of the $\dot{V}O_2$ max can be

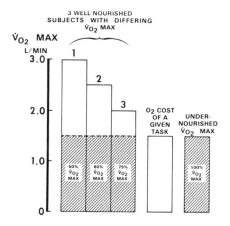

FIGURE 16: Theoretical data for 3 nutritionally normal subjects showing the relative work load of a given task in comparison to an undernourished individual. (Spurr 1983)

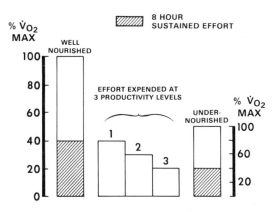

FIGURE 17: Theoretical data for a nutritionally normal subject (left scale) and an undernourished individual (shortened right scale to indicate reduced total $\dot{V}O_2$ max; see Fig. 8) showing effect on supposed productivity (no scale) of each subject working at the 40% maximum which can be sustained for 8 hours. (Spurr 1983)

sustained for an 8-hr work day (Astrand 1967b; Michael et al. 1961; Spurr et al. 1975) in individuals in good physical condition. Figure 17 attempts to show the relationship between the relative load sustained ($\%\dot{V}O_2$ max) and productivity in hard physical work. A well nourished subject willing to work at 40% of his $\dot{V}O_2$ max for 8 hours might have the highest productivity level while the lower productivity levels 2 and 3 would be achieved working at 30 and 20% of $\dot{V}O_2$ max, respectively. An undernourished subject is also shown at the right with a shortened scale of % $\dot{V}O_2$ max to indicate the reduced total $\dot{V}O_2$ max (Figure 15). Such a person, even utilizing the full 40% of his max for the 8 hours of work, would be able to produce only at the lowest level. Consequently, the undernourished with reduced work capacity cannot produce as much as the well-nourished. It must be emphasized that these concepts apply only to moderate to heavy physical labor and do not take into account the complexity of the work function and factors such as motivation, the work environment, or the advantage that small size might have in some work situations where body translation is involved (Viteri et al. 1981). However, since in the developing world the majority of the adult male work force is engaged in moderate to heavy work (Arteaga 1976; United Nations 1980), the implications for economic development are obvious (Berg 1973). Productivity in the more sedentary occupations has not been studied, if indeed it is measurable.

In gauging the effects of marginal malnutrition on adult productivity, how can these concepts be applied to the results obtained on rural children? Figure 18 presents the results of the measurements of $\dot{V}O_2$ max ($l \cdot min^{-1}$) in the nutritionally normal and W-H rural boys in terms of the O_2 cost of a task arbitrarily selected to be 40% of the maximum of the N group. The same task would represent 52% of $\dot{V}O_2$ max of the undernourished group and, therefore, a relatively more difficult work load which could be sustained for a shorter period with less productive results. With reduction in the total $\dot{V}O_2$ max ($l \cdot min^{-1}$) of adults, due either to malnutrition or restricted body size, the absolute level of energy expenditure ($\dot{V}O_2$) available to the worker at 40% of his $\dot{V}O_2$ max is likewise less and productivity is reduced. The worker may try to compensate by working in excess of 40% $\dot{V}O_2$ max but at a cost of more frequent rest stops or a shorter work day. The extrapolation of the $\dot{V}O_2$ max data on these rural children

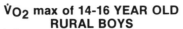

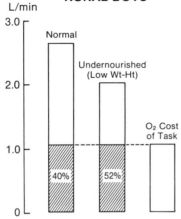

FIGURE 18: Average $\dot{V}O_2$ max of normal and low weight for height 14-16 yr old rural boys showing the relative work load in the latter of a task selected to be 40% of the $\dot{V}O_2$ max of the nutritionally normal group.

to their work potential as adults would seem to be justified from two standpoints. First, the growth spurt in the N boys had peaked and was at about peak by 15 years of age (Spurr et al. 1983b) when a significant difference between the N and W-H boys still existed (Figure 12). Thus, even with pubertal development, there is no apparent recovery in $\dot{V}O_2$ max in the nutritionally deprived group. Secondly, the curves in Figure 12 appear to be diverging when considering the N and W-H boys. This is supported by a statistically significant age-nutrition group interaction (F = 7.57; P <0.001) between N and W-H groups. It is impossible to state whether or not some sort of catch-up in $\dot{V}O_2$ max will not occur in the intervening years between this study and adulthood, but it seems unlikely in view of the small size of Latin-American adults (Figure 1).

In summary, there is a significant correlation between nutritional status and $\dot{V}O_2$ max and between the latter and work productivity. These observations, together with those of a number of other investigators, make it clear that poor nutritional status will result in low productivity in hard work. Chronic, marginal malnutrition in rural boys, with concomitant reduction in body size, augurs poorly for the physical work capacity and productivity of those who will engage in moderate to heavy physical work as adults. The data relating body size to productivity in both hard and moderate work also make it clear that bigger is better.

SUMMARY

In the developing countries of the world, where mechanization is at a minimum, agricultural workers make up a large percentage of the labor force. They are faced with a precarious supply of energy, and sometimes of protein, to fuel their productivity in work tasks which demand a high level of energy expenditure. Frequently the agricultural worker, either because of poor nutrition in childhood and a smaller adult body size and/or an inadequate diet in adulthood, finds himself disadvantaged in his ability to produce to his full potential had neither of these situations existed. Furthermore, the reduced energy available above the minimum required to sustain life, is largely expended in work tasks leaving little extra for those activities which might lead to a better quality of life for him and his family. Studies which have been carried out to date on the subject of "productivity," agricultural or otherwise, have been concerned almost exclusively with men. Despite the fact that in some cultures women are the primary food producers or gatherers, practically nothing is known about the added energy drains of child bearing and rearing on those variables which influence the work ability of women. In urban societies, the mother's energies may also have to be divided between the need to provide income and the care of the family. Studies on the physiological adjustment of women to malnutrition and physical work, therefore, might provide very useful information on human adaptability.

Agricultural productivity, like the productivity of other occupations which involve moderate to heavy physical work, is directly related to the physical work capacity of the individual, measured as the $\dot{V}O_2$ max. This physiological variable is related to body size (muscle mass), age, and sex and can be influenced by the degree of physical training (habitual activity) and nutritional status. There are also interrelations between habitual activity and nutritional status (or nutritional intake) so that a tripartite relationship exists among daily activity, nutritional status, and physical work capacity. The latter is the final common pathway which affects productivity in moderate to heavy physical work.

There is no question about the positive effect of physical training on PWC, and it is the subject of an enormous scientific literature. However, the influence of occupational activity on $\dot{V}O_2$ max is less clearly defined and is based largely on the negative changes which occur when individuals or populations become more sedentary in their life style. Few data exist on changes in physical work capacity when occupational intensity is increased over relatively long periods of time and at levels below those which produce a training effect ($> 50\%$ $\dot{V}O_2$ max). The scarcity of information on this question is related to the fact that the upward mobility so eagerly sought by most populations is associated with a decrease in labor intensity. Consequently, it may not be possible to carry out such studies except under laboratory conditions and only then with dedicated subjects and scientists.

A number of sources make it clear that malnutrition is associated with lower levels of daily energy expenditure both in terms of reduced BMR and habitual physical activity. Presumably this is an adaptive response which is protective of the individual in the face of reduced energy intake. With the exception of the studies made in Guatemala, the quantitation of the relationship under free-living conditions leaves much to be desired. Ideally, studies of malnutrition and habitual activity, in addition to the physiologic components such as fatigue, endocrinological and circulatory responses to work, state of muscle tissue, etc., should also include measurements of the psychological drives which motivate people to increase their activity under the adverse conditions in which poor nutrition exists. The difficulties of successfully carrying out such studies are obvious, but the research should be possible using the multi-disciplinary approach so common in recent years. Young and Torún (1981) have already called for investigations into the requirements for amino acids and total proteins in connection with the effects of chronic increases in habitual activity. How these might differ in malnourished subjects remains to be determined.

The effects of both acute and chronic malnutrition on physical work capacity as measured by $\dot{V}O_2$ max are well established. Poor nutritional status depresses $\dot{V}O_2$ max and the degree of depression is related to the severity of the malnutrition. The influence of mineral and vitamin deficiencies, as distinct from protein and calories, on work capacity remains to be determined although preliminary data indicate that a relationship does exist. The careful studies which are needed will probably have to be carried out in laboratory animals because of the complex nature of naturally occurring malnutrition.

The data available at the moment indicate that the reduced work capacity ($\dot{V}O_2$ max, $1 \cdot min^{-1}$) of both malnourished adults and marginally undernourished children is largely the result of reduced total muscle mass and not of a functional deficit in the skeletal muscle itself. Studies of malnourished animals however, have demonstrated a decrease in oxidative enzymes, and studies of hospitalized patients with undernutrition have shown reduced muscle function indicating deficiencies in energy liberation. Furthermore, studies by the author and colleagues on the endurance times at 80% $\dot{V}O_2$ max of chronically malnourished men do not show a relationship with the degree of nutritional compromise. This may be a result of the wide variability in the results of such studies. However, the surprising decrease in endurance times observed in severely malnourished subjects during dietary repletion is still unexplained. The whole question of the physiology of prolonged work in the malnourished remains to be investigated. Although these studies would be difficult to perform they would increase understanding of the physiological adaptation made by malnourished humans surviving under difficult environmental conditions. Such information might also improve knowledge of how best to supply the nutritional needs of the deprived.

Another question which arises is the effect that physical exercise training might have on the recuperation of malnourished adults during nutritional repletion. This is an important issue, particularly in view of the results obtained in Guatemala on the effect of increased physical activity in improving growth of children undergoing treatment for malnutrition. It may be that exercise coupled with dietary repletion will hasten an otherwise slow recuperation process and improve the quality of performance of the individual upon recovery. The association of chronic, severe malnutrition with the occurrence of cardiac myopathies and higher heart rates at relative submaximal work loads raises a question about circulatory responses, particularly cardiac output, to work and exercise and, indeed, about the degree of recuperation possible in these patients.

Finally, it is clear that agricultural or other types of productivity which involve heavy physical work are related to physical work capacity and body size. Since nutritional deprivation results in reduced work capacity and, when deprivation has occurred during the period of growth, in smaller adults, nutritional status is necessarily related to productivity. From studies in children it is possible to predict that the nutritionally deprived among them will develop into adults with lower working capacities. Obviously, this group is a prime target for nutritional help in developing their full potential as adults. But there is also no question that adult workers can benefit from improved nutrition in terms of productivity, to say nothing of the quality of life.

ACKNOWLEDGEMENTS

The original research from our laboratory which is reported here has been supported by Contract Nos. AID/CSD 1943 and AID/TA-C 1424 from the Office of Nutrition of the Agency for International Development, N.I.H. Grant No. HD10814, the Research Service, Wood V.A. Medical Center and the Fundación para la Educación Superior, Cali, Colombia. The work could not have been done without the collaboration of Mario Barac-Nieto, M.D., Ph.D., in all of the studies; M.G. Maksud, Ph.D., in the studies on adults; and Julio Cesar Reina, M.D., in the studies on children. The association with these investigators has been particularly rewarding. My gratitude is also expressed to Ms Therese Gauthier for her careful attention to detail in the typing of the manuscript.

REFERENCES

1.   Aghemo P, Limas FP and Sassi G (1971). Maximal aerobic power in primitive Indians. Int Z Angew Physiol 29:337-342.

2. Allen JG (1966). Aerobic capacity and physiologic fitness of Australian men. Ergonomics 9:485-94.

3. Andersen K (1964). Physical fitness - studies of healthy men and women in Norway. In Jokl E and Simon E (eds): "International Research in Sport and Physical Education," Springfield, IL: C.C. Thomas.

4. Apfelbaum M (1978). Adaptation to changes in caloric intake. Prog Fd Nutrition Sci 2:543-559.

5. Araujo J, Sanchez G, Gutierrez J and Perez F (1970). Cardiomyopathies of obscure origin in Cali, Colombia: clinical, etiologic and laboratory aspects. Am Heart J 80:162-170.

6. Areskog N-H, Selinus R and Vahlquist B (1969): Physical work capacity and nutritional status in Ethiopian male children and young adults. Am J Clin Nut 22:471-479.

7. Arteaga LA (1976). The nutritional status of Latin American adults. Basic Life Sci 7:67-76.

8. Astrand I (1967a). Aerobic working capacity in men and women in some professions. Forsvarsmedicin 3:163-166.

9. Astrand I (1967b). Degree of strain during building work as related to individual aerobic capacity. Ergonomics 10:293-303.

10. Astrand P-O and Rodahl K (1977). "Textbook of Work Physiology." New York: McGraw-Hill.

11. Awad el Karim MA, Sukkar MY, Collins KJ and Dore C (1981). The working capacity of rural, urban and service personnel in the Sudan. Ergonomics 24:945-952.

12. Banerjee B and Saha N (1970). Energy cost of some common daily activities of active tropical male and female subjects. J Appl Physiol 29:200-203.

13. Barac-Nieto M, Spurr GB, Maksud MG and Lotero H (1978a). Aerobic work capacity in chronically under-nourished adult males. J Appl Physiol:Respirat Environ Exercise Physiol 44:209-215.

14. Barac-Nieto M, Spurr GB, Lotero H and Maksud MG (1978b). Body composition in chronic undernutrition. Am J Clin Nut 31:23-40.

15. Barac-Nieto M, Spurr GB, Lotero H, Maksud MG and Dahners HW (1979). Body composition during nutritional repletion of severly undernourished men. Am J Clin Nut 32:981-991.

16. Barac-Nieto M, Spurr GB, Dahners HW and Maksud MG (1980). Aerobic work capacity and endurance during

nutritional repletion of severely undernourished men. Am J Clin Nut 33:2268-2275.

17. Benedict FG, Miles WR, Roth P and Smith HM (1919). Human Vitality and Efficiency under Prolonged Restricted Diet. Washington DC: (Publ No 280): Carnegie Inst.

18. Berg A (1973). "The Nutrition Factor. Its Role in National Development." Washington DC: The Brookings Inst.

19. Bergstrom J, Hermansen L, Hultman E and Saltin B (1967). Diet, muscle glycogen and physical performance. Acta Physiol Scand 71:140-150.

20. Brooks RM, Latham MC and Crompton DWT (1979). The relationship of nutrition and health to worker productivity in Kenya. E African Med J 56:413-421.

21. Brozek J, Grande F, Taylor HL, Anderson JT and Buzkirk ER (1957). Changes in body weight and body dimensions in men performing work on a low calorie carbohydrate diet. J Appl Physiol 10:412-420.

22. Brozek J (1963). Body Composition. Ann NY Acad Sci 110:1-1018.

23. Brun TA, Geissler CA, Mirbagheri I, Hormozdiary H, Bastani J and Hedayat H (1979). The energy expenditure of Iranian agriculture workers. Am J Clin Nut 32:2154-2161.

24. Buskirk E and Taylor HL (1957). Maximal oxygen intake and its relation to body composition, with special reference to chronic physical activity and obesity. J Appl Physiol 11:72-78.

25. Buzina R (1981). Marginal malnutrition and its functional consequences in industrialized societies. Prog Clin and Biol Res 77:285-303.

26. Consolazio CF, Nelson RA, Johnson HL, Matoush LO, Krzywicki HJ and Isaac GH (1967a). Metabolic aspects of acute starvation in normal humans: Performance and cardiovascular evaluation. Am J Clin Nut 20:684-693.

27. Consolazio CF, Matoush LO, Johnson HL, Nelson RA and Krzywicki HJ (1967b). Metabolic aspects of acute starvation in normal humans (10 days). Am J Clin Nut 20:672-683.

28. Correa P, Restrepo C, Garcia C and Quiroz A (1963). Pathology of heart diseases of undetermined etiology which occur in Cali, Colombia. Am Heart J 66:534-593.

29. Cotes JE, Berry G, Burkinshaw L, Davies CTM, Hall AM, Jones PRM and Knibbs AV (1973). Cardiac frequency during submaximal exercise in young adults; relation to lean body mass, total body potassium and amount of leg muscle. Quart J Exper Physiol 58:239-250.

30. Cumming GR and Bailey G (1974). Seasonal variation of cardiorespiratory fitness of grain farmers. J Occup Med 16:91-93.

31. Davies CTM (1973a). Physiological responses to exercise in East African children II. The effects of shistosomiasis, anaemia and malnutrition. J Trop Ped and Environ Child Health 19:115-119.

32. Davies CTM (1973b). Relationship of maximum aerobic power output to productivity and absenteeism of East African sugar cane workers. Brit J Industr Med 30:146-154.

33. Davies CTM, Chukweumeka AC and van Haaren JPM (1973). Iron-deficiency anaemia. Its effect on maximum aerobic power and responses to exercise in African males aged 17-40 years. Clin Sci 44:555-562.

34. Davies CTM, Brotherhood JR, Collins KJ, Dore C, Imms F, Musgrove J, Weiner JS, Amin MA, Ismail HM, El Karim M, Omer AHS and Sukkar MY (1976). Energy expenditure and physiological performance of Sudanese cane cutters. Brit J Industr Med 33:181-186.

35. Durnin JVGA (1982). Muscle in sports and medicine - nutrition and muscular performance. Int J Sprts Med 3:52-57.

36. Durnin JVGA and Passmore R (1967). "Energy, Work and Leisure." London: Heinemann.

37. Edgerton VR, Bryant SL, Gillespie CA, and Gardner GW (1972). Iron deficiency anemia and physical peformance and activity of rats. J Nut 102:381-400.

38. Edgerton VR, Gardner GW, Ohira Y, Gunawardena KA and Senewiratne B (1979). Iron deficiency anemia and its effect on worker productivity and activity patterns. Brit Med J 2:1546-1549.

39. Finch CA, Miller LR, Inamdar AR, Person R, Seiler K and Mackler B (1976). Iron deficiency in the rat. Physiological and biochemical studies of muscle dysfunction. J Clin Invest 58:447-453.

40. Gardner GW, Edgerton VR, Barnard JR and Bernauer EM (1975). Cardiorespiratory, hematological and physi-

cal performance responses of anemic subjects to iron treatment. Am J Clin Nut 28:982-988.

41. Gardner GW, Edgerton VR, Senewiratne B, Barnard JR and Ohira Y (1977). Physical work capacity and metabolic stress in subjects with iron deficiency anemia. Am J Clin Nut 30:910-917.

42. Gillanders AD (1951). Nutritional heart disease. Brit Heart J 13:177-196.

43. Gollnick PD, Piehl K, Saubert CW, Armstrong RB and Saltin B (1972). Diet, exercise and glycogen changes in human muscle fibers. J Appl Physiol 33:421-425.

44. Habicht J-P, Martorell R, Yarbrough C, Malina RM and Klein RE (1974). Height and weight standards for pre-school children. How relevant are ethnic differences in growth potential? Lancet 1:611-15.

45. Hanson DL (1967). Influence of the Hawthorne effect upon physical education research. Res Quart 38:723-724.

46. Hanson-Smith FM, Maksud MG and Van Horn DL (1977). Influence of chronic undernutrition on oxygen consumption of rats during exercise. Growth 41:115-121.

47. Hansson JE (1965). The relationship between individual characteristics of the worker and output of logging operations. Studia Forestalia Suecia No 29, Stockholm: Skogshogskolan, pp. 68-77.

48. Henschel A, Taylor HL and Keys A (1954). Performance capacity in acute starvation with hard work. J Appl Physiol 6:624-633.

49. Heymsfield SB, Stevens V, Noel R, McManus C, Smith J and Nixon D (1982). Biochemical composition of muscle in normal and semistarved human subjects: relevance to anthropometric measurements. Am J Clin Nut 36:131-142.

50. ICNND, Interdepartmental Committee on Nutrition for National Defense (1963a) Washington DC. US Gov't Printing Office Nutrition Survey (a) Ecuador: July 1959; (b) Chile: March 1960; (c) Colombia: May 1960; (d) Uruguay: March-April 1962; (e) North East Brazil: May 1963; (f) Venezuela; May 1963.

51. ICNND, Interdepartmental Committee on Nutrition for National Defense (1963b) Manual for Nutrition Surveys (2nd ed.) NIH:Bethesda.

52. Jansen WH (1917). Untersuchungen uber Stickstoffbilanz bei calorienarmer Ernahrung. Deutsch Arch f Klin Med 124:1-37.

53. Jelliffe DB (1966). The assessment of the nutritional status of the community. WHO Monograph Ser No 53: Geneva.
54. Johnson RE, Brouha L and Darling RC (1942). A test of physical fitness for strenuous exertion. Rev Canad Biol 1:491-503.
55. Keys A, Brozek J, Henschel A, Mickelsen O, and Taylor HL (1950). "The Biology of Human Starvation." Minneapolis: Univ Minn Press.
56. Keys A and Brozek J (1953). Body fat in adult man. Physiol Rev 33:245-325.
57. Koziol BJ, Ohira H, Edgerton VR and Simpson DR (1982). Changes in work tolerance associated with metabolic and physiologic adjustment to moderate and severe iron deficiency anemia. Am J Clin Nut 36:830-839.
58. Kozlowski S, Kirschner H, Kaminski A and Starnowski R (1969). The relationship between the predicted maximum oxygen uptake and the age of the workers employed in various professions. Polish Med J 8:1303-11.
59. Kraut HA and Muller EA (1946). Calorie intake and industrial output. Science 104:495-497.
60. Lohman TG, Boileau RA and Massey BH (1975). Prediction of lean body mass in young boys from skinfold thickness and body weight. Human Biol 47:245-262.
61. Lopes J, Russell DM, Whitwell J and Jeejeebhoy KN (1982). Skeletal muscle function in malnutrition. Am J Clin Nut 36:602-610.
62. Lukaski HC, Bolonchuk WW, Klevay LM, Milne DB and Sandstead HH (1983). Maximal oxygen consumption as related to magnesium, copper and zinc nutriture. Am J Clin Nut 37:407-415.
63. Lusk G (1921). The physiologic effects of undernutrition. Physiol Rev 1:523-552.
64. Maksud MG, Spurr GB and Barac-Nieto M (1976). The aerobic power of several groups of laborers in Colombia and the United States. Europ J Appl Physiol 35:173-182.
65. Malina RM (1980). The measurement of body composition. In Johnston FE, Roche AF and Sussan C (eds): "Human Physical Growth and Maturation: Methodologies and Factors," New York: Plenum, pp 35-49.
66. Martorell R, Lechtig A, Yarbrough C, Delgado H and Klein RE (1978). Small stature in developing nations:

Its causes and implications. In Margen S and Ogar RA (eds): "Progress in Human Nutrition, Vol 2," Westport, Conn: Avi Pub Co., pp 142-156.

67. Mayer J, Roy P and Metra KP (1956). Relation between caloric intake, body weight and physical work: Studies in an industrial male population in West Bengal. Am J Clin Nut 4:169-175.

68. Michael ED, Hutton KE and Horvath SM (1961). Cardiorespiratory responses during prolonged exercise. J Appl Physiol 16:997-1000.

69. Miller GJ, Cotes JE, Hall AM, Salvosa CB and Ashworth A (1972). Lung function and exercise performance of healthy Caribbean men and women of African ethnic origin. Quart J Exper Physiol 57:325-341.

70. Moore FD, Oleson KH, McMurrey JD, Parker HV, Ball MR and Boyden CM (1963). "The Body Cell Mass and Its Supporting Environment." Philadelphia: Saunders.

71. Morrison JF and Blake GTW (1974). Physiological observations on cane cutters. Europ J Appl Physiol 33:247-254.

72. Myrhage R and Hudlicka O (1978). Capillary growth in chronically stimulated adult skeletal muscle as studied by intravital microscopy and histological methods in rabbits and rats. Microvasc Res 16:73-90.

73. Ojikutu RO, Fox RH, Davies CTM and Davies TW (1972). Heat and exercise tolerance of rural and urban groups in Nigeria. In Vorster DJM (ed): "Human Biology of Environmental Change," London: Unwin Bros Ltd, pp 132-144.

74. Ohira Y, Kosiol BJ, Edgerton VR and Brooks GA (1981). Oxygen consumption and work capacity in iron-deficient anemic rats. J Nut 111:17-25.

75. Parizkova J (1977). "Body Fat and Physical Fitness." The Hague: Martinus Nijhoff BV.

76. Phillips PG (1954). The metabolic cost of common West African agricultural activities. J Trop Med Hyg 57:12-20.

77. Pollock ML, Wilmore JH and Fox SM (1978). "Health and Fitness Through Physical Activity." New York: John Wiley.

78. Raju NV (1974). Effect of early malnutrition on muscle function and metabolism in rats. Life Sci 15:949-960.

79. Ramana Murthy PSV and Belavady B (1966). Energy expenditure and requirement in agricultural labors. Ind J Med Res 54:977-979.

80. Ramana Murthy PSV and Dakshayani R (1962). Energy intake and expenditure in stone cutters. Ind J Med Res 50:804-809.

81. Reina JC and Spurr GB (1984). Daily activity levels of marginally malnourished school-aged girls: A preliminary report. In Pollitt E and Amante P (eds): "Energy Intake and Activity," New York: Alan R. Liss (In Press).

82. Rode A and Shephard RJ (1973). On the mode of exercise appropriate to an Artic community. Int Z angew Physiol 31:187-196.

83. Rueda-Williamson R, Luna-Jaspe H, Ariza J, Pardo F and Mora JO (1969). Estudio seccional de crecimiento, desarrollo y nutrición en 12,138 niños de Bogota, Colombia. Petriatr 10:337-49.

84. Saltin B, Blomquist G, Mitchell JH, Johnson RL, Wildenthal K and Chapman CB (1968). Response to exercise after bed rest and after training. Circ 38: Suppl 7.

85. Satyanarayana K, Nadamuni Naidu A, Chatterjee B and Narasinga Rao BS (1977). Body size and work output. Am J Clin Nut 30:322-325.

86. Satyanarayana K, Nadamuni Naidu A and Narasinga Rao BS (1978). Nutrition, physical work capacity and work output. J Med Res 68(Suppl): 88-93.

87. Satayanarayana K, Nadamuni Naidu A and Narasinga Rao BS (1979). Nutritional deprivation in childhood and the body size, activity and physical work capacity of young boys. Am J Clin Nut 32:1769-1775.

88. Shephard FJ (1978). "Human Physiological Work Capacity." New York: Cambridge Univ. Press.

89. Simopoulos AP (ed) (1982). Assessment of nutritional status. Am J Clin Nut 35:1089-1325.

90. Smil V (1979). Energy flows in the developing world. Amer Sci 67:522-531.

91. Spurr GB (1983). Nutritional status and physical work capacity. Yearbook of Physical Anthropology 26:1-34.

92. Spurr GB, Barac-Nieto M and Maksud MG (1975). Energy expenditure cutting sugar cane. J Appl Physiol 39:990-996.

93. Spurr GB, Maksud MG and Barac-Nieto M (1977a). Energy expenditure, productivity, and physical work

capacity of sugar cane loaders. Am J Clin Nut 30:1740-1746.

94. Spurr GB, Barac-Nieto M and Maksud MG (1977b). Productivity and maximal oxygen consumption in sugar cane cutters. Am J Clin Nut 30:316-321.

95. Spurr GB, Barac-Nieto M and Maksud MG (1977c). Efficiency and daily work effort in sugar cane cutters. Brit J Industr Med 34:137-141.

96. Spurr GB, Barac-Nieto M and Maksud MG (1978). Childhood undernutrition: Implications of adult work capacity and productivity. In Folinsbee LJ, Wagner JA, Borgia JF, Drinkwater BL, Gliner JA and Bedi JF (eds): "Environmental Stress: Individual Human Adaptations," New York: Academic Press, pp 165-181.

97. Spurr GB, Barac-Nieto M, and Maksud MG (1979). Functional assessment of nutritional status: heart rate response to submaximal work. Am J Clin Nut 32:767-778.

98. Spurr GB, Barac-Nieto N, Lotero H and Dahners HW (1981). Comparisons of body fat estimated from total body water and skinfold thicknesses of undernourished men. Am J Clin Nut 34:1944-1953.

99. Spurr GB, Reina JC, Barac-Nieto M and Maksud MG (1982). Maximum oxygen consumption of nutritionally normal white, mestizo and black Columbian boys 6-16 years of age. Human Biol 54:553-574.

100. Spurr GB, Reina JC, Dahners HW and Barac-Nieto M (1983a): Marginal malnutrition in school-aged Colombian boys: Functional consequences in maximum exercise. Am J Clin Nut 37:834-847.

101. Spurr GB, Reina JC and Barac-Nieto M (1983). Marginal malnutrition in school-aged Colombian boys: Anthropometry and maturation. Am J Clin Nut 37:119-132.

102. Stuart HC and Meredith H (1964). "Nelson's Textbook of Pediatrics (8th ed)." Philadelphia: Saunders.

103. Tasker K and Tulpule PG (1964). Influence of protein and calorie deficiencies in the rat on the energy-transfer reactions of the striated muscle. Biochem J 29:391-398.

104. Taylor HL, Buskirk ER, Brozek J, Anderson JT and Grande F (1957). Performance capacity and effects of caloric restriction with hard physical work on young men. J Appl Physiol 10:421-429.

105. Taylor HL, Henschel A, Mickelsen O, and Keys A (1954). Some effects of acute starvation with hard

work on body weight, body fluids and metabolism. J Appl Physiol 6:613-623.

106. Thomson AM (1968). The later results in man of malnutrition early in life. In McCance RA and Widdowson EM (eds): "Calorie Deficiencies and Protein Deficiencies," Boston: Little Brown, pp 289-299.

107. Torún B (1984). Physiological measurements of activity among children under free living conditions. In Pollitt E and Amante P (eds): "Energy Intake and Activity," New York: Alan R. Liss (In Press).

108. Torún B and Viteri FE (1981). Unpublished results quoted in Ref. 122.

109. United Nations (1980). Demographic Year Book (1979) Dept. Internat Econ and Social Affairs. New York: United Nations.

110. Van Graan CH, Wyndham CH, Strydom NB and Grayson JS (1972). Determination of the physical work capacities of urban and rural Venda males. In Vorster DJM (ed): "Human Biology of Environmental Change," London: Unwin Bros., Ltd., pp. 129-131.

111. Viteri FE (1971). Considerations on the effect of nutrition on the body composition and physical working capacity of young Guatemalan adults. In Scrimshaw NS and Altshull AM (eds): "Amino Acid Fortification of Protein Foods," Cambridge Mass: MIT Press, pp 350-375.

112. Viteri FE, Alvarado J, Luthringer DG and Wood RP (1968). Hematological changes in protein calorie malnutrition. Vitamins and Hormones 26:573-615.

113. Viteri FE and Torún B (1973): Anemia and physical work capacity. Clin in Haematol 3:609-626.

114. Viteri FE and Torun B (1975). Ingestion calorica y trabajo fisico de obreros agricolas en Guatemala. Efecto de la suplementacion alimentaria y su lugar en los programs de salud. Bol Of Sanit Panamer 78:58-74.

115. Viteri FE, Torún B, Galicia JC and Herreta E (1971). Determining energy costs of agricultural activities by respirometer and energy balance techniques. Am J Clin Nut 24:1418-1430.

116. Viteri FE, Torún B, Immink MDC and Flores R (1981). Marginal malnutrition and working capacity. In: Harper AE and Davis GK (eds): Nutrition in Health and Disease and International Development, New York: Alan R Liss, pp 277-283.

117. Wolgemuth JC, Latham MC, Hall A, Chester A and Crompton DWT (1982). Worker productivity and the nutritional status of Kenyan road construction laborers. Am J Clin Nut 36:68-78.
118. Wyndham CH (1966). Southern African adaptation to temperature and exercise. In Baker PT and Weiner JS (eds): "The Biology of Human Adaptability," Oxford: Clarendon Press, pp 201-244.
119. Wyndham CH, Strydom NB, Leary WP, Williams CG and Morrison JF (1966). Studies of maximum capacity of men for physical effort. Part III. The effects on the maximum oxygen intake of young males of a regime of regular exercise and an adequate diet. Int Z Angew Physiol 22:304-310.
120. Wyndham CH, Strydom NB, Morrison JF, Peter J, Maritz JS and Ward JS (1962). Influence of a stable diet and regular work on body weight and capacity for exercise of African mine recruits. Ergonomics 5:435-444.
121. Young VR (1981). Skeletal muscle and whole-body protein metabolism in relation to exercise. Internat Ser Sports Sci 11A:59-74 .
122. Young VR and Torún B (1981). Physical activity: Impact on protein and amino acid metabolism and implications for nutritional requirements. Prog Clin Biol Res 77:57-85.

Energy Intake and Activity, pages 263–283

DAILY ACTIVITY LEVEL OF MARGINALLY MALNOURISHED
SCHOOL-AGED GIRLS: A PRELIMINARY REPORT

J.C. Reina and G.B. Spurr

Departamento de Pediatría, División de Salúd
Universidad del Valle; Cali, Colombia

Department of Physiology, Medical College of
Wisconsin; Milwaukee, WI 53226

INTRODUCTION

It has been estimated that in developing countries 80-90% of the pre-school children in the poor segments of the populations are malnourished (Reddy 1981). While estimates of the incidence of undernutrition in school-aged children in the same population do not seem to be available, it is clear from studies in Colombia (Spurr et al. 1983a; 1983b) that a large segment is at least marginally malnourished, or has been through a period of nutritional deprivation earlier in life which has curtailed their normal growth pattern.

In recent years a number of studies have focused on determination of daily energy expenditure in normal children. Study methods have included time budget and questionnaire techniques (Leighton et al. 1981; Rutenfranz et al. 1974; Satyanarayana et al. 1979; Seliger et al. 1974) and, in free ranging children, the heart rate recording method (Cunningham et al. 1981; Gilliam et al. 1981; Griffiths et al. 1976; Spady 1980; Warnold and Lenner 1977). The latter was described in great detail in a symposium on the assessment of typical daily energy expenditure (Bradfield 1971). However, there have been few attempts to assess daily energy expenditure in malnourished children. Chavez and Martinez (1979) observed that undernourished pre-school children were more passive than similar children who were receiving nutritional supple-

mentation. Although preliminary attempts have been made
(Heywood and Latham 1971), there appear to be only two
studies which attempt to document this reduction in
daily energy expenditure in malnourished pre-school children, and only one which has attempted to relate activity to
nutritional status in school-aged children. Rutishauser and
Whitehead (1972) reported that many young Ugandan children (1-3 yrs. of age), on energy intakes 70% or less of
recommended levels, were able to gain weight and height at
rates similar to those of children on much higher energy
intakes. These data suggested that less energy intake was
required for growth in these children. Pradilla (1981) has
raised a question about the appropriateness of existing
recommended daily allowances based on similar considerations. Alternatively, because Ugandan children appeared to
be less active than European children (Welbourn 1955),
Rutishauser and Whitehead (1972) suggested that the former
were compensating for their reduced intakes by concomi-
tantly reducing their daily energy expenditures. Indeed,
measurements of daily activity, using a diary technique,
indicated that Ugandan children with reduced intakes spent
significantly less time than European children in activities
involving relatively high rates of energy expenditure, such
as walking and running (Rutishauser and Whitehead 1972).
Viteri and Torun (1981) also reported decreased spontaneous physical activity in preschool children associated with
reduced energy intake. The results of a study by
Satyanarayana et al. (1979), in undernourished teen-aged
boys, showed a statistically significant positive, low level
correlation ($r = 0.38$) between physical activity status and
body weight. Habitual physical activity in their studies
was determined by questionnaire.

The studies to be discussed were undertaken because
of the general lack of information on daily physical activity
in undernourished school-aged children. The data presented here are preliminary in nature, and are the result of the
first round of measurements in an ongoing study. They
include measurements of anthropometry, basal metabolic rate
(BMR), daily energy expenditure, and maximum oxygen
consumption (VO_2 max).

METHODS

The methodology common to all the above mentioned measurements is presented in this section. That peculiar to each variable is presented under the appropriate heading. All of the laboratory measurements were made in a mobile, air-conditioned unit constructed in a 30-foot truck-trailer. Contacts were made with the parents through the neighborhood public schools. After explanation of the purpose of the study, informed consent was obtained in every case.

Subject Selection and Groups

All subjects were girls selected from volunteers in 2 schools located within 5 blocks of each other, in the same economically deprived neighborhood of Cali, Colombia. The subjects were classified as control or undernourished based on their achieved weight for age and weight for height in comparison to the data of Rueda-Williamson et al. (1969) for the reference population, upper socioeconomic children in Bogota. Those who fell in the range 95-110% of these norms for weight for age and height were classified as nutritionally normal and served as the control subjects (n=27). Those who were < 95% of the reference population for both weight for age and height were considered to be currently undernourished (n=22). These girls all attended one school while the control subjects attended the other. The two groups were separated in this manner because the experimental design called for the opening of a school restaurant in one school to supply extra calories to the undernourished subjects. This supplementation program occurred after the results reported here.

Following selection for inclusion in the study, every child underwent a thorough physical examination which included a 12 lead resting electrocardiogram and medical history by a team pediatrician. Any acute disease or condition (cardiac, cardiorespiratory musculo-skeletal or hypertensive) which might interfere with a subject's performance on the treadmill during the testing for maximum oxygen consumption resulted in exclusion from the study and, where indicated, referral to a physician or neighborhood medical clinic.

Anthropometry, Hemoglobin, and Hematocrit

    Body weights were obtained on a Homs beam balance
($\pm$25 gm) with the subject wearing a pair of shorts and a
light blouse, and heights were measured as described
previously (Spurr et al. 1983). Triceps, subscapular and
abdominal (right of umbilicus) were taken in triplicate with
a Lange Skinfold Calipers. Mid-upper arm and head circumference measurements were made with a flexible tape
measure. The same two trained observers made all anthropometric measurements throughout the study. Mid-arm
muscle area was calculated from triceps skinfold and
mid-upper arm circumference as described by Frisancho
(1974). The DuBois (1916) formula was used to calculate
the body surface area.

    Blood hemoglobin and hematocrit values were obtained
on finger-tip blood using the cyanmethemoglobin and
microhematocrit techniques, respectively.

Pulmonary Ventilation ($\dot{V}_E$), Oxygen Consumption ($\dot{V}O_2$),
Carbon Dioxide Production ($\dot{V}CO_2$) and Heart Rate (f_H)

    These variables were determined in several of the
procedures to be described. $\dot{V}_E$ was measured by means of
a Parkinson-Cowan Dry Gas Meter (Model CD-4). $\dot{V}O_2$ and
$\dot{V}CO_2$ were calculated from $\dot{V}_E$ and the concentrations of O_2
and CO_2 obtained from a mixing chamber in the expiratory
line. A Costill-Wilmore sampling device and Beckman Gas
Analyzers (OM-14 and LB-2, respectively) were used.
These analyzers were calibrated with gases standardized by
the Scholander technique. During the exercise testing of
the subjects in the laboratory, heart rates were recorded
on a Gilson Recorder using precordial lead CM_5.

Statistical Analysis

    Unless otherwise indicated the data are presented as
means $\pm$ standard deviation in the text, and as means $\pm$
standard errors of the mean in the illustrations. Comparisons between groups were done simply on the basis of
unpaired Student "t" analyses. The null hypothesis was
rejected at the 0.05 level of probability.

RESULTS AND DISCUSSION

Nutritional Status

The averaged data of age, weight and height for the control and undernourished girls are presented in Figure 1. The average age of the two groups was the same, 9.6 yrs. The undernourished girls weighed significantly less and were shorter than the controls. This is a reflection of the process of selection. The data for weight and height were compared to the Colombian data of Rueda-Williamson et al. (1969) and to those of the U.S. National Center for Health Statistics (NCHS). The control subjects were about 100% of Colombian norms for weight and height for age, and about 94 and 99%, respectively, of the NCHS norms. In weight for height the nutritionally normal girls were 98% of U.S. norms and about 97% of the norms for the reference population. In weight for age the undernourished girls were 81% of the Colombian normative data and 76% of the NCHS figures, in height for age they were 96 and 93%, and in weight for height, 88 and 92% respectively. The group averages of the control subjects for weight and height for age, and weight for height, were on or only slightly below the 50th percentile for NCHS data. In the case of the

Physical Characteristics

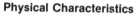

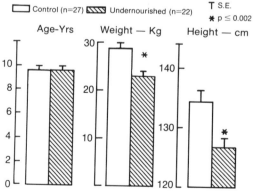

FIGURE 1. Average age, weight and height of nutritionally normal (control) and marginally undernourished girls.

undernourished girls, height for age fell on the 5th percentile, weight for age below the 5th percentile and weight for height below the 25th percentile of the NCHS data curves.

Other anthropometric measures which delineate the nutritional status of the two groups of girls are summarized in Figure 2 and compared to reference populations of North American children. The control girls were 97-101% of the 50th percentile values of the reference populations where these are available (Frisancho 1974; McCammon 1970). The undernourished girls had values for all measures which were significantly less (p<0.001) than the control subjects and whose values varied from 76 to 96% of the reference populations. Consequently, from the results of the anthropometric measures, there is no doubt about the retarded growth of the undernourished girls (Figures 1,2), or about the latter having less subcutaneous fat and muscle mass, as indicated from the skinfold measurements and estimates of upper arm muscle area. These results are similar to those

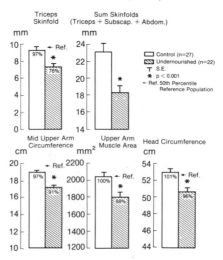

FIGURE 2. Nutritional anthropometry in control and marginally malnourished school-aged girls. The 50th percentile reference standards for triceps skinfold, mid-upper arm circumference and muscle area are from Frisancho (1974) and head circumference from McCammon (1970). Percentages in bars are observed/reference standard.

reported from studies of boys recruited from the same socioeconomic circumstances and point to the existence of a state of marginal malnutrition (Spurr et al. 1983).

The results of the analyses for blood Hemoglobin (Hb) and hematocrit showed that the control and undernourished girls had an average Hb of 13.5 ± 1.0 and 13.3 ± 0.6 $g \cdot dl^{-1}$, respectively, and hematocrit of 41.7 ± 2.6 and $40 \pm 1.8\%$. There was no statistically significant difference in hemoglobin, but the lower value for hematocrit in the nutritionally deprived group of girls was statistically significant ($t=2.70$; $p=0.01$). The Hb values fell on the 50th percentile of the data presented by Garn et al. (1981) for American females. Although there is a statistically significant difference between control and undernourished girls in the value for hematocrit, it is difficult to make any case for a physiological significance because of its small magnitude, and the two groups of girls are considered to be normal in regard to the O_2 carrying capacity of their blood.

Basal Metabolic Rate

The basal metabolic rate is another aspect of daily energy expenditure which has not been investigated in detail in the school-age population. It is widely accepted that adult undernutrition, even in acute episodes, is accompanied by a reduction in BMR (Benedict et al 1919). Indeed, Apfelbaum (1978) states that every investigator since the turn of the century has found this decrease. In malnourished infants and pre-school children with marasmus or kwashiorkor, various investigators have reported a decreased (Montgomery 1962), increased (Fleming 1921; Talbot 1921), or normal (Monckeberg et al. 1964) basal metabolic rate. It is likely that these discrepancies can be resolved by detailed studies of body composition and/or by measuring BMR at the same stage of disease or recovery (Montgomery 1962). There are few studies of BMR in school-age children. The studies available in the older literature point to a normal BMR, but one which is higher than normal when expressed in terms of body weight, with a gradual reduction as weight is gained during recovery (Blunt et al. 1921; Wang et al. 1926; 1929). In spite of these discrepancies there seems to be a general consensus that, at least in severely malnourished young children, there is depressed metabolic activity (Viteri and Torún 1980; Waterlow and Alleyne 1971).

In the present study BMR was determined, in most cases on two separate days, by having the technical team go to the child's home at 6:30-7:00 a.m. and obtain the requisite data. Parents were instructed not to allow the child to get up or to eat prior to the team's arrival. Usually the child had to be awakened by a team member. After appropriate flushing procedures, a 10 min sample of expired air was collected in a 200 L. meteorological balloon. During the period of collection, duplicate heart rates were obtained by palpation and an aliquot of room air taken in a 50 ml glass syringe. Immediately upon termination of the 10 min collection, duplicate aliquots of the mixed expired air were obtained in syringes for subsequent analysis at the laboratory (0.5-1 hr after data collection). Measurements of resting metabolic rate (RMR) were made in the laboratory with the child seated comfortably. Using 2 min. collection periods, the $\dot{V}O_2$ was measured every 10 min until stable, minimal values were obtained.

The results of the measurements of BMR and RMR are presented in Figure 3 together with the RMR/BMR ratio. The undernourished girls had significantly reduced values for BMR and RMR in terms of Cal·hr^{-1}, but the differences disappeared when expressed in terms of body surface area (Figure 3) or body weight ($Kg^{0.75}$). The BMR in Cal· $24hr^{-1}$ ·$Kg^{-0.75}$ was 89.3 ± 9.2 for the control subjects and 94.2 ± 9.0 for the undernourished girls. The ratio of

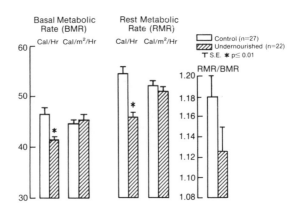

FIGURE 3. Average values of basal and resting metabolic rates and the ratio of the two in control and marginally undernourished school-age girls.

RMR/BMR was 1.18 ± 0.13 and 1.12 ± 0.12 in the 2 groups respectively and, since there was no statistically significant difference in the ratio, the average was 1.15 ± 0.12 when combined. When compared to the norm as estimated by the Harris-Benedict equation (1919) the average % deviation was -1.7% and -6.8% for control and undernourished groups respectively, and there was no statistically significant difference between the 2 groups. In other words, while the BMR (Cal·Hr) was significantly depressed in the under-nourished girls, this was a result of their smaller size (Figures 1-2) and the BMR of both groups was essentially normal.

Daily Energy Expenditure

The estimation of total daily energy expenditure (TDEE) included measurements of BMR, RMR and energy expenditure while the children were engaged in their usual free-ranging activities. The latter is a two-step procedure involving first the calibration of each child and then measurement of the heart rate during the day.

Subject Calibration

Subject calibration was carried out 2.5-3 hrs after the most recent meal as suggested by Schutz et al. (1981). Beginning at a treadmill speed of 1.5 mph and 0° grade, the grade and speed were changed every 2 minutes, and measurements of $\dot{V}O_2$ and f_H were made during the last 30 seconds of each activity period, until an f_H = ~150 was achieved. The f_H and $\dot{V}O_2$ values obtained in the BMR measurement were used as the resting values because of the inordinately high f_H values obtained for rest while in the sitting or standing position (Payne et al. 1971). A typical calibration curve for a subject is shown in Figure 4, to-gether with the average and standard deviations of the slopes and intercepts of the least squares regression lines and the correlation coefficients of the two groups of sub-jects. There were no statistically significant differences in slopes or intercepts between the two subject groups.

Heart Rate Monitoring

Immediately following the termination of the BMR measurement, the precordial bipolar leads for the heart rate monitor (UFI, Moro Bay, CA) were attached. Heart rate recording was begun and the time noted. At the end of the day, close to the girl's bedtime, a member of the technical team again went to the child's home to record the time and the accumulated heart rate. The girl's mother was instructed to note the time the child went to bed. The average $f_H \cdot min^{-1}$ was then calculated for the time of the monitoring and mean $\dot{V}O_2$ obtained from the calibration curve (Figure 4). In converting $\dot{V}O_2$ to caloric expenditure, 4.9 was used as the caloric equivalent for O_2. In 25 cases the TDEE was measured on 2 consecutive days. The average coefficient of variation for these 25 children was 6.8% (S.D. = 5.8).

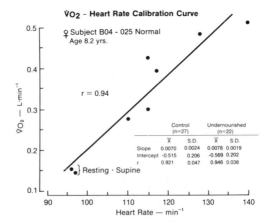

FIGURE 4. Typical calibration curve in one subject with averages of slopes, intercepts and correlation coefficient (r) in control and marginally malnourished school-age girls.

Calculations

The TDEE was then estimated as follows:

$$TDEE = (ST \times BMR) + (MT \times EE) + (ET \times RMR) = Cal \cdot 24 \ hr^{-1}$$

where ST = sleep time (hrs), MT = monitor time on heart beat accumulator, EE = average energy expenditure calculated from the calibration curve (Figure 4) and ET = extra time not accounted for by ST and MT (ST + MT + ET = 24 hrs). Since the time awake (TA) is

$$TA = MT + ET$$

then the maintenance energy expenditure (MEE) is

$$MEE = (ST \times BMR) + (TA \times RMR)$$

and the energy available for activity (EAc) is

$$EAc = TDEE - MEE.$$

The average sleep time was 9.8 ± 0.6 and 9.7 ± 0.5 hrs in the control and undernourished girls respectively. The girls wore the heart monitor for 12-13 hours on each day of measurement of TDEE.

There are few published data with which to compare those obtained on control girls, but some do exist. Using similar techniques to those employed in the present study, Spady (1980) reported the results of measurements of daily energy expenditure in healthy free-ranging Canadian boys and girls 8-11 years of age. Some comparisons with his data are presented in Figure 5. The children in the Colombian study were of approximately the same age, weighed less, and were slightly shorter than the Canadian girls, but there were no statistically significant differences between the two groups. In terms of various parameters of energy expenditure there also were no statistically significant differences in total daily calorie expenditure ($Cal \cdot Kg^{-1} \cdot 24$ Hr^{-1}), or in calories spent in activity above the maintenance level. However, the average f_H during the day was significantly higher (t = 2.07; p = 0.047) in the Colombian (f_H = 109.5 $\pm$ 9.5) than the Canadian girls (f_H = 103.1 $\pm$ 7.5). From the data of Gilliam et al. (1981) it is possible to estimate that the average f_H of their female subjects 7 years of age in Michigan was 105 $\cdot min^{-1}$ during 12 hours of measurement. So the average f_H in the Colombian girls is slightly higher than their North American counterparts. This may be partially related to the altitude. Cali is located 1000m above sea level, and it is known that even resting heart rates are higher in altitude natives (Forster et al. 1974).

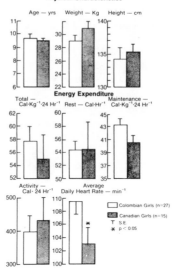

FIGURE 5. Comparison of average values of the control subjects in the present study and those obtained by similar procedures on normal Canadian girls by Spady (1980).

The results of the estimations of TDEE, MEE and EAc are presented in Figure 6. The total daily energy expenditure was 1639 ± 330 Cal·24 Hr^{-1} in the control subjects and 1532 ± 325 Cal·24 Hr^{-1} in the undernourished girls, and the 107 Cal·24 hr^{-1} difference was not statistically significant. The cost of MEE was significantly less in the undernourished girls (p < 0.001), but this was due to the difference in body size since the difference disappeared when the MEE was expressed in terms of body weight (Figure 6). In addition, there were no significant differences between the two groups when EAc and TDEE were expressed in terms of Kg of body weight, although both TDEE and EAc were slightly higher in the undernourished girls. Total calories spent for activity were 422 ± 310 and 496 ± 310 Cal·24 Hr^{-1} for the control and undernourished groups, respectively, compared to 434 ± 218 Cal·24 Hr^{-1} observed by Spady (1980) for his female subjects. In order to get some idea of the applicability of the recommended allowances to the needs of the children, the TDEE was also expressed as a percentage, based on body weight, of the recommended daily energy allowance (Pardo 1981) for these girls

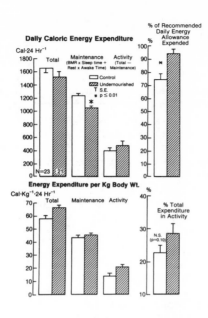

FIGURE 6. Daily energy expenditure values in control and marginally malnourished school-age girls.

(Figure 6). The control girls were expending about 75% of the RDA while the undernourished girls expended 93%. The difference was significant (p < 0.01). It is clear that the RDA's are sufficient for the two groups and that there is a tendency for the undernourished girls to expend more energy when expressed in terms of body weight. The FAO/WHO Expert Committee on Energy and Protein Requirements (1973) estimated that 9-10 year old boys would expend about 26% (640 Cal.) of their caloric intake on activity. In the absence of intake data we have expressed energy expended in activity as percent of total expenditure (Figure 6). This amounted to 23% and 29% for the control and undernourished girls respectively. The difference was not statistically significant. Spady (1980) reported values of 31% and 25% for normal Canadian boys and girls, respectively.

Payne and Waterlow (1971) have pointed out that the daily energy expended for maintenance is remarkably similar in a wide variety of species, including man, when expressed per Kg of body weight to the power of 0.75 ($Kg^{0.75}$). Without regard to sex they found this value to be about 105 $Cal \cdot Kg^{0.75}$. Study values for this variable were 99.3 ± 9.7 and 100.5 ± 8.4 $Cal \cdot Kg^{0.75}$ in the two groups of girls as compared to 95.6 ± 7.5 $Cal \cdot Kg^{0.75}$ in the normal Canadian girls studied by Spady (1980). Payne and Waterlow (1971) further indicated that in the same units the daily BMR of the same animals is 70 $Kg^{0.75}$, so that the ratio of MEE/BMR is 1.5. However, in children the BMR is much higher than 70 $Cal \cdot Kg^{0.75}$ Using Talbot's (1938) table of standard BMR values it is easy to calculate that a girl with a body weight of 29 Kg (the average weight of the study control girls) would have a coefficient of 89.6 $Cal \cdot Kg^{0.75}$ and for a girl of 23.3 Kg (malnourished mean weight), a coefficient of 90.1 $Cal \cdot Kg^{0.75}$; i.e., much higher than the value of 70 for adults. Thus, in young girls of this weight range, the value is about 90 $Cal \cdot Kg^{0.75}$ and, since 105 $Cal \cdot Kg^{0.75}$ seems to be a reasonable value for MEE even in children, the ratio MEE/BMR would be 1.17 rather than 1.50 as in the case of adults (Payne and Waterlow 1971). The ratio for the study data was 1.11 ± 0.08 and 1.08 ± 0.08 $Cal \cdot Kg^{0.75}$ for the control and undernourished girls. These are close to the theoretical value (1.17) for young girls at this age. In any event, there were no statistically significant differences in MEE/$Kg^{0.75}$ or the ratio MEE/BMR between the control/and poorly nourished girls in these preliminary studies.

Two major difficulties are associated with use of the heart beat accumulation method in this study, one concerns quantification of energy expenditure and the other an inability to qualify the kinds or intensities of activities in which the subjects engaged. The use of 24 hr periods of measurement has generally been judged inappropriate because average heart rates for the period are usually only slightly above resting levels (Christensen et al. 1983). In addition, at low heart rates a different relationship appears to exist between heart rate and VO_2 than at the higher heart rates obtained during usual calibration procedures (Warnold and Lenner 1977). For this reason, heart rates were measured only during waking hours in the present study. A question still exists about low heart rates in periods of rest during the day. Gilliam et al. (1981) found that the 7 year old children in their study spent only about 5% of the 12 hr measurement period at heart rates below 80 min^{-1}. Even though their study was carried out during the summer months, when activity levels might be presumed to be higher than while attending school, the average 12 hr heart rates of their female subjects was about 105 min^{-1}, which is quite comparable to the authors' data and well within the applicable linear portion of the calibration curves (Figure 4).

The problem of determining variation in intensity of activities by the heart rate method may be approached by the application of equipment which allows for storage of averaged heart rates every 10, 6 or even one minute during the period of measurement (Baharestani et al. 1979). The kinds of activities in which children participate must still be determined by direct observation.

Maximal Oxygen Consumption

The maximal aerobic power of an individual is measured by the maximum ability to consume oxygen ($\dot{V}O_2$ max) while exercising at sea level (Astrand and Rodahl 1977) and is the best overall measure of an individual's physical condition (Shephard 1978).

The $\dot{V}O_2$ max was measured by the open circuit technique in the air conditioned (22-24°C) mobile laboratory using the modified Balke-Ware (1959) treadmill procedure described previously (Spurr et al. 1983). The results of the maximum exercise testing are shown in Figure 7. The average f_H max values were 208 ± 6 and 204 ± 6 min^{-1} in the control and undernourished girls, respectively. Total $\dot{V}O_2$ max was 1.22 ± 0.16 and 1.01 ± 0.17 L·min^{-1} in the two groups, and the difference was statistically significant (p<0.001). The difference in $\dot{V}O_2$ max disappeared when expressed in terms of body weight (Figure 7).

Except for the magnitude, these results are similar to those reported for nutritionally normal and marginally undernourished boys (Spurr et al. 1983). The reduced total $\dot{V}O_2$ max (L·min^{-1}) is the result of the smaller size of the undernourished girls in comparison to the control subjects.

Boys of the same age as the girls in Figure 7 have an average aerobic power of 57.4 ml·kg^{-1}·min^{-1} (Spurr et al. 1983). Grouping all of the girls in the present study, their average aerobic power is 43.6 ml·kg·min^{-1} or 76% of that found in males (Spurr et al. 1983). This ratio is

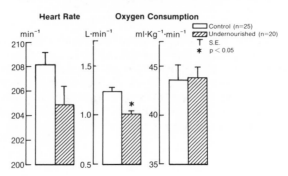

FIGURE 7. Maximum oxygen consumption and heart rate in control and marginally malnourished school-age girls.

similar to the 79% found by Dill et al. (1972) for sedentary American teenagers, and to the 75% reported by Metheny et al. (1942) for non-athletic young adults. Only a part of this difference is due to the difference in body composition of the 2 sexes. For example, in Dill et al. (1972), the aerobic capacity of the female teenage subjects increases to 87% of the males when both are expressed in terms of lean body weight. The remainder is believed to be the result of differences in habitual physical activity, i.e., females are more sedentary than males.

The point of emphasizing these differences in habitual physical activity between boys and girls is that it may be more difficult to detect differences in daily energy expenditure between control and undernourished girls, particularly at the marginal level of malnutrition, when neither group is particularly active. It may be easier to detect such differences, if they exist, in boys whose levels of daily activity are higher (Gilliam et al. 1981; Spady 1980).

SUMMARY

The studies reported here are preliminary and do not permit definitive conclusions of a general nature. The data show that in 22 marginally malnourished girls, the observed reduction in basal metabolic rate and maintenance energy

expenditure is a result of their smaller body size in comparison to 27 nutritionally normal girls of the same average
age (9.6 yrs). Total daily energy expenditure measured by
means of heart rate accumulation in individually calibrated
subjects and the energy expended in physical activity were
not significantly different in the two groups. While not
statistically significant, there was a tendency for the undernourished girls to expend more energy in activities on a
per Kg body weight basis. This lack of significant difference in activity may be the result of peer pressure to keep
up with whatever the cultural standards of the group define
as "normal" activity (school, games, after-school play,
etc.). If a difference in physical activity levels exists in
marginally malnourished children it may not be possible to
reveal such differences with the techniques employed in this
study. Furthermore, the wide variability in the data found
in this preliminary study points to the need for larger
numbers of subjects measured over periods of time longer
than 1-2 days. But before they are abandoned, the
authors believe that it is important to expand these studies
to include older girls and, more importantly, boys. The
reason for the latter is the difference in level of daily
activities. Observations of lower VO_2max values in girls
than boys, described in the study reported here and in
other sources, make it clear that boys are more active than
girls. Consequently, if there is a reduction in physical
activity in marginally malnourished school-age children, as
might be hypothesized from the results obtained in more
severely malnourished pre-school children, it should be
easier to detect in more active groups of subjects.

ACKNOWLEDGMENT

Supported in part by a grant from the United Nations
University; also by the Research Service of the Wood VA
Medical Center and the Fundación para la Educación Superi-
or, Colombia.

REFERENCES

1. Apfelbaum M (1978). Adaptation to changes in caloric
    intake. Prog Fd Nut Sci 2:543-559.
2. Astrand P-O and Rodahl K (1977). "Textbook of Work
    Physiology." New York: McGraw-Hill.

3. Baharestani H, Tomkins WJ and Webster JG (1979). Heart rate recorder. Med Biol Eng and Comput 17:719-723.

4. Balke B and Ware W (1959). An experimental study of physical fitness of Air Force personnel. US Armed Forces Med J 10:675-688.

5. Benedict FG, Miles WR, Roth P and Smith HM (1919). Human Vitality and Efficiency under Prolonged Restricted Diet. Washington DC: Carnegie Institute, Publ No 280.

6. Blunt K, Nelson A and Oleson HC (1921). The basal metabolism of underweight children. J Biol Chem 49:247-262.

7. Bradfield RB (ed) (1971). Assessment of typical daily energy expenditure. Am J Clin Nut 24:1111-1192; 1405-1493.

8. Chavez A and Martinez C (1979). Consequences of insufficient nutrition on child character and behavior. In Levitzky DA (ed): "Malnutrition, Environment and Behavior," Ithaca, NY: Cornell Univ Press, pp. 238-255.

9. Christensen CC, Frey HMM, Foenstelien E, Aadland E, and Refsum HE (1983). A critical evaluation of energy expenditure estimates based on individual O_2 consumption/heart rate curves and average daily heart rate. Am J Clin Nut 37:468-472.

10. Cunningham DA, Stapelton JJ, MacDonald IC and Paterson DH (1981). Daily energy expenditure of young boys as related to maximal aerobic power. Canad J Ap Sport Sci 6:207-211.

11. Dill DB, Myhre LG, Greer SM, Richardon JC and Singleton KG (1972). Body composition and aerobic capacity of youth of both sexes. Med Sci in Sports 4:198-204.

12. DuBois D and DuBois EF (1916). A formula to estimate the approximate surface area if height and weight be known. Arch Interm Med 17:863-867.

13. FAO/WHO Expert Committee (1973). Energy and Protein Requirements FAO, Rome.

14. Fleming GB (1921). An investigation into the metabolism in infantile atrophy, with special reference to the respiratory exchange. Quart J Med 14:171-186.

15. Forster HV, Dempsey JA, Vidruk E, and DoPico G (1974). Evidence of altered regulation of ventilation during exposure to hypoxia. Resp Phys 20:379-392.

16. Frisancho AR (1974). Triceps skin fold and upper arm muscle size norms for assessment of nutritional status. Am J Clin Nut 27:1052-1058.
17. Garn SM, Ryan AS, Abraham S and Owen G (1981). Suggested sex and age appropriate values for "low" and "deficient" hemoglobin levels. Am J Clin Nut 34:1648-51.
18. Gilliam TB, Freedson PS, Geenen DL and Shahraray B (1981). Physical activity patterns determined by heart rate monitoring in 6-7 year old children. Med Sci Sport and Exercise 13:65-67.
19. Griffiths M and Payne PR (1976). Energy expenditure in small children of obese and non-obese parents. Nature 260:698-700.
20. Harris JA and Benedict EG (1919). "A Biometric Study of Basal Metabolism in Man." Washington, DC: Carnegie Inst., Pub No 279.
21. Heywood PF and Latham MC (1971). Use of the SAMI heart-rate integrator in malnourished children. Am J Clin Nut 24:1446-1450.
22. Leighton CK, Shapiro LR, Crawford PB and Huenemann RL (1981). Body composition and physical activity in 8-year-old children. Am J Clin Nut 34:2770-75.
23. McCammon RW (1970). "Human Growth and Development." Springield: CC Thomas.
24. Metheny E, Boruha L, Johnson RE and Forbes WH (1942). Some physiologic responses of men and women to moderate and strenuous exercise: a comparative study. Am J Phys 137:318-326.
25. Monckeberg F, Beag F, Horwitz I, Dabancens A and Gonzalez M (1964). Oxygen consumption in infant malnutrition. Pediatrics 33:554-561.
26. Montgomery RD (1962). Changes in the basal metabolic rate of the malnourished infant and their relation to body composition. J Clin Invest 41:1653-1663.
27. Pardo F (1981). Recommendaciones de Consumo de Calorías y Nutrientes para la Población Colombiana. Programa de Educación Nutr, Bogotá.
28. Payne PR and Waterlow JC (1971). Relative energy requirements for maintenance, growth and physical activity. Lancet 2:210-211.
29. Payne PR, Wheeler EF and Salvosa CB (1971). Prediction of daily energy expenditure from average pulse rate. Am J Clin Nut 24:1164-1170.

30. Pradilla AG (1981). Nutrition interventions: the role of international agencies and the prospectives for the future. In Harper AE and Davis GK (eds): "Nutrition in Health and Disease and International Development," New York: Alan R. Liss, pp. 611-618.

31. Reddy V (1981). Protein energy malnutrition. An overview. In Harper AE and Davis GK (eds): "Nutrition in Health and Disease and International Development," New York: Alan R. Liss, pp. 227-235.

32. Rueda-Williamson R, Luna-Jaspe H, Ariza J, Pardo F, Mora JO (1969). Estudio seccional de crecimiento, desarrollo y nutrición en 12,138 niños de Bogotá, Colombia. Pediatr 10:337-49.

33. Rutenfranz J, Berndt I and Knauth P (1974). Daily physical activity investigated by time budget studies and physical performance capacity of school boys. Acta Ped Belg 28(suppl) 79-86.

34. Rutishauser IHE, and Whitehead RG (1972). Energy intake and expenditure in 1-3 year-old Ugandan children living in a rural environment. Brit J Nut 28:145-152.

35. Satyanarayana K, Nadamuni Naidu A, Narasinya Rao BS (1979). Nutritional deprivation in childhood and the body size, activity and physical work capacity in young boys. Am J Clin Nutr 32:1769-1775.

36. Schutz Y, Bray GA and Margen S (1981). Effect of a meal on the oxygen consumption-heart rate relationship. Am J Clin Nut 34:965-966.

37. Seliger V, Trefny Z, Bartunkova S and Pauer M (1974). The habitual activity and physical fitness of 12 year old boys. Acta Ped Belg 28:(Suppl) 54-59.

38. Shephard RJ (1978). "Human Physiological Work Capacity." Cambridge: Cambridge Univ Press.

39. Spady DW (1980). Total daily energy expenditure of healthy, free ranging school children. Am J Clin Nut 33:766-775.

40. Spurr GB, Reina JC and Barac-Nieto M (1983a). Marginal malnutrition in school-aged Colombian boys: Anthropometry and maturation. Am J Clin Nut 37:119-132.

41. Spurr GB, Reina JC, Dahners HW and Barac-Nieto M (1983b). Marginal malnutrition in school-aged Colombian boys: Functional consequences in maximum exercise. Am J Clin Nut 37:834-847.

42. Talbot FB (1921): Severe infantile malnutrition. Am J Dis Child 22:358-370.

43. Talbot FB (1938). Basal metabolism standards for children. Am J Dis Child 55:455-459.
44. Viteri FE and Torún B (1980). Protein-calorie malnutrition. In Goodhart PS and Shils ME (eds): "Modern Nutrition in Health and Disease (6th ed)," Philadelphia: Lea and Febiger.
45. Viteri FE and Torún B (1981). Nutrition, physical activity and growth. In Ritzen M, Aperia A, Hall K, Larsson A, Zeherberg A and Zeterstrom (eds): "The Biology of Normal Human Growth," NY: Raven Press, pp. 265-273.
46. Wang CC, Kern R, Frank M and Hays BB (1926). Metabolism of undernourished children. II Basal metabolism. Am J Dis Child 32:350-359.
47. Wang CC, Kern B and Kaucher M (1929). Metabolism of undernourished children IX. A study of the basal metabolism, caloric balance and protein metabolism during a period of gain in weight. Am J Dis Child 38:476-480.
48. Warnold I and Lenner RA (1977). Evaluation of the heart rate method to determine the daily energy expenditure in disease. A study in juvenile diabetics. Am J Clin Nut 30:304-315.
49. Waterlow JC and Alleyne GAO (1971). Protein malnutrition in children. Advances in knowledge in the last 10 years. Adv Prot Chem 25:117-241.
50. Welbourn HF (1955). Danger period during weaning; study of Uganda children who were attending child welfare clinics near Kampala, Uganda. J Trop Ped 1:98-111.

Energy Intake and Activity, pages 285–302
© *1984 Alan R. Liss, Inc., 150 Fifth Avenue, New York, NY 10011*

PHYSICAL ACTIVITY AND MOTOR DEVELOPMENT/PERFORMANCE IN POPULATIONS NUTRITIONALLY AT RISK

Robert M. Malina

Department of Anthropology
The University of Texas

Austin, Texas 78712

INTRODUCTION

Physical activities are an essential component of the behavioral repertoire of children and youth, and of many adults. They make up the substrate of performance, i.e., motor tasks, muscular strength, and physiological capacities in energy production and work output. Activities occur in many contexts - at home, during leisure, at work or in school, and in a variety of forms - play, games, sports, subsistence, exercise per se, and so on.

Motor or movement skills are integral to physical activities, and the development and refinement of skillful performance in motor activities is a major developmental task of childhood and youth. Further, it is through the medium of fundamental and special movement patterns and skills that many childhood experiences, especially learning and inter-personal experiences within a specific culture, are mediated.

Many factors influence activity habits and motor performance, including age, sex, size, physique, body composition, health status, nutritional status, and a host of socio-cultural circumstances. This paper focuses only on nutritional status and considers physical activity and motor development/performance in populations nutritionally at risk. The nutritional risk factor is largely dependent upon protein and energy intake and, therefore, is substantial in the majority of developing countries where protein-energy malnutrition (PEM) is prevalent.

ACTIVITY, GROWTH AND MATURATION IN WELL NOURISHED CHILDREN

A certain level of physical activity is apparently necessary to support normal growth, and to maintain functional efficiency and the integrity of bodily tissues. Just how much physical activity is necessary during the growing years is not known with certainty, and individual variation presumably is great. Physical activity, however, is only one of many factors that may affect growth and maturation, so that the precise role of properly graded activity programs in influencing these processes is not completely understood. More detailed discussions of problems in defining and quantifying activity and/or training, study designs, and the effects of activity programs on body size and composition, selected tissues and functions, and biological maturation have been reviewed elsewhere (Malina 1979; 1980; 1983a).

Data on the effect of activity on the growth of children living under poor or marginal nutritional circumstances would be relevant, but such data are unavailable. Under conditions of PEM, for example, bone growth is inhibited and maturation is delayed (Himes 1977), but the response apparently varies with the intensity and timing of the nutritional stress. The superimposition of vigorous physical activity upon such nutritional circumstances may exaggerate the stress. Clinical observations on a sample of Japanese children from an economically poor and nutritionally substandard background (Kato and Ishiko 1966), for example, suggest premature closure of the epiphyses of the lower extremities due to excessive loads carried on the shoulder and resultant stress across the epiphyses. Hence, stature of the children was reduced. Suboptimal nutritional circumstances and excessive physical activity may interact to interfere with skeletal growth.

MOTOR DEVELOPMENT AND PERFORMANCE

The development and refinement of movement capacities are the domain of motor development and performance. Motor development is a continuous process through which a child acquires basic movement patterns and skills. It is a process of modification based upon the interactions of the genetically controlled rate of neuromuscular maturation, residual effects of prior experiences, and new motor experiences. It is a major developmental task of infancy and early childhood, for by six or seven years of age fundamental motor patterns (walk, run, jump, hop, kick, throw, etc.) are ordinarily developed. After these ages, no new basic patterns appear in the child's movement repertoire; rather, the quality of performance continues to improve as the fundamental patterns are refined and integrated into more complex sequences.

Developmental scales used to appraise the mental abilities of infants and preschool children incorporate motor items, several have specific motor subscales, and in a few cases the mental and motor scales are distinct from one another. Such scales are essentially schedules of sensory and motor achievements during the first two years of life. As the child grows older, test items become more specific. In contrast to the developmental emphasis of these scales during in the preschool years, more emphasis is placed on performance during the school ages. Motor performance is viewed in the context of tasks which are performed under specified conditions and which are amenable to more or less precise measurement, e.g., distance an object is thrown, distance jumped, number of errors in a coordination task, amount of force exerted against resistance, and so on. The last mentioned refers to muscular strength, which is a component of the motor performance process. Age trends and sex differences in motor development and performance, and factors which influence motor development and performance, have been presented in more detail elsewhere (Bouchard and Malina, 1983; Malina 1975; 1977;1980b; 1980c; 1982; 1983b).

UNDERNUTRITION AND PHYSICAL ACTIVITY

Clinical descriptions of PEM often indicate reduced levels of, and interest in, physical activities. The same is generally true in animals placed on calorically restricted diets (Elias and Samonds 1974). More specific data on levels of physical activity associated with undernutrition are not extensive. In part this is related to difficulties in quantifying physical activities in field situations.

Chávez and colleagues studied Mexican rural infants who did and did not receive a nutritional supplement. The physical activity index for non-ambulatory infants was based on the frequency of foot contacts with the supporting surface; the index for mobile infants was based on the number of steps taken. They reported significantly reduced levels of physical activity among the children who were unsupplemented but "not clearly malnourished" in contrast to 19 supplemented children, 4 to 24 months of age, from the same peasant community (see Chávez and Martinez, this volume).

Activity differences between the groups was already apparent at four months of age and generally increased with age, reaching a maximum at 24 months of age when the supplemented group was about six times more active than the non-supplemented group. More detailed observations of the children emphasized the role of maternal-child interactions in addition to nutritional and size differences between the two samples. The more active infants and young children made more demands on their mothers, thus increasing the frequency and quality of mother-child interactions and, in turn, the stimuli to further physical activity. The supplemented group also scored consistently higher on motor and adaptive items (largely fine motor tasks) of the Gesell scales. In contrast, mothers of the non-supplemented children seemed limited, more or less, to three kinds of interactions with their children: placing youngsters in a cradle or rocking them, carrying the youngsters on their backs, and holding the youngsters in their arms for feeding (Chávez and Martinez 1975; Chávez et al. 1975). These observations thus suggest a significant role for factors other than nutritional status per se in influencing levels of physical activity in young children.

Generally consistent results have been reported for West Bengali and Nepalese children (Graves 1976; 1978). Youngsters 7 to 18 months of age, classified as undernourished and well-nourished on the basis of anthropometric characteristics, differed in exploratory and vigorous activity. The well-nourished youngsters showed significantly greater activity scores than the undernourished, and also spent significantly more time in play. Maternal behavior varied in the two studies. In the West Bengali study (Graves 1976), mothers of undernourished youngsters showed significantly lower scores for maternal responsiveness and distance interaction,[1] while in the Nepalese study (Graves 1978), maternal behavior was generally similar in both the well-nourished and undernourished groups. The differences may reflect cultural variation in expectations and attitudes. Nevertheless, undernourished youngsters in both studies were less active, showed a greater need for physical closeness to the mother, and had noticeably lower distance interaction scores.

Viteri and Torun (1981) reported markedly reduced levels of activity (e.g., walking, running, tricycling, other games), as assessed by time-motion studies, in six preschool Guatemalan children under conditions of reduced energy intake (with other dietary components and feeding conditions the same). The level of energy intake during the experimental period (70-90 Kcal kg/day) was equivalent to that observed in dietary surveys of Guatemalan preschool children. Similar observations were made on 18 protein-energy supplemented and 18 non-supplemented adult male Guatemalan agricultural workers (Viteri and Torun 1975). At the conclusion of a work period involving similar activities for the two groups, the non-supplemented workers spent most of their time resting and sleeping while the supplemented group engaged in various activities. Under conditions of semi-starvation in the Minnesota experiment (Keys et al. 1950), reduction in physical activity was at least 50%.

A subsequent study of boys 2 to 4 years of age recovering from PEM compared the effects of a six week mild activity program on recovery and growth (Viteri and Torun 1981). The "active" group (n=11) participated in games and other activities which raised the heart rate by approximately 26 beats/minute above resting and required an energy expenditure of 50 Kcal/hour. The "normal" group (n=9) participated in activities requiring very little physical activity, i.e., a mean heart rate about 17 beats/minute above resting levels and an energy expenditure of about 38 Kcal/hour. The "active" group made significantly greater gains in height and in protein repletion over the six week

---

[1]Distancing refers to "...behavior or events which separate the child cognitively from the immediate behavioral environment..." (Graves, 1978, p. 548). It is postulated that distancing contributes to cognitive stimulation and development.

program. The mild activity program apparently contributed in a positive manner to the recovery process. Circumstantial data from three day-care nutrition centers in Guatemala seem to corroborate the preceding. Using as criteria variation among centers in terms of facilities for play and physical activity and mean time to discharge, Viteri and Torun (1981) noted that the time required for discharge from the nutrition centers varied inversely with the opportunity for physical activity.

The observations of the few available studies emphasize the reductions in physical activity with PEM and a favorable role for physical activity in the nutritional recovery process. The data, however, are limited to the preschool ages. If limited energy intake is associated with reduced physical activity in school age children, it may indirectly influence the development of proficiency in motor skills. Reduced physical activity may function to limit and/or prevent the practice of motor skills in play and games, and thus contribute to perceptual-motor and gross motor performance deficiencies. There appears to be, however, more concern for quantifying the energy expenditure of school children living under marginal nutritional conditions than for the quality of activity and movement experiences relevant to the development of proficiency in motor skills.

MOTOR DEVELOPMENT AND PERFORMANCE IN SEVERE PEM

Severely undernourished (marasmus and kwashiorkor) infants and young children usually present delayed psychomotor development, including measures of personal-social, language, adaptive or fine motor, and gross motor responses. This section focuses only on motor responses which are almost universally delayed in severe PEM. Motor development, in general, and the attainment of such motor milestones as sitting, standing alone and walking independently are delayed in severe PEM. Retarded motor development is also one of the constant signs of kwashiorkor (Jelliffe 1966).

The role of organic change in the central nervous system, as it relates to delayed or retarded motor development, requires consideration if a relationship between such changes and neuromuscular development is assumed. Reduced motor nerve conduction velocities are commonly observed in severe PEM (Sachev et al. 1971; Engsner and

Woldemariam 1974; Kumar et al. 1977a), while in healthy, well-nourished children motor nerve conduction velocities improve from birth to three or four years when adult levels are attained. In contrast, some evidence indicates no change in distal latencies in children with PEM (Kumar et al. 1977b). It would appear that severe PEM influences the conduction of impulses along the motor nerve, but does not influence the transmission of impulses at nerve terminals and neuromuscular junctions. Severe PEM apparently influences the process of myelinization and may result in alterations of the myelin sheath (Engsner and Woldemariam 1974; Kumar et al. 1977b).

Changes in the muscular system, the substrate of movement, are also associated with PEM. Evidence indicates a reduction in muscle mass, fiber size, muscle potassium, energy metabolism, estimated "cell" size, and satellite cells in severe PEM (Malina 1978).

It is reasonable to assume that changes in peripheral nerves and muscle tissue on one hand, and motor development on the other, are related. The persistence of the changes associated with PEM most likely varies with the timing, severity and duration of the nutritional stress and may also vary with the system involved. For example, children with kwashiorkor, placed on a nutritional rehabilitation program, showed rapid normalization in motor nerve conduction velocities (Engsner and Woldemariam 1974). On the other hand, studies of severely malnourished children who had undergone subsequent rehabilitation did not show complete recovery in muscle tissue measurements, e.g., estimated "cell" size (Cheek et al. 1970) and fiber size (Hansen-Smith et al. 1979).

Data for motor development after rehabilitation also indicate persistent deficits. In a sample of 200 infants hospitalized for severe undernutrition, Colombo and Lopez (1980) noted, as expected, severely delayed motor development. After nutritional rehabilitation for an average of 180 days, motor development showed no recovery. Follow-up studies, done on the average 180 days after release from the nutritional recovery center, indicated that "... the deficit in the motor area appears as irrecoverable" (p. 76). Celedon and de Andraca (1979) noted similar results. After five months of nutritional and psychological treatment 24 marasmic children, 5 to 19 months of age on admission, made virtually no progress in gross motor performance, while fine motor coordination improved significantly. The authors related these observations to the syndrome of dissociated motor performance, in which gross motor development is delayed while fine motor coordination appears as expected.

Results of nutritional rehabilitation studies must be evaluated carefully. The type of rehabilitation program is important. Pollitt and Granoff (1967), for example, noted more severe motor retardation in youngsters, 11 to 32 months of age, kept in metabolic beds (n=8) compared to those in convalescent units (n=11). A primary difference between the two was in motor activity. Those in the metabolic units were more restricted motorically than those in the convalescent units. These clinical observations should be related to those of Viteri and Torun (1981), who noted a more rapid nutritional recovery in severely malnourished youngsters who were placed on a mild, regular physical activity program. Nevertheless, in the study of Pollitt and Granoff (1967), both groups of youngsters were delayed in motor development after treatment for PEM.

Long term follow-up studies of children hospitalized in the first year of life for severe PEM are variable. Monckeberg (1968), for example, noted that motor development was still retarded three to six years after nutritional recovery in 14 severely malnourished children. Bartel and colleagues (1978), on the other hand, compared the motor performance of 31 urban Soweto children, 6 to 12 years of age, who were hospitalized for kwashiorkor during the first 27 months of life, to that of non-hospitalized siblings and yard-mates of a similar age. The results indicated no significant differences among the three groups. The children did not differ in physical development, but height, weight and age were not statistically controlled in the analysis, and these exert a significant influence on motor performance (Malina 1975). Furthermore there are reasonable sibling similarities in strength and motor performance, and the age difference between siblings influences the correlation (Malina and Mueller 1981).

Hoorweg and Stanfield (1976) reported lower Lincoln-Oseretsky motor development and spatial-perceptual scores in 60 rural Kampala children, 11 to 17 years of age, who were hospitalized for PEM between 8 and 27 months of age. In a group of 20 Cape Town youth followed since hospitalization for undernutrition during infancy, Stoch and Smythe (1976) noted marked deficits in visual-motor perception at 15 to 18 years of age. It may be of interest that all but five of the index cases were living under the same conditions as control subjects, so that the impaired visual-motor perception of the index cases may reflect deficits in the central neurosensory integration level acquired early in life.

The influence of nutritional inadequacy early in life on motor development may be related to the brain growth spurt described by Dobbing and Sands (1973). The spurt is a period of rapid brain growth which begins at about mid-pregnancy and continues through three or four years of age. The extent of the spurt, however, varies with region of the brain, and the unique pattern characteristic of the cerebellum is relevant to motor development. The cerebellum starts its growth spurt later than the other parts of the brain, but completes the spurt earlier, i.e., it is getting its growth faster and over a shorter period of time. Functions of the cerebellum include the development and maintenence of neuromuscular coordination, balance, and muscle tone. Equilibrium reactions (righting reflexes) normally appear between 6 and 12 months of age and aid the child to regain balance when it is lost. These reflexes play an important role in the development of motor control and lead to erect posture, locomotion, and other motor skills. Hence, potential interference with the growth spurt of the cerebellum through prenatal and postnatal nutritional inadequacy may interfere with the development of normal motor control. Studies of adult rats undernourished during most of gestation and all of lactation indicate poor motor performance attributable to impaired motor coordination. The undernourished rats also had smaller cerebella (Lynch et al. 1975). These data suggest a differential vulnerability of the cerebellum to early nutritional stress, with resulting impairments in motor coordination. Implications for the motor development and performance of young children thus seem reasonable.

MOTOR DEVELOPMENT AND PERFORMANCE IN MILD-TO-MODERATE PEM

What level of motor development and performance might we expect for children reared under marginal nutritional circumstances and not hospitalized? It may be safe to assume that this population, which survived an infancy and early childhood of mild-to-moderate PEM, experiences changes in muscle metabolism and mass, and perhaps in neurointegrative processes. These children, who subsequently comprise the school age and eventually the productive adult population, are shorter and lighter than better nourished individuals, have a reduced muscle mass, and reduced working capacity (see Spurr, this volume). Since strength of a muscle is proportional to its cross-sectional area, reduced muscle mass in undernourished individuals results in an absolute reduction in static and dynamic muscular strength (Malina and Buschang, submitted for publication). Dynamic strength (power) underlies performance in many motor tasks, e.g., dashes, jumps, and throws, and involves motor coordination in addition to strength.

There is a reasonably extensive cross-cultural literature which considers motor development during the first two years of life (Freedman 1974; Leiderman et al. 1977; Malina 1977; Freedman and De Boer 1970; Super 1979). After two years of age, the cross-cultural motor data are extremely limited, perhaps reflecting the orientation of the researchers. The focus is largely on cognitive development, mother-child attachment and interaction, caretaking and caregiving practices, etc.; the motor items of the infant scales are less emphasized as they show a reduced correlation with other items in the scales as children get older. Furthermore, the disciplines involved in studies of a cross-cultural nature, e.g., anthropology, psychology, and medicine, generally show little interest in the motor development and performance of children at older ages, and the majority of the normative motor performance research beyond the first two or three years of life is done by physical educators.

The cross-cultural evidence, nevertheless, indicates satisfactory motor development in most groups and precocity in a few during the first year. A developmental lag towards the end of the first year and during the second year is commonly observed in samples from developing areas of the world and is related to the break in continuity of rearing at weaning, the effects of marginal nutritional status, and reduced levels of physical activity. It is also towards the end of the first year and during the second year that stunting in physical growth becomes especially apparent.

Ashem and Janes (1978) and Rocha-Ferreira (1980) reported consistently poorer motor performance in under-nourished preschool children in Ibadan and São Paulo respectively. However, these studies grouped the children into nutritional categories by stature and weight. Thus, given the significant effect of stature and weight on motor performance (Malina 1975), the results are somewhat confounded.

Among rural Guatemalan Ladino children living under conditions of moderate malnutrition, Lasky et al. (1981) considered the relationships of several anthropometric dimensions to scores of children 6, 15 and 24 months of age, on the motor subscale of a Composite Infant Scale. After controlling for length and weight, none of the other anthropometric variables added significantly to describing the variation in motor development at these three ages. Weight appeared to have a greater effect on motor development than length, and for the same length, heavier youngsters tended to perform better than lighter youngsters. In a longitudinal subsample of these Guatemalan infants, earlier measurements of length and weight were not significantly related to motor development once current size was statistically controlled.

Since the growth status of children is related to a number of factors in the child's immediate environment, Lasky et al. (1981) also evaluated the effects on motor development of such factors as gestational age, parity, hypoxia and trauma at birth, socioeconomic status, nutrient intake, parental weights, and morbidity. None of these factors added significantly to the variation in motor performance indicated by the relationship between body size and motor performance.

At older ages, Malina and Buschang (submitted for publication) considered motor performance relative to body size of Zapotec Indian children, 6 to 16 years of age, raised under conditions of chronic mild-to-moderate undernutrition in southern Mexico. Their absolute body size and levels of performance, in tests of running, jumping, throwing and grip strength, were significantly below those for better nourished American children. When motor performance was corrected for the size difference between the undernourished and better nourished samples, i.e., plotted relative to stature or weight rather than age, strength, running, and jumping performance were commensurate with the smaller body size of Zapotec children, especially at the younger ages (6-11 years). At the older ages, performance was considerably poorer than expected for body size. In contrast, performance of the Zapotec children in the ball throw for distance was greater than expected for their reduced body size. It should be emphasized that performance on such motor tests is influenced by motivational factors, and subtle cultural differences may play a significant role.

The pattern of partial correlations between motor performance and age, height, and weight in Zapotec children was similar to that for well-nourished children (Malina 1975). After controlling for the effects of age and weight, stature had a low, positive, significant correlation with performance on three of the tasks in both sexes. When controlling for age and stature, partial correlations between performance and weight existed only for the dash. This indicated a low, significant, negative relationship and seems to suggest, even in moderately malnourished children, a small negative effect of body weight on running speed. Weight had a low, significant, positive correlation with grip strength in both sexes but, after controlling for age and stature, weight correlated with the distance throw only in boys older than 9 years of age. This would seem to emphasize the role of absolute body mass in strength and in power tasks such as ball throwing for distance. The effects of other body dimensions (e.g., specific lengths, breaths, circumferences and skinfolds) on the motor performance of the Zapotec school children were also considered. After removing the effects of age, stature, and weight, other anthropometric dimensions did not add significantly to describing the remaining variation in motor performance. Hence, body size was the significant factor influencing performance of school children living under marginal nutritional circumstances. These observations are consistent with those for rural Guatemalan children, 6-24 months of age (Lasky et al. 1981).

Data for the strength and motor performance of adults reared under marginal nutritional circumstances are quite limited. Grip strength of Zapotec adults from the same community as the children described earlier was absolutely less than that of better nourished adults (Malina et al. 1982). However, when expressed per unit body weight the difference disappeared. For example, in the 20-29 year age group of Zapotec males, mean strength per unit body weight was 0.70 kg/kg and in the 30-39 year age group it was 0.62

kg/kg. Corresponding values for well nourished males in the same age range and calculated from means were 0.71 kg/kg and 0.62 kg/kg, respectively. Among Zapotec women 20 to 29 years of age, mean strength per unit body weight was 0.52 kg/kg, while an estimated value for college age women in the United States based on a different dynamometer was 0.60 kg/kg.

Studies of previously well-nourished adults who underwent an acute period of semi-starvation also show reductions in grip strength. The reduction was 8-9% in the Carnegie Nutrition Laboratory experiment (Benedict et al. 1919), and was more marked, 28% after 24 weeks, in the Minnesota experiment (Keys et al. 1950). After a 12 week nutritional rehabilitation period in the Minnesota experiment, grip strength showed minimal recovery; subjects had recovered about one-third of the strength lost. After 20 weeks recovery in strength was not yet complete; approximately 64% of the starvation loss had been regained. More recently, Wirths (1969) reported an average reduction of about 27-28% in dynamometric strength of the arms and legs in males and females subjected to limited activity (seclusion in a narrow room) and restricted intake of calories and proteins over a period of only two weeks duration.

The subjects of the Minnesota experiment also experienced a significant reduction in speed and coordination of movement, although not as marked as that observed for muscular strength (Keys et al. 1950). After 12 weeks of nutritional rehabilitation, tapping speed recovered completely, while manual speed and two measures of coordination recovered 85%, 53%, and 63%, respectively, of the performance lost during the semi-starvation period.

SUMMARY

Youngsters with severe PEM show changes in peripheral nerves and muscle tissue, the substrate of physical activity and motor performance. Hence, it is no surprise that they show reduced levels of physical activity and delayed motor development. The deficits in motor development and perceptual motor performance incurred early in life persist after nutritional rehabilitation.

Youngsters and adults living under conditions of chronic mild-to-moderate undernutrition also show reduced levels of physical activity, motor performance, and muscular strength. The latter two are related in part to the reduction in body size and muscle mass associated with chronic PEM.

Results of experimental studies of previously well-nourished adults suggest greater deterioration in strength (which is dependent upon the state of the musculature) than in speed and coordination (which are dependent upon central nervous system factors). Although the studies were conducted on individuals who had not been previously exposed to undernutrition, implications for field studies of populations nutritionally at risk are obvious. Periodic bouts of acute nutritional deficiency are probably quite common in the life of individuals from the lower social strata, both urban and rural, of developing countries. The cumulative effects of such acute bouts of nutritional stress, in addition to chronic mild-to-moderate undernutrition, on the growth, development and physical performance of children, and physical performance of adults may be significant.

REFERENCES

1.   Ashem B, Janes MD (1978). Deleterious effects of chronic undernutrition on cognitive abilities. J Child Psychol Psychiat 19:23.
2.   Bartel PR, Griesel RD, Burnett LS, Freiman I, Rosen EU, Geefhuysen J (1978). Long-term effects of kwashiorkor on psychomotor development. S Afr Med J 53:360.
3.   Benedict FG, Miles WR, Roth P, Smith HM (1919). Human vitality and efficiency under prolonged restricted diet. Carnegie Inst Washington Publ No 280.
4.   Bouchard C, Malina RM (1983). Genetics of physiological fitness and motor performance. Ex Sport Sci Rev 11:306.
5.   Celedon JM, de Andraca I (1979). Psychomotor development during treatment of severely marasmic infants. Early Human Dev 3:267.
6.   Chávez A and Martinez C (1984). Behavioral measurements of activity in children and their relation to food intake in a poor community. In Pollitt E and

Amante P (eds): "Energy Intake and Activity," New York: Alan R. Liss. (In press).

7. Chávez A, Martinez C (1975). Nutrition and development of children from poor rural areas. V. Nutrition and behavioral development. Nutr Rep Int 11:477.

8. Chávez A, Martinez C, Bourges H (1972). Nutrition and development of infants from poor rural areas. II. Nutritional level and physical activity. Nutr Rep Int 5:139.

9. Chávez A, Martinez C, Yaschine T (1975). Nutrition, behavioral development, and mother-child interaction in young rural children. Fed Proc 34:1574.

10. Cheek DB, Hill DE, Cordano A, Graham GG (1970). Malnutrition in infancy; changes in muscle and adipose tissue before and after rehabilitation. Pediatr Res 4:135.

11. Colombo M, Lopez I (1980). Evolution of psychomotor development (developmental quotient and areas), in severely undernourished infants submitted to an integral rehabilitation. Pediatr Res 14:76.

12. Dobbing J, Sands J (1973). Quantitative growth and development of human brain. Arch Dis Child 48:757.

13. Elias MF, Samonds KW (1974). Exploratory behavior and activity of infant monkeys during nutritional and rearing restriction. Am J Clin Nutr 27:458.

14. Engsner G, Woldemariam T (1974). Motor nerve conduction velocity in marasmus and in kwashiorkor. Neuropadiatrie 5:34.

15. Freedman DG (1974). "Human Infancy: An Evolutionary Perspective." New York: Wiley.

16. Freedman DG, DeBoer MM (1979). Biological and cultural differences in early child development. Ann Rev Anthropol 8:579.

17. Graves PL (1976). Nutrition, infant behavior, and maternal characteristics: a pilot study in West Bengal, India. Am J Clin Nutr 29:305.

18. Graves PL (1978). Nutrition and infant behavior: a replication study in the Katmandu Valley, Nepal. Am J Clin Nutr 31:541.

19. Hansen-Smith FM, Picou D, Golden MH (1979). Growth of muscle fibers during recovery from severe malnutrition in Jamaican infants. Br J Nutr 41:175.

20. Himes JH (1978). Bone growth and development in protein-calorie malnutrition. Wld Rev Nutr Diet 28:143.

21. Hoorweg J, Stanfield JP (1976). The effects of protein energy malnutrition in early childhood on intellectual

and motor abilities in later childhood and adolescence. Dev Med Child Neurol 18:330.

22. Jelliffe DB (1966). "Assessment of the Nutritional Status of the Community." Geneva: World Health Organization.

23. Kato S, Ishiko T (1966). Obstructed growth of children's bones due to excessive labor in remote corners. In Kato K (ed): "Proceeding of International Congress of Sport Sciences," Tokyo: Japanese Union of Sport Sciences, p 479.

24. Keys A, Brozek J, Henschel A, Mickelsen O, Taylor HL (1950). "The Biology of Human Starvation." Minneapolis: University of Minnesota Press.

25. Kumar A, Ghai OP, Singh N (1977a). Delayed nerve conduction velocities in children with protein-calorie malnutrition. J Pediatr 90:149.

26. Kumar A, Ghai OP, Singh N (1977b). Failure of marasmus and kwashiorkor to affect distal latencies in infancy and childhood. Dev Med Child Neurol 19:790.

27. Lasky RE, Klein RE, Yarbrough C, Engle PL, Lechtig A, Martorell R (1981). The relationship between physical growth and infant behavioral development in rural Guatemala. Child Dev 52:219.

28. Leiderman PH, Tulkin SR, Rosenfeld A (eds): (1977). "Culture and Infancy: Variations in the Human Experience." New York: Academic Press.

29. Lynch A, Smart JL, Dobbing J (1975). Motor coordination and cerebellar size in adult rats undernourished in early life. Brain Res 83:249.

30. Malina RM (1975). Anthropometric correlates of strength and motor performance. Ex Sport Sci Rev 3:249.

31. Malina RM (1977). Motor development in a cross-cultural perspective. In Landers DM, Christina RW (eds): "Psychology of Motor Behavior and Sport. Volume II. Sport Psychology and Motor Development," Champaign, Illinois: Human Kinetics Publishers, p 191.

32. Malina RM (1978). Growth of muscle tissue and muscle mass. In Falkner F, Tanner JM (eds): Human Growth. 2. Postnatal Growth," New York: Plenum, p. 273.

33. Malina RM (1979). The effects of exercise on specific tissues, dimensions, and functions during growth. Stud Phys Anthropol 5:21.

34. Malina RM (1980a). Physical activity, growth, and functional capacity. In Johnston FE, Roche AF,

Susanne C (eds): "Human Physical Growth and Maturation: Methodologies and Factors," New York: Plenum,
p 303.
35. Malina RM (1980b). Biosocial correlates of motor development during infancy and early childhood. In Greene
LS, Johnston FE (eds): "Social and Biological Predictors of Nutritional Status, Physical Growth, and Neuro-
logical Development," New York: Academic Press,
p 143.
36. Malina RM (1980c). Growth, strength, and physical
performance. In Stull GA (ed): "Encyclopedia of
Physical Eduction, Fitness, and Sports: Training,
Environment, Nutrition and Fitness," Salt Lake City:
Brighton, p 443.
37. Malina RM (1982). Motor development in the early
years. In Moore SG, Cooper CR (eds): "The Young
Child: Reviews of Research," Washington, DC: National Association for the Education of Young Children,
p 211.
38. Malina RM (1983a). Human growth, maturation, and
regular physical activity. Acta Med Auxol 15:5
39. Malina RM (1983b). Socio-cultural influences on physical activity and performance. Bull Soc Roy Belge
Anthrop Prehist 94:155.
40. Malina RM, Buschang PH (submitted for publication).
Growth, strength and motor performance of children
living under conditions of mild-to-moderate
undernutrition.
41. Malina RM, Buschang PH, Aronson WL, Selby HA
(1982). Aging in selected anthropometric dimensions in
a rural Zapotec-speaking community in the Valley of
Oaxaca, Mexico. Soc Sci Med 16:217.
42. Malina RM, Mueller WH (1981). Genetic and environmental influences on the strength and motor performance of Philadelphia school children. Hum Biol 53:163.
43. Monckeberg F (1968). Effect of early marasmic malnutrition on subsequent physical and psychological development. In Scrimshaw NS, Gordon JE (eds):
Malnutrition, Learning, and Behavior," Cambridge,
Mass: MIT Press, p 269.
44. Pollitt E, Granoff D (1967). Mental and motor development of Peruvian children treated for severe malnutrition. Rev Interam Psicol 1:93.
45. Rocha-Ferreira MB (1980). "Estado Nutricional e
Aptidao Fisica em Pre-Escolares," Master's Thesis,
University of Sao Paulo.

46. Sachdev KK, Taori GM, Pereira SM (1971). Neuromuscular status in protein-calorie malnutrition. Neurology 21:801.
47. Spurr GB (1984). Physical activity, nutritional status, and physical work capacity in relation to agricultural productivity. In Pollitt E and Amante P (eds): "Energy Intake and Activity," New York: Alan R. Liss. (In press)
48. Stoch MB, Smythe PM (1976). 15-year developmental study on effects of severe undernutrition during infancy on subsequent physical growth and intellectual functioning. Arch Dis Child 51:327.
49. Super CM (1979). Behavioral development in infancy. In Munroe RL, Munroe RH, Whiting BB (eds): "Handbook of Cross-Cultural Human Development," New York: Garland Press.
50. Viteri FE, Torún B (1975). Ingestion calorica y trabajo fisico de obreros agricolas en Guatemala. Bol Of Sanit Panam 78:58.
51. Viteri FE, Torún B (1981). Nutrition, physical activity, and growth. In Ritzen M, Aperia A, Hall K, Larsson A, Zetterberg A, Zeterstrom R (eds): "The Biology of Normal Human Growth," New York: Raven Press, p 265.
52. Wirths W (1969). Muskelfunktionsprunfungen mit Hilfe von Dynamometermessungen unter Einfluss mangelnder Aktivitat und restriktiver Calorien-und Eiweissaufnahme. Int Z Angew Physiol 27:116.

Energy Intake and Activity, pages 303–321
© *1984 Alan R. Liss, Inc., 150 Fifth Avenue, New York, NY 10011*

BEHAVIORAL MEASUREMENTS OF ACTIVITY IN CHILDREN
AND THEIR RELATION TO FOOD INTAKE
IN A POOR COMMUNITY

Adolfo Chávez and Celia Martinez

Instituto Nacional de Nutrición Mexico
Mexico 140, Tlalpan D.F., Mexico

INTRODUCTION

A large portion of those engaged in manual labor in
developing countries suffer nutritional deficiencies. This
results in a paradox in which those with the greatest need
for energy have the least access to it. This population
works in the primary sector of the economy, and their
efficiency depends on the socio-economic development of the
country. It is important, therefore, to define the functional consequences of specific nutritional problems, in terms of
general malnutrition or specific nutrient deficiencies, in
order to safeguard the health and well-being of individuals
and to clarify cost-benefit equations relating to nutritional
intervention programs.

Several studies indicate that deficient diets, especially
where anemia is present and where the diet is low in energy, decrease work productivity (Basta et al. 1974; Spurr
1982; Viteri et al. 1981), but the malnutrition-work productivity relationship continues to be poorly defined. The
difficulty of measuring both factors of the relationship with
precision, and the presence of number of intermediate
variables which are characteristic of underdevelopment, add
confusion of the equation. It is clear that limitations in
natural resources may be the main restrictions on operating
at full capacity (Correa 1969).

Low productive yields among poorly nourished populations do not necessarily imply a direct relationship between

low energy intake and low work output. The process of adaptation may be in operation, i.e., those who survive malnutrition in early life acquire certain metabolic and social characteristics related to energy saving. These characteristics can result in a cycle of deficient productivity, low earnings, insufficient food consumption and, consequently, limited energy output.

This adaptation to low intake also may be transgenerational in nature and have cultural and genetic components as well. In populations demonstrating severe nutritional limitations, those with the greater adaptive capacity have certain advantages. Undoubtedly, the most apt survive, but these are not necessarily the strongest, the most active, or those with greatest capacity for growth. Rather, they are most probably those who have the greatest endurance, who are most resistant to scarcity, and who have the greatest ability to economize nutrients; that is, those who do not grow, who develop slowly, and who do not expend energy needlessly. There must also be a cultural adaptation that, from generation to generation, selects survivors from the most intense periods of deprivation as well as from periods of seasonal hunger. Those who are habituated to saving energy also are able to transmit these protective mechanisms to succeeding generations. In Mexico the well known figure of a man, wearing a sombrero and a serape, sleeping with his head on his knees, is probably the best representation of this "cultural adaptation" to low energy consumption. Those who maintain such a pose during periods of hunger or dry seasons, when there is no productive work available, have a greater likelihood of survival than those who are active.

STUDY DESCRIPTION

In 1968 the authors initiated a study in a small, poor, agricultural community to establish the relationship between food consumption and behavior in early life (Chávez and Martinez 1981a). The hypotheses were that the level of energy consumption determines the activity level of the child, and that the role of activity is much wider than had been thought previously, and could be the principal mediating factor between nutrition and behavior (Chávez and Martinez 1973).

Food supplementation was administered to one group while the control group continued in its normal state. Children born in 1968 have been observed longitudinally and without modification, and have been fed according to the customs of the town. Thus, for 8 to 10 months they received breast milk only, after which time the mothers provided modest quantities of supplementary feeding, mainly maize products. The women who became pregnant during 1969 received a milk based supplement of 350 calories a day beginning on the 45th day of pregnancy. Subsequently, the children of these women began receiving good quality supplementary feeding between the third and fourth month of life, in quantities comparable to those of a child from an urban family.

Measurement of Food Consumption

Both variables, food consumption and physical activity of young children in free living conditions, are difficult to measure: consumption because of maternal breast feeding, and activity because of long periods of sleep and short periods of non-directed activity.

Lactation was measured longitudinally during a period of 72 consecutive hours, by determining the difference in the weight of the child before and after each breast feeding (Martinez and Chávez 1982). These measurements were recorded at 2,8,16,24, and 36 weeks, and at 13 and 18 months of age. In each case and in each of the surveys, every time a child sought the mother's breast a waterproof diaper was placed on him, and he was weighed on a precision scale. After the feeding he was again weighed and the difference was regarded as the amount of the child's consumption or the mother's production.

Studies of Physical Activity

While the lactation studies were carried out, observations were made of activity, behavior, and mother-child interaction. The dietary survey was the vehicle for having the observer in the house; the time the researcher waited between feedings was used for observation. Several methods were used, most of them based on time samplings. Children were observed in open field tests; time-motion

observations of mothers were made over 12 hour periods;
and, more recently, a combination of observation-
interrogation was used.

Systematic Observation Samplings of 10 Minutes every
Hour. This method was designed for young children who
sleep for various periods during the day. A period of
10 minutes during an hour was selected at random, and
this was systematically repeated 12 times during the
subsequent hours in order to gather information covering
120 minutes. For example, if the initial observation was
from 7:20 to 7:30 am, subsequent observations took place
at the same portion of every hour from then until 6:20-6:30
pm. The number of contacts with the surface of support
was the main indicator of activity level (Chávez et al.
1972). Observations were made by a specially trained
aide who was present every hour and used a manual counter
to record the number of times one of the child's feet
touched the bed, the crib, the ground, the mat, etc.

Periodic instantaneous samplings. These observations
were designed to document mother-child interaction. They
covered a period of 90 minutes each in the morning and
afternoon, and during these periods observations were
recorded every 30 seconds. An aide positioned herself so
that she could observe the child unobtrusively and, while
appearing to read a book, she made notations. Every 30
seconds she looked up and, like a camera, captured a scene
(mother-child interaction, activity of mother or child, or
specific behavior characteristics). She then made a nota-
tion on a sheet containing a list of expected activities. In
this project the list contained 17 areas into which
mother-child interaction activities were divided (Chávez et
al. 1975).

A variant of this method was used to define the activities of the children of school age while they were in class.
A type of periscope was inserted in a wall and was focused
on the child to be observed. Resorting to momentary
observations, notations were made recording the number of
times the child was found to be asleep, playing, fighting,
distracted, etc. (Chávez and Martinez 1981b).

Random samplings in time. During the day random
minutes were selected and observations made of the activity
being carried on by the individual or family. This method,

although less precise, is easier. It was designed to evaluate the father's presence in the house and, to a certian degree, his activity (Chávez and Martinez 1975).

Open field tests. The "field" used for these tests was 3 meters square and was ringed by railing 60 cm high. The floor had lines 30 cm apart drawn in each direction, like the pattern on a chess board. Upon beginning a test, the child was placed in the center of the square, the mother on one side, toys on another side, and two observers on the third and fourth sides. Using forms on which the pattern of the square was drawn, the observers marked the path of the child's movements during two consecutive sessions of ten minutes each. This procedure measures level of activity by evaluating the number of times the child crosses lines while either crawling or walking (Chávez et al. 1974). At the same time, it measures other behavior characteristics such as dependence on or independence from the mother. This is indicated by the number of times the child crosses lines in the area near the mother compared with its movements in the area near the toys or near the observers. This method offers other possibilities for observation since the system allows for the expression of several behavior characteristics in addition to those noted here (Viteri et al. 1981).

Time-Motion Studies. This format was used to observe the activities of the mother throughout the day. The subject was followed during 12 non-consecutive hours. Observations were made for three to four hours and, when the mother or the aide became tired, the observations were discontinued. On the following day the observations began again at the hour they had stopped on the previous day. The aide, who had received special training, described each activity; subsequently, the activities were categorized by specialized personnel (Martinez and Chávez 1982).

At the present time another study is being carried out on the subject of functional manifestations of malnutrition. It is experimenting with a similar method, but interrogation is also being included. That is, there is an observation period and a question period during which previous activities, including the time, are defined. In a pilot sampling of 30 women evaluated through a 48 hour quantitative diet survey (Allen et al. 1982 this method had a correlation (r) of 0.61 between intensity of activity and energy consumption. There is now a program to evaluate this system using longitudinal monitoring of pulse frequency.

Levels of Calorie-Protein Consumption

Difference in nutrient consumption between the two groups of children grew progressively divergent a few months after birth. In the case of most of the non-supplemented mother-child pairs, breast milk consumption/production began to decrease shortly after the third month (Chávez et al. 1975). This decrease reflects the fact that malnourished mothers are unable to increase or even sustain a satisfactory level of milk secretion. Mothers in the supplemented group, on the other hand, maintained a satisfactory level for a slightly longer time (at least four months). At this point, following the program plan, administration of mashed food and bottles ad libitum were initiated.

Figure 1 compares consumption between the non-supplemented and supplemented groups. The upper curves indicate that maternal feeding in the non-supplemented children is insufficient after two or three months, and that inadequate supplementary feeding takes place under customary conditions in the home. This is totally discordant with the increasing necessities of the child. The curves for supplemented children show that consumption is progressive and reaches levels twice as high as the levels for the unsupplemented children. At 18 months of age the non-supplemented children receive about 550 calories, half from mother's milk and the other half from foods, especially maize products. The supplemented children, on the other hand, consume 1120 calories, all from a mixed diet which includes milk.

Differences in protein consumption are even more marked, although they follow the same pattern as caloric consumption. The non-supplemented children show a drop after reaching a maximum peak of production-consumption of mother's milk, and because of the poor quality of the other foods given to them, do not recuperate well until the 18th month. In the supplemented group, protein consumption may even be described as excessive; because of the administration of cow's milk, it reaches almost 50 g a day at 18 months of age.

**Figure 1 The calorie-protein consumption of non-supplemented
children increases very slowly in comparison with
supplemented children.**

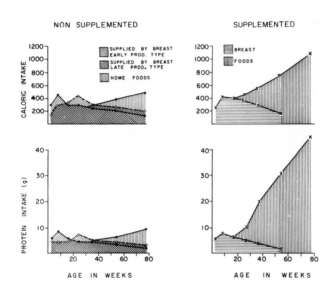

Intensity of Physical Activity

As a consequence of the difference in levels of consumption, there are undoubtedly great differences in physical activity between the two groups (Figure 2). During the
first eight months of age no differences were detected, but
when the children began to crawl, the supplemented group
was much more active.   Differences became greater with
time so that by two years of age the supplemented children
were six times more active than the non-supplemented ones
(Chávez et al. 1972). The levels of activity among the
non-supplemented children increased very slowly with age
as compared with the first months of life.   On the other
hand the supplemented children showed a very sharp rise.

Types of Activities

The instantaneous time samplings designed to study
types of activity were done only during daytime hours

Figure 2 Non-supplemented children are much less active since they make fewer foot contacts with the surface of support.

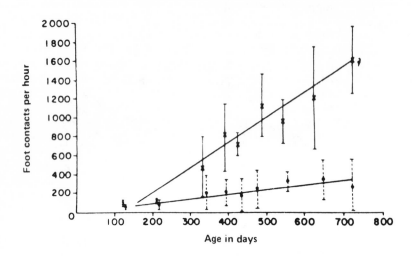

Figure 3 After the 40th week the undernourished child remains in crib more than 10% of the time observed.

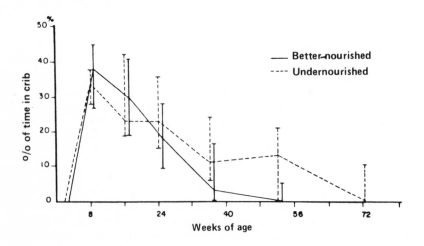

(Chávez and Martinez 1975; 1979; 1981b; Chávez et al. 1974; 1975). Figure 3 indicates that, after the eighth month, the non-supplemented children remain in their cribs for longer periods of time than do the supplemented children; the latter, at this age, spend virtually no time in their cribs. Several factors may influence this situation. The supplemented children, because they are more active, move around more and, in view of the fact that the cribs are small and are hung from the ceiling, a danger is present. Another factor may be related to the length of time that the children sleep. A difference between the groups becomes evident at the age of six months (Figure 4). At one year of age only a few of the supplemented children were asleep occasionally while most of the non-supplemented children were asleep for a considerable amount of time.

Figure 4 The undernourished child sleeps longer during the day; differences from the better-fed children are significant from the age of 6 months.

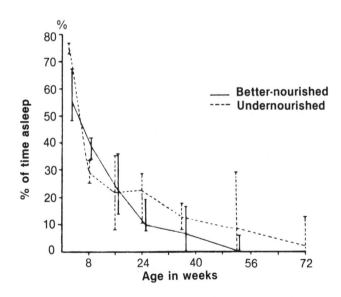

Undoubtedly both factors explain, in part, the differences in the time that the two groups spend outside the house (Figure 5). Beginning at an early age the supplemented children disliked being left inside the house for long

Figure 5 The undernourished child spends more time indoors, especially at about 6 months of age.

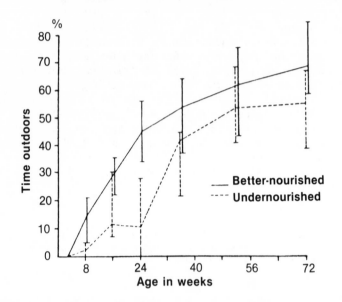

periods of time. These children were found to have a higher body temperature and this may make them feel uncomfortable inside a warm house during the daytime. At a very early age their mothers placed them on mats in the shade outside the house. They were always under the care of an older brother of sister since the children frequently tried to crawl toward the periphery of the house.

It is probable that the same factors that are related to the differences in level of activity and in body temperature influence the differences in the time that both groups are carried on their mothers' backs (Figure 6). Most of the differences that are found between the two groups after 6 months of age are due, to a great extent, to the children themselves. The supplemented children often rejected being wrapped in the mother's shawl and being carried on the mother's back; they frequently kicked or cried, indicating that they were uncomfortable. The supplemented children were also larger, weighed more and, in addition, they frequently moved around a great deal. In contrast, the poorly nourished children liked being tied to the mother

Figure 6 During the second semester of life, the undernourished child is carried on the mother's back for longer periods time. The differences are very noticeable at about 8 months of age.

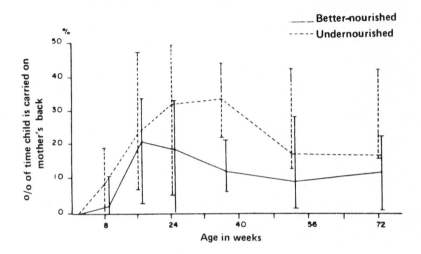

Figure 7 Non-supplemented children begin playing almost six months later than supplemented children. They also exhibit a delay in the appearance of a more elaborate form of play.

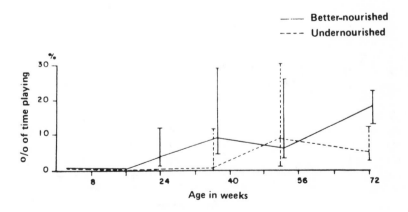

and, in spite of the mother's constant movements, almost always slept when being carried in this way. At the age of 8 to 12 months differences in the children being carried in this manner were three times greater among the non-supplemented than among the supplemented.

The play habits were different in both groups of children (Figure 7). The supplemented children, at the age of 6 months, began a relatively simple form of play, using their crib or the mother's shawl. They soon changed to some other form of play, which they did systematically when they reached the age of one year. In the non-supplemented children, the first form of play appeared late and the second form of play did not appear during the first 18 months of life. Other important differences between the non-supplemented and the supplemented children were the frequency with which each was observed to be babbling (Figure 8) or crying (Figure 9).

The supplemented children progressively increased the noises they made, the beginnings of language. This was clear at one year of age. At no time did the non-supplemented children attempt to do this; rather, they resolved problems by crying. This last feature is very

Figure 8 The undernourished children seldom babble or talk, while the supplemented children do so increasingly from the 40th week on.

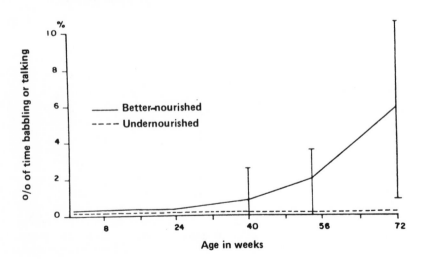

**Figure 9 The non-supplemented children cry more after the 8th
week and especially after the 36th week.**

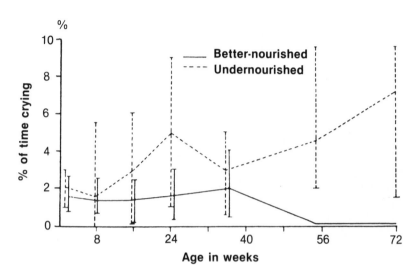

characteristic of non-supplemented children; at about 6
months the non-supplemented children cry a great deal,
probably because of hunger which they certainly must feel.
Later the hunger decreases because malnutrition begins and
leads to anorexia. Eventually the children manifest another
type of crying, which increases progressively until they
reach the age of 18 months. This is undoubtedly related to
psychological phenomena (insecurity and mother dependency) which are characteristic of malnutrition.

Use of open field tests in a portion of the study was
designed to test experimentally, under a regulated situation, the differences between the two groups of children
with regard to their levels of activity and some characteristics in the mother-child relationship. The behavioral differences between the two groups were evident when the
children were placed on the "field" described earlier. Even
at a late age 2 or at 3 years of age, the non-supplemented
children nearly always moved around very little, went
toward the mother, and cried (Figure 10). It was clear
that they felt either fear at finding themselves in a strange
environment, anxiety because the mother was separated
from them, anger because the mothers did not pick them

Figure 10 The undernourished children move toward the mother,
cry, and they do not explore the environment.

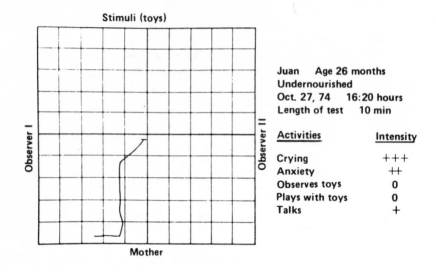

Juan   Age 26 months
Undernourished
Oct. 27, 74   16:20 hours
Length of test   10 min

Activities	Intensity
Crying	+++
Anxiety	++
Observes toys	0
Plays with toys	0
Talks	+

Figure 11 The better-nourished child is more active, seeks the
toys, and talks with the observer.

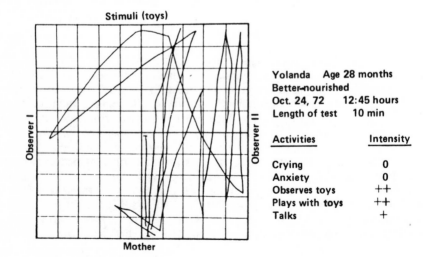

Yolanda   Age 28 months
Better-nourished
Oct. 24, 72   12:45 hours
Length of test   10 min

Activities	Intensity
Crying	0
Anxiety	0
Observes toys	++
Plays with toys	++
Talks	+

up, or a mixture of all these feelings. Moreover, they were not interested in the toys.

The better fed children felt more confident and moved around a great deal beginning at a very early age. It was typical for them to pick up a toy and show it to the mother or to the research aides. Figure 11 illustrates a typical activity pattern for a child from the better nourished group. Comparison of this pattern with that in Figure 10 illustrates the wide differences between the supplemented and non-supplemented groups.

Differences in the classroom behavior of well nourished and poorly nourished school age children was studied effectively using the method of instantaneous samplings every 30 seconds (Table 1) (Chávez and Martinez 1981b). In general, the poorly nourished child is distracted a great deal--three fourths of the time--and spends the rest of the time in passive attitudes, sleeping or writing. This child is active only a small percentage of the time; he is not a participant to any great extent since he spends the time either playing, talking with his classmates, or crying. It

TABLE 1

CLASSROOM BEHAVIOR IN NON-SUPPLEMENTED
AND SUPPLEMENTED CHILDREN

Percent of 3240 observations during first year

Activities Observed	Non-Supplemented	Supplemented
1. Goofing Around	74.5%	48.9%
2. Playing	3.6%	12.7%
3. Being Attentive to the Teacher	3.1%	10.0%
4. Writing or Drawing	6.5%	13.4%
5. Repeating Sentences or Instructions	1.3%	2.6%
6. Asking Questions to the Teacher	0.1%	1.3%
7. Talking to Classmates	2.8%	4.6%
8. Out of Seat	1.3%	7.2%
9. Fighting	0.4	1.0%
10. Asleep	5.7%	0.7%
11. Crying	4.7%	0.6%

is incredible to note that only one of every thirty observations shows the child to be looking at the teacher attentively and that it is even rarer to observe him obeying instructions. In the case of the better nourished child the situation while different, is not very good. This is an indication of the inefficiency of the rural school system. Nevertheless, during at least half the time the better nourished child is doing something. He spends more time than the undernourished child in activities that are characteristic of school activities, but he also spends a great deal of time in activities such as playing and fighting. When the complete picture was analyzed it was found that the poorly nourished child is passive and inactive while the supplemented child is more of a participant, is more interested, and much more restless.

Value of Time Sampling Versus Time-motion Studies

Direct observation methods used to measure physical activity are difficult and imprecise. Prolonged observation often influences subjects' behavior. If observation is combined with questioning, interference may be lessened, but precision is lost. It was out to the ordinary that, in a pilot study using this method, such a high correlation ($r = 0.61$) was found between energy consumption and recall of physical activity (Allen et al. 1982).

Time sampling for intermittent observations are, in reality, indicators, but it is the experience of the authors that they can be both useful and precise. They can be combined with time-motion observations such as those used to quantify the activity of the small children during 10 minute observations periods every hour, or in a periodic instantaneous fashion such as that used to qualitatively define activity by observations made every 30 seconds. Time sampling proved to be ideal when it was used with school age children within the classroom. It was noteworthy how this method was able to differentiate between well and poorly nourished children and, above all, how it was able to define the level and the type of activity. The method also can be structured with lapses of various lengths between observations. For example, random minutes of the day were selected for sampling when the effect of the father's presence in the house, and his relationship with the child, was to be evaluated.

Unfortunately, on a world-wide basis, few publications document the value of time sampling, nor are there comparisons between this system and the time-motion method. The experience of the authors is that time sampling has many possibilities and that the information it provides can attain the same certainty as statistical sampling systems of any other kind. It can also function in a controlled environment; it merely requires creating and standardizing the conditions, something which is not difficult to do with young children. The method identified the significant differences between the supplemented and nonsupplemented groups and facilitated quantification of measures of activity. Until now a similar method has not been attempted among students, adolescents, or adult men and women, but it could be done without great difficulty.

SUMMARY: NUTRITION, PHYSICAL ACTIVITY, AND DEVELOPMENT OF BEHAVIOR

The close relationship between nutrition and activity is clear since modifying nutrition also proportionally modified activity. It is difficult to prove, however, that this change in activity has important effects on performance capacity on mental tests and on other characteristics of behavior. It has long been maintained that malnutrition damages the brain organically or functionally, but this mechanism is doubtful or unimportant when malnutrition is moderate. For this reason many researchers in this area of study have insisted on the view that low performance on mental tests is not the direct consequence of malnutrition, but rather of its always accompanying social deprivation.

This study emphasizes another mechanism, one which is perhaps more important. Malnutrition depresses activity which, in turn, isolates the individual from contact with the environment, from necessary interaction with the mother and the family, and from all sources of stimuli that are of vital importance to the functional development of the brain. A small child, weak and asleep most of the time, to whom virtually no one talks, and with whom almost no one plays, can hardly be expected to achieve optimum development of his abilities.

AKNOWLEDGMENTS

Partially sponsored by National Institutes of Health of U.S. and the Mexican Council of Science and Technology (CONACYT).

REFERENCES

1.   Allen L, Pelto P and Mata A (1982). Preliminary Report on Pilot Group Study. Mimeographed edition. Solis Project, Mexico.
2.   Basta SS, Soekirman, Karyadi C and Scrimshaw NS (1974). Iron deficiency anemia and productivity of adult males in Indonesia. Am J Clin Nutr 32:916-925.
3.   Chávez A and Martinez C (1973). Nutrition and development of children from poor rural areas 111. Maternal nutrition and its consequences in fertility. Nut Rep Intern 7:1.
4.   Chávez A and Martinez C (1975). Nutrition and development of children from poor rural areas III EEE. Nutrition and behavioral development. Nutr Rep Intern 11:477.
5.   Chávez A and Martinez C (1979). Consequences of insufficient nutrition on child character and behavior. In Levitsky DA (ed): "Malnutrition, Environment and Behavior," Ithaca, New York: Cornell University Press, pp 238-256.
6.   Chávez A and Martinez C (1981a). "Growing Up in a Developing Community." Guatemala: INCAP-UNU, pp 5-11.
7.   Chávez A and Martinez C (1981b). School performance of supplemented and unsupplemented children from a poor rural area. In Harper AE and Davis GK (eds): "Nutrition in Health and Disease and International Development," New York: Alan R. Liss, pp 393-402.
8.   Chávez A, Martinez C and Bourges H (1972). Nutrition and development of infants from rural area II. Nutritional level and physical activity. Nutr Rep Intern 5:139.
9.   Chávez A, Martinez C and Bourges H (1975). Role of lactation in the nutrition of low socioeconomic groups. Ecol Food and Nutr 4:159.
10.   Chávez A, Martinez C and Yaschine T (1974). Nutrition, behavioral development and mother-child interaction in young rural children. Fed Proc 34:1575.

11. Chávez A, Martinez C and Yaschine T (1975). Nutrition, behavioral development and mother-child interaction in young rural children. Fed Proc 34:1575.
12. Correa H (1969). Nutrition, working capacity, productivity and economic growth. In: "Proc Western Hemisphere 11," Chicago: AMA, pp 188-192.
13. Martinez C y Chávez A (1982). Proyecto de investigación sobre nutrición materna, lactancia y actividad fisica. Mexico: Edición mimeografiada CONACYT, pp 12-18.
14. Spurr GB (1982). Nutritional status and physical work capacity. Mimeographed Report, Veterans' Administration Medical Center, Wood Wisconsin, USA.
15. Viteri FE, Torun B, Immink MDC and Flores R (1981). Marginal malnutrition and working capacity. In Harper AE and Davis GK (eds): "Nutrition in Health and Disease and International Development," New York: Alan R. Liss, pp 277-283.

Energy Intake and Activity, pages 323–327
© 1984 Alan R. Liss, Inc., 150 Fifth Avenue, New York, NY 10011

SLEEP, NUTRITION AND METABOLISM DURING DEVELOPMENT

Piero Salzarulo

INSERM U3, 47, Bd de l'Hopital, Paris 13.

INTRODUCTION

The link between nutrition and sleep, as well as the regulation of metabolism during sleep, has been a topic of wide interest in human studies. This paper will explore certain aspects of this relationship from a developmental perspective.

If sleep is regarded as being part of a rhythm constituted by the alternation of waking and sleeping, one may ask whether the feeding rhythm contributes to the development of the waking-sleeping rhythm. Moreover since sleep patterns are an expression of a brain function, and variations of nutrient supply can modify both function and development, it is of interest to investigate the role of the nutrient supply (particularly, as in malnutrition, its reduction or absence) in the maturation of brain activity during sleep.

INFLUENCE OF NUTRITION MODALITIES ON THE WAKING-SLEEPING RHYTHM

There is a long standing acceptance, especially by pediatricians and physiologists, of the relationship between either the rest-activity rhythm (or waking-sleeping rhythm) and the feeding rhythm. Some (Hellbrugge 1968) have stressed the role of feeding in the fluctuation of motility, which becomes greater just before expected feeding time or at the end of the night. An investigation carried out on infants who were fed continuously from birth (Salzarulo et al. 1979) showed that cycles of motility exist even in the absence of meals and that at the end of the night motility increases sharply just as it does in infants with normal oral feeding. The analysis of the waking-sleeping rhythm in the continuously fed infants showed results similar to those observed in infants fed orally: at night (as opposed to daytime) the amount of sleep was greater, the period of uninterrupted sleep was longer, and the distribution of sleep onset in the 24-hour period was similar (Fagioli et al. 1981b).

The literature indicates that the effect of the quality of nutrients has been studied on infants only through "clinical" approaches which lacked precise experimental recordings. It has been found that the introduction of solid foods, particularly cereals, is not related to the establishment of uninterrupted night sleep. Similarly, no differences were found in the night hours of sleep between infants on meat and on cereal feeding schedules (Parmelee et al. 1964; Kleitman and Engelmann 1953; Beal 1969). It has not yet been determined if the quality of nutrients influences the characteristics of the sleep states and the length of the sleep cycle following the meal. The conclusion seems to be that neither the rhythm nor the quality of feeding is a decisive factor in the establishment of motility and of waking-sleeping rhythms.

EARLY MALNUTRITION AND MATURATION OF SLEEP PATTERNS

It is well established that early malnutrition provokes disturbances of central nervous system (CNS) development, i.e., cellular growth, waking EEG frequency, evoked potentials, etc., and that sleep organization closely reflects functional changes in CNS activity (see references in Salzarulo et al. 1982). The following are the results of an investigation carried out in infants severely malnourished from birth who were polygraphically recorded for a 24-hour period. First, neither the total amount of sleep per 24-hours (and, conversely, hours of waking) nor the amount of rapid eye movement (REM or paradoxical) sleep were modified by malnutrition. In contrast, the amount of non-rapid eye movement (NREM or quiet) sleep was clearly reduced, but only in those infants older than 4 months. The reduction in the amount of quiet sleep is due to the shortening of the phases which, in the malnourished infant, last about 17 minutes, instead of about 27 minutes as in the controls. As a consequence of the shortening of the NREM phases, the sleep cycles of the older malnourished infants are shorter than the sleep cycles of controls of the same age (Salzarulo et al. 1982). Disturbances of the cardiac rhythm are also observed. These are more frequent during NREM than during the other states, and are more frequent in malnourished compared to controls, regardless of state (Fagioli et al. 1983).

The changes in sleep patterns mentioned above are not only a functional effect of malnutrition; they also can play a role in the metabolic regulation of the malnourished child. There is a growing field of data, as well as increased specu-lation, concerning the role of sleep, particularly NREM, in energy metabolism and protein synthesis. According to these hypotheses, energy expenditure is reduced and protein synthesis is enhanced during NREM. Accordingly, malnour-ished infants, who have less NREM and shorter sleep cycles, should be in jeopardy. They require increased amounts of NREM to reduce energy expenditure.

METABOLISM AND SLEEP

There is a paucity of data on metabolic processes related to sleep during development, but the behavioral state appears to have an important role in energy expenditure from birth on. During REM (paradoxical) sleep, O_2 consumption is higher than during NREM (quiet) sleep (Strothers and Warner 1977). The results of this study should be replicated and expanded so that they cover a greater period of time and explore different epochs of the nyctemeron. Nevertheless, the work done thus far does have certain implications: it suggests the importance of taking into account the proportions of REM and NREM sleep, which change during early infancy (Wolff 1973), when calculating the energy expenditure per day in each epoch of development.

Anabolism constitutes one of the most important aspects of body processes during development. For this reason the theoretical framework of Adam and Oswald (1977) about the role of sleep in the anabolic process is particularly interest-ing. The approach of Salzarulo and colleagues to this problem involved an investigation of the relationship between weight changes and sleep organization in infants being treated with parenteral nutrition, a feeding technique which provides precise measurements of nutrients introduced into the blood stream. When only the amounts of each type of sleep were considered, this study (Fagioli et al. 1981a) showed a correlation between weight gain and total sleep time, REM sleep, or NREM sleep. This data has been interpreted as indicating a possible relationship betwen anabolic processes and sleep.

The interpretation appears to be supported by preliminary laboratory findings in an investigation using nitrogen balance as an indicator of protein turnover. Children continuously fed by catheter were recorded polygraphically all night, and urine samples were collected separately for daytime and nightime periods. The amount of nitrogen oxidized was determined by the difference between the known intake and the amount of nitrogen which was retained. Nitrogen retention during night time periods appears to increase when there is a high proportion of sleep cycles relative to the total duration of sleep. These results indicate that protein turnover is related to sleep organization: the better the sleep organization (i.e., the higher the proportion of sleep cycles), the greater the nitrogen retention.

CONCLUSION

In infants, the contribution of nutrition to sleep organization primarily relates to the building up of behavioral states (mainly NREM sleep) which require an adequate nutritional intake for development or, as in the case of previous nutritional deficiency, for recovery. The presence of well organized sleep, also contributes to a strengthening of the anabolic processes. In contrast, feeding rhythm appears to have little influence on the development of the waking-sleeping rhythm. It is difficult, however, on the basis of actual knowledge, to identify the critical factor(s) in the regulation of waking-sleeping rhythm.

ACKNOWLEDGMENTS

I. Fagioli, F. Salomon, C. Ricour, G. Putet, and F. Bes participated in the research reported in this chapter. P. Ktonas revised the English.

REFERENCES

1. Adam K, Oswald I (1977). Sleep is for tissue restoration. J Roy Coll Physicians 11:376-388.
2. Beal VA (1969). Termination of night feeding in infancy. Journal of Pediatrics 75:690-692.
3. Fagioli I, Ricour C, Salomon F and Salzarulo P(1981a). Weight changes and sleep organization in infants. Early Hum Dev 5:395-399.
4. Fagioli I, Salomon F and Salzarulo P (1981b). L'endormissement chez l'enfant en nutrition continue: enregistrements de vingt-quatre heures. Rev EEG Neurophysiol 11:37-44.
5. Fagioli I, Salzarulo P, Salomon F and Ricour C (1983). Sinus pauses in early human malnutrition during waking and sleeping. Neuropediatrics 14:43-46.
6. Hellbrugge T (1968). Ontogenese des rythmes circadiens chez l'enfant. In: Ajuriaguerra j de (ed): "Cycles biologiques et psychiatrie," Geneve: George et C, p 159.
7. Kleitman N and Engelmann TG (1953). Sleep characteristics of infants. J Appl Physiol 6:269-282.
8. Parmelee AH, Wenner WH and Schulz H (1964). Infant sleep patterns: from birth to 16 weeks of age. Journal of Pediatrics 65:576-582.
9. Salzarulo P, Fagioli I, Salomon F, Duhamel JF and Ricour C (1979). Alimentation continue et rythme veille-sommeil chez l'enfant. Arch Franc Pediatr (suppl.) 36:26-32.
10. Salzarulo P, Fagioli I, Salomon F and Ricour C (1982). Developmental trend of quiet sleep is altered by early human malnutrition and recovered by nutritional rehabilitation. Early Hum Dev 6:257-264.
11. Stothers JK and Warner RM (1977). Oxygen consumption and sleep state in the newborn. J Physiol 269:57-58.
12. Wolff PH (1973). Organization of behavior in the first three months of life. Bio and Environ Determinants of Early Dev. 51:132-153.

CONSEQUENCES

Energy Intake and Activity, pages 331–353
© 1984 Alan R. Liss, Inc., 150 Fifth Avenue, New York, NY 10011

THE ROLE OF MOTOR ACTIVITY IN HUMAN COGNITIVE AND SOCIAL DEVELOPMENT

Arnold J. Sameroff
Susan C. McDonough

Institute for the Study of Development Disabilities, University of Illinois at Chicago

INTRODUCTION

Despite the documented physical effects of mild to moderate malnutrition it is surprising that corollary behavioral effects have been difficult to identify. While there have been claims for the identification of a variety of deficiencies contemporary to the malnutrition, long term negative consequences have been far less evident. Determining the relationship of malnutrition to the later social and cognitive behavior of the child is an example of the more general problem of understanding the developmental relationship between biological and behavioral processes.

This attempt to explore the relationship between activity level and social and cognitive functioning will be in three parts. The first will review the evidence for effects of early malnutrition on later cognitive and social functioning. The second will examine the factors that do seem to have important consequences for children's social and cognitive functioning. The final section will include a discussion of the theoretical models for understanding developmental relationships and an agenda for future research directions.

EARLY ACTIVITY AND LATER CHILD COMPETENCE

A number of reviews of the connection between chronic malnutrition and child behavior have concluded that strong relationships are not evident (Barrett et al. 1982; Pollitt and

Thomson 1977). Physical consequences have been found in the relationship between undernutrition and reduced physical and cranial development, but behavioral consequences have only been found for children with severe malnutrition in infancy (MacLaren et al. 1973). However, in those studies which did find later deficits it was not clear whether the deficits were the result of the malnutrition or were accompanying correlates of poverty, such as low SES and impoverished learning and socialization environments. Lloyd-Still (1976) reviewed 13 studies of the effects of malnutrition on cognitive development. If poverty or economic deprivation did not accompany the malnutrition there were no lasting effects on intelligence test scores. In all the studies reviewed the differences in intelligence scores between malnourished and control children decreased over time.

While the studies of cognitive functioning have been inconclusive at best, there has been a major lack of research on social and emotional consequences. Barrett et al. (1982) investigated the existence of such a relationship. They pointed out that most such investigations were restricted to the period of infancy.

> From the research a consistent pattern of behavioral characteristics of malnourished infants appears, including impaired attentional processes (Lester, 1975); reduced social responsiveness (Brazelton, Tronick, Lechtig, Lasky, & Klein, 1977; Mora et al. 1979); heightened irritability and inability to tolerate frustration (Mora et al. 1979); and low activity level, reduced independence, and diminished affect (Chávez & Martinez, 1979). (p. 542)

Barrett et al. (1982) went on to propose that such at-risk infants could develop disordered social interaction patterns that would inhibit the development of interpersonal skills and consequently reduce social and emotional competence later in childhood. In a study of 6 to 8-year-old children who had received nutritional supplements during various periods of infancy, they found that low supplementation was associated with passivity, dependency on adults, and anxious behavior. They argued that adequate energy uptake in infancy was important for later adequate social-emotional development. This relationship, however, was mediated by effects of malnutrition on both the behavior of the child and the child's caretakers. The affected children developed behaviors that insulated them from the social and non-social environment and inhibited the later development of appropriate patterns of social interaction.

The cycle of dysfunctional responses that led to unsatisfying caregiver-child interactions was elaborated by Lester (1979). He argued that early malnutrition affects energy expenditure so that the child is less likely to respond to and stimulate caregivers, thus reducing the likelihood of developing a normal interaction pattern. The problems are further exacerbated if the caregivers are also malnourished and living in an impoverished social-emotional milieu. This transactional view (Sameroff and Chandler 1975) is that behavioral outcomes can never be explained by characteristics of the child taken alone at one point in development. Instead, outcomes are always the product of the child's characteristics and the child's experiences. Without knowing both, developmental predictions or explanations are impossible.

Read (1982) points out that while severe malnutrition early in life may alter brain structure, there are a variety of other routes which are not biologically mediated through which learning can be effected by even mild malnutrition. The malnourished child lives in a restricted environment and has less energy to respond to those stimuli that are available. Changes in personality, emotionality, and behavior also interfere with the interpersonal relationships necessary for learning. Read describes a negative transactional cycle leading to developmental failure.

> The hungry child is apathetic, disinterested, and irritable when confronted with difficult tasks. He tends to live in a world of his own, relatively independent of the world around him. To the extent that his parents or teachers respond negatively to his behaviors his isolation is increased. . . being hungry in a world where others are not decreases one's sense of self worth, further stigmatizing the child in his own eyes and those of his teachers. Thus, he fails to learn for social and psychological reasons, not for biological or neurological ones. (p. 290)

Initial attempts to modify the outcomes for malnourished children intervened primarily in the nutritional domain. Almost immediately it was observed that positive changes in outcome were accompanied by corollary behavioral changes in the childrearing environment. Chávez and Martinez (1979) found that supplemented infants became more active. These more active children made more demands on their mothers, increasing the amount and quality of mother-child interactions, and thus increasing the mother's stimulation of the children to further physical activity. Mothers of the more passive nonsupplemented children restricted their interactions to either holding, carrying, or rocking them.

Later studies with malnourished children added educational components to provide a comprehensive biobehavioral intervention. In the analysis of a major study that included both nutritional supplementation and educational intervention Bejar (1981) found that changes in the cognitive functioning of the children could be completely attributed to the educational program. Bejar makes the interesting point that "whether nutritional supplementation can restore normal cognitive development to malnourished children depends on whether malnutrition was the cause of the problem in the first place." (p. 66)

Zeskind and Ramey (1981) used only an educational intervention when they tested a transactional model in an exploration of the effects of fetal malnutrition on later intelligence. In a lower SES sample, half of whom were in an educational intervention program, they were able to examine the impact of an underweight (i.e., low ponderal index) infant on the developmental system. As a group, the developmental quotients (DQ) of infants without educational intervention declined within 3 to 18 months of age and continued to be lower on tests at 36 months of age. However, within that group the low ponderal index babies showed a much greater decline into the retarded range. Their lower DQs were associated with lower levels of maternal involvement. In contrast, in the group of families that received educational intervention the malnourished infants who had scored significantly lower than the rest of the group at 3 months were doing as well as the others by 18 months. Zeskind and Ramey concluded that the educational program had interrupted the negative transaction found in the control group. Low social status mothers usually would be put off by the characteristics of a fetally malnourished infant thus contributing to a worsening developmental outcome. Intervention, however, fostered the relationship between mother and child, thereby leading to an above average outcome.

In the transactional model the child and the environment are seen as actively engaged with one another, changing and being changed by their interactions. Past developmental research has found that children's behavior is organized in complex structures. Current developmental research is finding that the childrearing environment is equally structured in terms of norms, values and institutions. The Rochester Longitudinal Study (Sameroff et al. 1982) offers an opportunity to examine more fully the factors that contribute to childhood social and cognitive competence.

ROCHESTER LONGITUDINAL STUDY

The Rochester Longitudinal Study (RLS) has been conducted since 1970, and investigates the role of parental mental illness, social status, and other family cognitive and social variables that create risk factors in the development of children from birth through 4 years of age. The study is one of many begun in the last 15 years which were explicitly concerned with the impact of parental factors on the development of children. A recent monograph reported findings from this longitudinal study through 2½ years of age (Sameroff et al. 1982). This report will add analyses of factors contributing to child outcomes at age 4.

The RLS was designed originally to determine the impact of emotionally disturbed parents on their young children but, because of the number of assessments on a heterogeneous sample, more general developmental issues could be addressed as well. Of specific relevance are analyses of the relative impact of a variety of risk factors, especially the environmental factors that mediate much of early child development.

In previous analyses comparing children from various groups of mothers it was demonstrated that both parental mental illness and social status factors were directly related to child performance (Sameroff et al. 1982). While these results are meaningful, they do not fully address the issue of what psychological mechanisms are responsible for the individual and group variation observed in the children's development. The next step in addressing the complex interactions of risk factors was the examination of additional groups of measures that might explain the broad social status and mental illness factors (Sameroff and Seifer 1983). These included the cognitive capacities, attitudes, beliefs, and values of the mother, as well as the stresses that impact on the family. The measures used in these multivariate analyses and the characteristics of the RLS sample are summarized below.

Study Sample

When the children of the RLS were 4 years of age there were 215 families participating in the study. These families were heterogeneous in many dimensions. All five of Hollingshead's SES levels were represented; there were 15 in SES I, 19 in SES II, 39 in SES III, 77 in SES IV, and 65 in SES V. There were 131 white families, 79 black families, and 5 Puerto Rican families. Family size ranged from 1 to 10 children; 64 families had 1 child, 65 had 2, 47 had 3, 18 had 4, and the remainder had 5 or more children. The mothers' ages ranged from 15 to 40 at the time of the children's birth and their education ranged from completion of third grade to advanced degrees. Most of the women were married when their child was born but 37 had never married and 17 were separated or divorced. Finally, 122 of the children were boys and 93 were girls.

Outcome Measures

The outcome criteria of particular interest for this publication were assessments of the cognitive and social-emotional competence of the child. The competence measures used as criteria were the Wechsler Pre-School Scales of Intelligence (WPPSI) Verbal Intelligence Quotient (VIQ) for cognitive competence, and the Rochester Adaptive Behavior Inventory (RABI) Global Rating for social-emotional competence of the child in areas of family life, social interaction, and solitary behavior (Seifer et al. 1981). This measure was developed during the course of the RLS and consisted of a 90 minute interview of the mother, by a trained interviewer, about the adaptive behavior of her child. The global rating is a summary score given by the interviewer on a 5-point scale where 1 indicates superior adjustment and 5 indicates clinical disturbance.

Risk Variables

From the set of variables assessed during the RLS, 11 variables were selected that were hypothesized to be related to either cognitive or social-emotional competence. These variables were:
  1) Severity of Maternal Mental Illness
  2) Chronicity of Maternal Mental Illness
  3) Maternal Anxiety
  4) Parental Perspectives
  5) Maternal Interactive Behaviors
  6) Maternal Education
  7) Occupation of Head of Household
  8) Minority Group Social Status
  9) Family Social Support
  10) Stressful Life Events
  11) Family Size
Each of these variables was used to form a low risk group and a high risk group as described in Table 1.

TABLE 1

Summary of risk variables

Risk Variable	Low Risk	High Risk
Severity of Illness	No Symptoms	Symptoms
Chronicity of Illness	0-1 Contact	More than 1 Contact
Anxiety	75% Least	25% Most
Parental Perspectives	75% Highest	25% Lowest
Spontaneous Interaction	75% Most	25% Least
Education	High School	No High School
Occupation	Skilled	Semi- or Unskilled
Minority Status	White	Nonwhite
Family Support	Father Present	Father Absent
Stressful Life Events	75% Fewest	25% Most
Family Size	1-3 Children	4 or More Children

Effects of Risk Factors

The low risk and high risk groups for all 11 risk variables were compared on the two outcome criteria of WPPSI-VIQ and RABI global rating.

All comparisons for the VIQ scores were significantly different, and in all cases the low risk group had higher scores than the high risk group. The largest absolute difference was for race (about 18 points) but most differences were about 7 to 10 IQ points, about 1/2 to 2/3 of a standard deviation.

On the RABI global rating the low risk group performed significantly better than the high risk group for all but one of the comparisons. This exception was for mother-child interaction where no difference was found. The differences between groups on these comparisons was generally about ½ of a standard deviation.

While there are many differences on the individual risk factors there are two major shortcomings in such analyses. First, there is a wide range of outcomes within each of the risk groups so that the discrimination between the two groups is not large enough to accurately predict poor outcome on the basis of a single risk factor. Second, it is not clear statistically whether the many risk factors are overlapping in their effects or whether there are unique additive components when these risk variables are viewed in unison.

In an attempt to be more accurate in predicting outcomes, a multiple risk score was created by summing the single risks for each family. The actual multiple risk scores ranged from 0 to 9. Since only one family had a score of 9, it was combined in all analyses with those whose score was 8. The largest resulting group contained 36 families and the smallest group had 10 families.

Multiple Risk Scores and Outcomes

The relation between the multiple risk classification and the 4-year IQ outcome criterion is summarized graphically in Figure 1. A linear trend analysis of the IQ scores was significant with no reliable deviation from linearity, indicating that as the number of risk factors increased, performance decreased for children at 4 years of age.

FOUR YEAR VERBAL INTELLIGENCE

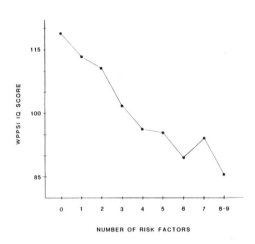

FIGURE 1

In addition to the clear downward linear trend, the size of the effect for multiple risk factors was much larger than for individual risk factors. For the IQ scores, the difference between the lowest and highest risk groups was about 2 standard deviations. This compares with a 1/2 to 2/3 standard deviation difference for most of the individual risk factors.

The relation between the total risk scores and the RABI global rating is shown in Figure 2. The linear trend was significant here also, with no reliable deviations from linearity. For the RABI, the difference in the multiple risk analysis was about 1-1/3 standard deviations compared with the ½ standard deviation differences found in the single risk analyses. Thus the combination of risk factors resulted in a nearly three-fold increase in the magnitude of differences found among groups of children.

FOUR YEAR SOCIAL-EMOTIONAL COMPETENCE

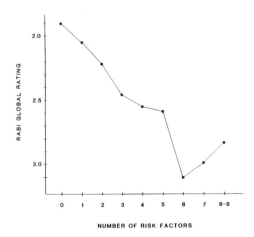

FIGURE 2

The analyses of these results leads to the conclusion that prediction of developmental outcome is a complex enterprise. Because of the dynamics of the developmental system, the effects of single risk factors can be moderated by other positive aspects of the childrearing environment. Where there is economic deprivation, competent interactive parents can make up for the deficit. Where there is a high level of environmental stress, parental coping skills can reduce the impact on the child, and where there is a low level of stressful events, poor parental coping is irrelevant. However, where compensating mechanisms are deficient and stress levels are high, problems for the child will be much more likely.

The combination of risk factors into a single score has shown the strongest relationship to child intellectual and social-emotional competence. More risk factors produce a heavier load on the system. By examining a population that is admittedly biased toward developmental problems, as in the RLS, one can examine a large array of risk factors that would not be evident in a more homogeneous sample. It is clear that there are many children who are suffering severe deficits in competence. To the extent that any one of the identified risk factors is increased in the general population, we can expect to see increases in the number of children who will suffer the consequences.

This paper has been limited to an analysis of environmental influences that explain variations in the competence of pre-school children. While it might be expected that previous assessments would have made a major contribution to explaining these variations in competence, this has not been the case with earlier analyses of data (Seifer and Sameroff 1982) or with similar studies. The biology and behavior of the child are necessary conditions for their pre-school competence, but assessments of these factors explain little of the variance in that competence (Broman et al. 1975).

DEVELOPMENTAL MODELS

This paper began by stating that the relationship of malnutrition to later cognitive and social behavior of the child was another example of the more general problem of understanding the developmental relationship between biological and behavioral processes. This general problem will now be addressed. Many longitudinal research projects, such as those mentioned above, have presented compelling evidence that there are few continuities between infant physical status and later behavioral status (Sameroff and Chandler 1975). Whenever a biological condition has been identified, whether it is risk from perinatal complications or actual chromosomal anomalies, children with the same initial condition have developed quite differently. The range of intellectual outcomes for children with Down syndrome, for example, is much greater than the range for children without the syndrome (Ryders et al. 1978). As with the research on effects of nutrition, most of these studies have only sampled development at various points in time. At each of these points outcome measures are compared for children that differ in a variety of risk factors. The data from the RLS presented above is an example of such logitudinal studies. What is not revealed by such analyses is the developmental process by which early deficits are either eliminated or augmented. It has been argued already that experience plays a key role in this developmental process.

Sameroff and Chandler suggested that the <u>self-righting</u> tendencies which operated biologically in the embryological system to produce a physically normal infant (Waddington 1966) might operate postnatally through social systems to produce a psychologically normal child. The biological self-righting tendencies are coded in a genetic system that monitors biochemically the status of the developing embryo and introduces regulatory processes to maintain a normative condition. Sameroff (1983) suggested that similar self-righting tendencies are located in the caregiving environment organized around behavioral norms and coded into social institutions and cultural heritages. In a society that endures over several generations there must be a codified system of childrearing and socialization into appropriate roles to assure the continuity of that society.

In defining the developmental risk associated with any specific child, the characteristics of the child must be related to the ability of the environment to provide experiences that regulate the development of the child toward social norms. In extreme cases of massive biological abnormality such regulations may be ineffectual. At the other extreme, disordered social environments might convert biologically normal infants into caretaking casualties.

In the developmental biological model, changes in an organism are viewed as a joint function of the previous activity of the organism and the context in which that activity occurs. The importance of context can be seen even in genetics where, despite the fact that each cell has an identical genetic structure, these genes will express themselves differently because each cell provides a unique chemical environment. Moreover, as the organism develops, these changes result in reorganizations in which higher-order coordinations come into play. The importance of reorganizations can be seen in embryology, where the initial fertilized cell begins a process of cell division that leads first to a ball of morphologically similar cells, and then through a folding process into a morphologically dissimilar organization of three cell layers that will each take a uniquely different course to form different organs of the body.

Developmental reorganizations also characterize behavioral development. Piaget, especially, has identified stages of cognitive organization that build upon one another, the achievements of each previous phase becoming the substrate of each succeeding phase. Continuity and discontinuity of handicap can be interpreted within such a model. Continuity is provided by the fact that each previous stage is required for each later one. Developmental achievements occur in a dependent sequence. Discontinuity is provided by the fact that each previous stage does not depend on all the achievements of the previous one. In cognitive development the achievement of object permanence results from the coordination of the activity of sensory modalities on an object. However, the combination of modalities can be different for each object. In the case of blind infants, all such achievements are without the visual activity that characterizes object permanence for most sighted children. However, blind infants can go on to the conceptual and logical structures that characterize later stages of cognitive development. There is a discontinuity in the performance of blind children since sensory handicaps at one level need not become cognitive handicaps at another. On the other hand there is a continuity in that they are still blind no matter what there level of cognitive development.

Methodologies must be developed to separate the various aspects of child behavior that contribute to cognitive and social development. It is not ethically possible to manipulate the activity level of groups of children to determine the effects of motor behavior on intelligence; however, certain natural experiments permit an approximation of such manipulations.

DEVELOPMENT OF HANDICAPPED CHILDREN

The study of the development of handicapped children can throw light on a variety of developmental processes. This section will explore how contrasts between children with a number of handicaps can help us to understand the factors that contribute to the development of normal children. In the present case, where the interest is on the developmental impact of low activity level, children with Down syndrome can serve as an interesting contrast group since they, too, have lower activity levels because of hypotonicity.

Motor Activity and Cognition

Investigations of the intellectual progress of children with Down syndrome (DS) show a progressive retardation beginning soon after birth and resulting in a rate of development that is about 50% that of normal infants. By two years of age, the DS child is functioning at about one year level (Hanson 1981). This average lag is not universal for all DS children. The range of test IQ scores reported for DS children is from 9 to 120 (Rynders et al. 1978), a far wider range than the fifty points for normal and borderline children, i.e., 75 to 125. The reason for this variation has been attributed to many factors including the specific nature of the chromosomal anomaly, motivational level, extent of hypotonicity, temperament, socialization, and educational intervention.

Of most concern here are the motoric, affective, and cognitive components of intellectual functioning and their interplay in development. Although the typical focus in DS research has been on tests of intelligence, recent work has been studying the correlates of intellectual development in emotional and motor domains. DS children have been found to lag significantly in the timing and the strength of emotional expression (Emde et al. 1978). These delays in affective display have been tied to delays in cognitive development (Cicchetti and Sroufe 1976). Furthermore, the children in these studies who showed the greatest lags in affective and cognitive development had the poorest levels of motor tones. The unresolved issue in these studies is the causal connection between these factors.

Are the delays found in cognitive, affective, and motor performance the direct expression of some common biological factor in DS, or are they connected in some chain of sequential causes where a biological factor reduces muscle tone that, in turn, reduces the capacity for affective involvement that, in turn, retards learning and intellectual progress?

The role of motor capacities can be viewed from two perspectives. The first sees motor performance as an expression of the same source of motivation that underlies emotional displays either in a causal connection, i.e., motivation energizes muscles which then energize affect expression, or a correlative connection, i.e., the same motivation energizes muscles and affect expression through separate pathways. The second view sees motor activity as a necessary part of cognitive development (Piaget 1952). From this view it is the coordination of sensory-motor activity that produces higher levels of cognitive functioning. Intellectual retardation in this view would be the result of the reduced number of activities engaged in by the hypotonic DS infant rather than the reduced level of involvement in each activity.

In order to explore these interrelationships between cognition, affect, and motor performance, populations and measures must be utilized that separate these functions. Assessments of cognitive development should be used that are free from motor and affective factors, as much as possible, as well as measures that involve affective and motor factors. In addition, groups of children should be studied in which these factors can be dissociated. Assessments that can fill these needs have been found and are described below. Samples cannot be identified that permit a dissociation between affective and cognitive behavior but they can be found at different developmental levels in these areas, e.g., DS vs normal infants. It is possible to successfully separate motor from cognitive and affective factors by using infants handicapped motorically, e.g., cerebral palsy or spina bifida, who display a range of intellectual achievements not correlated with the motor disability.

Perceptual-Cognitive Development

Although a great deal is known about visual attention, memory, and information processing in normal infants, there is little information about these processes in handicapped infants. One reason may be that whether traditional infant scales (e.g., Bayley, Gesell), or more experimental paradigms (e.g., object permanence) are used, the tasks generally require the infants to respond motorically. Given the severe motor impairments present in many of these infants, it is difficult to interpret their performance, particularly if it is poor. To what extent does it result from an underlying perceptual or cognitive deficit, and to what extent from difficulty in making the proper motor response?

There is evidence that in normal infants, specific markers or ages exist below which most infants will process information one way and above which they will process it in a different way. Techniques have been developed for assessing, relatively independently, the process of visual attention, memory, and discrimination or information processing. One such technique is the habituation-dishabituation paradigm. This paradigm requires a minimum amount of movement and yet has been effective with normal (Cohen and Gelber 1976), high-risk (Sigman and Parmelee 1974), cerebral palsied (McDonough and Cohen 1983), and Down syndrome infants (Cohen 1981).

The habituation-dishabituation procedures require little if any movement from the infant; the infant merely looks from a blinking light to a visual stimulus. The task requires only that the infant be able to move his eyes approximately 15 degrees; hold his head erect, with adult support if necessary; fixate on a stationary visual stimulus; and remain seated on his parent's lap for 6 to 8 minutes.

Even though the procedure is simple and the motor requirements are minimal, it can provide a wealth of information about attention, memory, and information-processing. For instance,it allows for independent assessments of what Cohen (1972) has called Attention Getting and Attention Holding. The Attention Getting process determines whether and how often an infant will turn to look at a pattern, while the Attention Holding process controls how long fixation will continue once the infant has turned to look at the pattern. Cohen asserts that Attention Getting is influenced by certain stimulus parameters such as size and distance, whereas Attention Holding is influenced by the amount of information in the stimulus such as complexity or novelty. Thus, Attention Holding is a more sensitive measure of the infant's memory and information-processing than Attention Getting.

Regarding the assessment of the perceptual-cognitive abilities of motorically impaired infants, the separability of these two processes provides a reflection of both the infant's motoric and intellectual functioning. Through the Attention Getting process, as measured by latency to turn, one can acquire some indication of the severity of the infant's motor problems. Even if the infant experiences some difficulty in turning, the Attention Holding process, as measured by fixation duration, provides information regarding the infant's ability to fixate differentially on novel versus familiar stimuli, i.e., the ability to process visual information.

Affective-Cognitive Development

Affective behavior, in the most general sense, is made up of the observable expressions of an individual that are interpreted as reflecting feelings or emotions. Positive affect is more than a social response or a simple response to pleasure. Instead, there are indications that ordered, developmental changes in affect occur over time in the infant and that smiling may be a key human response system.

The role of affect in the development of a child has not been investigated with the same intensity as that of cognition. However, recent work has indicated that affective behavior has its origins in, and follows developmentally, the cognitive changes of the infant and could be considered a reflection of underlying cognitive processes and cognitive growth (Cicchetti and Sroufe 1976; Sroufe and Wunsch 1972; Zelazo and Komer 1971). Affect and cognition appear to develop in a parallel and interactive fashion, each playing a complementary role to the other (Piaget 1952; Lewis and Rosenblum 1978).

In a study that examined the affective responsiveness of DS infants, Cicchetti and Sroufe (1976) hypothesized that if affect and cognition are parallel phenomena, (a) they should follow similar developmental pathways; (b) affective responses of infants should change with cognitive development and not change solely as a function of chronological age; and (c) delayed cognitive development should show corresponding delay in development of affective responses. They reported that the pattern of affective responses of DS infants showed a developmental delay and that the delay was associated with level of cognitive functioning, not simple with chronological age. Furthermore, the children who were the most unresponsive i.e., who laughed and smiled least and who showed the greatest age delay for laughter, were the children who demonstrated the lowest performance on the Bayley Scales.

Further, Cicchetti and Sroufe speculated on a relationship between degree of hypotonia and affective responses in handicapped children. It was found that in DS infants affect was diminished in degree of response level, i.e., they smiled instead of laughed and that the most hypotonic children lagged behind the normally developing children in the onset and frequency of laughter.

Expanding on this work Gallagher (1979) established that multiply handicapped/mentally retarded infants demonstrated similar relationships between cognitive status and affective expression. Developmentally older children responded to different stimuli than did developmentally younger children, and the older children's affective responses were more intense (i.e., they laughed more than younger children).

The importance of muscle tone for laughing was suggested initially by Cicchetti and Sroufe (1976), who found that the DS child expressed affect less intensely than did normally developing children. Studies with DS children, normally developing children (Sroufe and Wunsch 1972), and multiply handicapped/mentally retarded children (Gallagher et al. 1983) have shown consistent results: as the infant develops cognitively, smiling and laughing at specific groups of stimuli are increased. Laughing is not simply a phenomenon that develops as a function of age, but appears to have a direct link with evolving cognitive abilities.

Gallagher (1979) believes that previous research into the development of affect has revealed these findings: (a) affect and cognition are interdependent, neither superseding the other; (b) stages in affective development are congruent with stages in cognitive development; and (c) the ability to respond affectively to external stimuli is not only cognitive in nature but its expression may also have physiological determinants. With normally intact infants it is virtually impossible to assess separately the contribution made by such development upon the total development of the child. With the handicapped, developmental processes are often slowed sufficiently so that the researcher can view the interrelationships that exist among critical developmental components (e.g., affect, cognitive states, and physical status).

In the growth of the non-handicapped child, the development of motor, emotional, and intellectual processes appear to be so highly coordinated that casual connections are difficult or impossible to identify. The correlation between mental and motor scales on most IQ tests, especially in infancy, are very high. It is only by the study of children that are delayed in one or more of these areas that some hope emerges for a causal analysis that would be applicable not only to the targeted population, but also to other populations, biologically handicapped or normal.

SUMMARY AND IMPLICATIONS

Human behavior is nested in a hierarchy of contexts changing from biological substrates to levels of cognitive and affective exchanges within an environment primarily structured by social institutions. In general, few linear relationships have been identified between early biological factors and later behavioral variables. Where biological deficits exist there are many opportunities for their reduction or exacerbation at points of developmental transformation.

Motor behavior provides the basis for the infant's interactions with the environment. The experiences gained from such interactions are the basis for cognitive advances in the sensorimotor period. Environments that provide different experiences to infants produce infants that advance through the sensorimotor period at different rates (Hunt 1976) although all intact infants eventually reach major developmental milestones. Experimental manipulations of motor experience is difficult or unethical with normal children. In the case of motorically impaired infants, however, the effects of major differences in motor capacities on cognitive development can be examined.

Common assessments of cognitive development (Scales of Infant Development or the Uzgiris-Hunt Ordinal Scales) require motor performance for the majority of items. In the case of handicapped infants it is often difficult to determine if low scores are the result of intellectual deficits or the inability to perform the necessary motor response. By using techniques of cognitive assessment that do not depend on motor performance, it is possible to separate intellectual from motor deficits in young infants. Using a visual fixation technique with cerebral palsied children, it was possible to identify those with severe motor deficits who, nevertheless, showed normal information processing skills on the visual fixation tasks.

Using methodologies that separately assess contributors to scores on developmental assessments will make it possible to evaluate the effects of reduced activity levels on subsequent development. Theoretical models have been developed which can test alternative hypotheses about such relationships. For example, does reduced activity effect intellectual development through the lack of motor interaction with the environment, or through reduced motivational levels that hinder learning. Analogs of this work with handicapped children can be utilized with children experiencing differing degrees of malnutrition to help untangle the relationship between activity level, motor behavior, and subsequent intellectual performance.

Complex experimental models will be necessary to tease apart the influences of hunger, energy level, and activity level on cognitive and social development. While the characteristics of children may influence their course of development, and should be studied, it must be emphasized that social and cultural factors have already been shown to have much stronger influences on the cognitive and social outcomes for children. Any further study of activity level must take into account the more compelling variables of the environmental context.

Acknowledgements

Research reported in this paper was supported by grants from the National Institute of Mental Health, W. T. Grant Foundation, and March-of-Dimes Birth Defects Foundation. The Authors wish to acknowledge the help of Pat Gallagher in formulating some of the ideas in this paper.

REFERENCES

1. Barrett DE, Radke-Yarrow M and Klein RE (1982). Chronic malnutrition and child behavior: Effects of early caloric supplementation on social and emotional functioning at school age. Child Dev 18:541-556.
2. Bejar IJ (1981). Does nutrition cause intelligence? A reanalysis of the Cali experiment. Intelligence 5:49-68.
3. Brazelton TB, Tronick E, Lechtig A, Lasky RE, and Klein RE (1977). The behavior of nutritionally deprived Guatemalan infants. Dev Med and Child Neur 19:364-372.
4. Broman SH, Nichols PL and Kennedy WA (1975). Preschool IQ: prenatal and early developmental correlates. New York: Erlbaum.

5.   Chávez A and Martinez C (1979).   Consequences of insufficient nutrition on child character and behavior. In Levitsky DA (ed.): "Malnutrition, environment and behavior," Ithaca, NY: Cornell University Press.
6.   Cicchetti D and Sroufe LA (1976).   The relationship between affective and cognitive development in Down's syndrome infants.   Child Dev 46:920-929.
7.   Cohen LB (1972).   Attention getting and attention holding processes of infant visual preferences.   Child Dev 43:869-879.
8.   Cohen LB (1976).   Habituation of infant visual attention.   In Tighe TJ and Leaton RN (eds.):   "Habituation: Perspectives from child development, animal behavior, and neurophysiology," Hillsdale, NJ: Erlbaum.
9.   Cohen LB (1981).   Examination of habituation as a measure of aberrant infant development.   In Friedman S and Sigman S (eds.): "Pre-term birth and psychological development."   New York: Academic Press.
10. Cohen LB and Gelber ER (1975).   Infant visual perception.   In Cohen L and Salapatek P (eds.):   "Infant perception: From sensation to cognition: Basic visual processes Vol. 1,"   New York: Academic Press, 347-403.
11. Emde RN, Katz EL and Thorpe JK (1978).   Emotional expression in infancy: II. Early deviations in Down's syndrome.   In Lewis M and Rosenblum LA (eds.): "The development of affect," New York: Plenum Press.
12. Gallagher RJ, Jens KG, and O'Donnell KJ (1983).   The effect of physical status on the affective expression of handicapped infants.   Infant Behav and Dev 6:73-77.
13. Gallagher RS (1979).   Positive affect in multiply handicapped infants: Its relationship to developmental age, temperament, physical status and setting.   Unpublished doctoral dissertation, University of North Carolina at Chapel Hill.
14. Hanson MJ (1981).   Down's syndrome children: Characteristics and intervention research.   In Lewis M and Rosenblum LA (eds.):   "The uncommon child," New York: Plenum Press.
15. Hunt J McV (1976).   Environmental programming to foster competence and prevent mental retardation in infancy.   In Walsh RN and Greenough WT (eds.): "Environments as therapy for brain dysfunction," New York: Plenum Press.

16. Lewis M and Rosenblum LA (1978). Introduction: Issues in affective development. In Lewis M and Rosenblum LA (eds.): "The development of affect," New York: Plenum Press.

17. Lester BM (1975). Cardiac habituation of the orienting response in infants of varying nutritional status. Dev Psychology 11: 432-442.

18. Lester BM (1979). A synergistic process approach to the study of prenatal malnutrition. Internat J of Behav Dev 2:377-394.

19. MacLaren DS, Yaktin US, Kanawati A, Sabbagh S and Kadi Z (1973). The subsequent mental and physical development of rehabilitated marasmic infants. J Mental Def Res 17:273-281.

20. McDonough SC and Cohen LB (1983). Attention and memory in cerebral palsied infants. Infant Behav and Dev 6:73-77.

21. Mora JO, et al (1979). Nutritional supplementation, early stimulation, and child development. In Brozek J (ed.): "Behavioral effects of energy and protein deficits," Bethesda, Md.: Department of Health, Education and Welfare. (Cited in Barrett et al., 1982).

22. Piaget J (1952). The origins of intelligence in children. New York: International Universities Press, Inc.

23. Pollitt E and Thomson C (1977). Protein-calorie malnutrition and behavior: A view from psychology. In Wurtman RJ and Wurtman JJ (eds.): "Nutrition and the brain, Vol. 2," New York: Basic Books.

24. Read MS (1982). Malnutrition and behavior. Appl Res in Mental Retard 3:279-291.

25. Ryders JE, Spiker D and Horrobin JM (1978). Underestimating the educability of Down's syndrome children: Examination of methodological problems in recent literature. Am J Mental Def 82:440-448.

26. Sameroff AJ (1983). Systems of development: Contexts and evolution. In W. Kessen (ed.): "Handbook of child psychology, Vol. 4". New York: John Wiley.

27. Sameroff AJ and Chandler MJ (1975). Reproductive risk and the continuum of caretaking casualty. In Horowitz FD, Hetherington M, Scarr-Salapatek S, and Siegel G (eds.): "Review of child development research, Vol. 4," Chicago : University of Chicago Press.

28. Sameroff AJ and Seifer R (1983). Familial risk and child competence. Child Dev 54:1254-1268.

29. Sameroff AJ, Seifer R and Zax M (1982). Early development of children at risk for emotional disorder. Monographs of the Society for Research in Child Development 47 (7, Serial No 199).

30. Seifer R and Sameroff AJ (1982). A structural equation model analysis of competence in children at risk for mental disorders. Prev Hum Serv No. 4:85-96.

31. Seifer R, Sameroff AJ and Jones FH (1981). Adaptive behavior in young children of emotionally disturbed women. J Appl Dev Psych 1:251-276.

32. Sigman M and Parmelee AH (1974). Visual preferences of four-month-old premature and full-term infants. Child Dev 45:959-965.

33. Sroufe LA and Wunsch JP (1972). The development of laughter in the first year of life. Child Dev 43:1326-1344.

34. Waddington CH (1966). "Principles of development and differentiation." New York: MacMillan.

35. Zelazo PR and Komer JM (1971). Infant smiling to non-social stimuli and the recognition hypothesis. Child Dev 42:1327-1339.

36. Zeskind PS and Ramey CT (1981). Preventing intellectual and interactional sequels of fatal malnutrition: A longitudinal, transactional, and synergistic approach to development. Child Dev 52:213-218.

Energy Intake and Activity, pages 355–376
© 1984 Alan R. Liss, Inc., 150 Fifth Avenue, New York, NY 10011

MICROECONOMIC CONSEQUENCES OF ENERGY DEFICIENCY
IN RURAL POPULATIONS IN DEVELOPING COUNTRIES

Maarten D.C. Immink*
Fernando E. Viteri**
Rafael Flores***
Benjamin Torun***

*School of Public Health, The University of
Texas Health Science Center at Houston,
Texas

**Pan American Health Organization, Washington,
D.C.

***Institute of Nutrition of Central America
and Panama, Guatemala

INTRODUCTION

This paper examines some of the microeconomic consequences of energy deficiency among rural populations in
developing countries. Evidence relating indicators of chronic
and acute energy deficiency to physiological and cognitive
parameters is relatively abundant, as demonstrated by some
of the chapters in this volume (Spurr 1984; Malina 1984;
Sameroff 1984), but a great deal of work remains to be done
to analyze these results in economic terms. As has been
argued elsewhere, physiological and cognitive outcomes of
energy deficiency interact with physical, cultural, and
socioeconomic settings to produce economic effects (Viteri et
al. 1981). For example, the biological consequences of mild
to moderate energy deficiency interact with wage and other
economic incentives and with managerial and physical factors
to produce, or impede, specific work performance effects.
Ultimately it will be necessary to provide policy makers and
planners in developing countries with estimates of the economic costs of energy deficiency and of the economic returns

on investment in programs designed to reduce its prevalence.

CONCEPTUAL FRAMEWORK

A simple household production model, adopted from a body of economic literature referred to as "the new home economics" (Evenson 1981; Becker 1965), will serve as a starting point. The household is seen as both a production and a consumption unit, and home production is emphasized. Rural households engage in market production (wage labor or self-employment) and in home production. Home production activities can be separated into:

a. production of goods and services (e.g., food processing and preparation, house repair, child care);
b. leisure production, or non-work activities (playing soccer, attending a film showing); and
c. human capital formation activities (formal and non-formal schooling, participation in MCH programs).

Market goods, purchased with income from market production, are combined with time inputs to produce home goods. Households maximize utility and minimize total cost by choosing optimal combinations of home goods. Marginal costs of home goods production, which depend on the value of home production time (i.e., market wage rates) and on the prices of market goods, form the constraints to the optimization process. Households then choose optimal quantities of market and home goods, and allocate their time among market and home production activities. Total household income ("full income") is defined as the sum of monetary income and the value added component in the total value of home production. An expanded definition of household income also includes the net present value of those increased future earnings of all household members which are attributable to human capital formation. Behaviorally this income component is only relevant when it can be converted into current monetary income. This implies perfect access to capital markets, something which is generally not the case for rural households in developing countries.

Only a few studies examine the whole range of activities undertaken by rural households and describe the relationship between changes in time allocation and energy expenditure and changes in energy-protein availability and/or in economic incentives. Time allocation studies have been undertaken by many anthropologists (Minge-Klevana 1980; Nag et al. 1978) and by some economists (Evenson 1978). These cross-sectional studies provide little insight into how rural households re-allocate time and energy among market and home production activities in response to changes in economic incentives. Studying a small group of rural women in Guatemala, McGuire (1979) found that when engaged in market production these women expended more energy (per kg of body weight) in work activities outside the home than in domestic chores. On these days time was re-allocated from resting and food handling to market production activities, while other home production activities, such as child care and breastfeeding, were unaffected. Popkin (1980) has shown that when mothers' participation in market work is incompatible with child care, the net effect is negative for the nutritional status of preschool age children in the rural Philippines. Gross and Underwood (1971) demonstrated that when agricultural development represents a shift from subsistence farming to cash crop production, a detrimental effect on the nutritional status of non-productive household members can result. This appears to be an example of human capital formation being adversely affected even when the supply of market goods (foods) to the households may have increased.

In the absence of empirical data, the economic consequences of low energy intake levels can only be hypothesized. Previously presented evidence suggests that nutritional levels are associated with a reduction in marginal productivity in market production among rural workers (Spurr 1984). Agricultural wage income often depends on work efficiency. When the marginal labor productivity of low energy intake workers engaged in market production is low, the value of home production time will be reduced correspondingly. The outcome is likely to be less market production, lower monetary income, and increased home production and leisure. If the low energy intake worker does not engage in home production of goods, or if his/her marginal productivity in home goods production is reduced, the result will be increased leisure production. Moreover, because optimal combinations of goods and time inputs are not possible under severe market income constraints, decreased efficiency in home production may be an additional result. The total effect, then, is a lower level of full income. The effect of the lower market income is likely to result in decreased leisure production and increased rural labor force participation by other household members.

A second conceptual model in the economics literature focuses on the relationship between productivity in rural wage employment and food or energy intake. The theory was first proposed by Leibenstein during the 1950's as part of the controversy about the existence or non-existence of underemployment in the rural areas of developing countries (1957; 1958). Since then the efficiency-wage theory has been expanded and its ramifications investigated in terms of rural income distributions, resource allocations in the rural sector, effects of rising rural populations on agricultural production, etc. (Mirrlees 1976; Stiglitz 1976). A comprehensive review of the theory was undertaken by Bliss and Stern (1978a), before they went on to examine some of the empirical evidence in relation to the productivity-food consumption relationship (1978b).

Figure 1

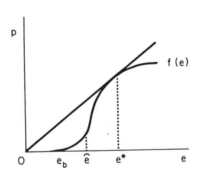

The efficiency curve of the efficiency wage hypothesis

The relationship of productivity to energy intake is defined in specific terms (Figure 1). Productivity is expressed in standardized work units (such as weight of coffee beans picked, pre-measured area weeded with a machete). It is postulated that after daily energy intake (e) covers basal metabolic energy requirements (e_b), the remainder is allocated first to work activities. Over a certain range (e_b - ê), there will be increasing (more than proportional) productivity returns in response to higher levels of daily energy intake. Beyond this range diminishing (less than proportional) returns set in. Rural employers will pay a real wage equivalent to e* ("efficiency wage"), because at that wage their average wage cost per unit of work equals the marginal cost of a work unit, and thus they maximize profits.

The strength of the productivity-food consumption relation, or efficiency curve, will depend on the types of work to be undertaken. In rural areas these will vary among different occupations, different seasons of the agricultural cycle, etc. In setting wages, rural employers must be aware of the productivity-energy intake link, and must be able to internalize the productivity benefits resulting from higher energy intakes by workers. The latter calls for long-term labor contracts, or other labor-tying arrangements.

The efficiency-wage hypothesis does not consider the wage laborer as a member of a household unit; therefore, its application is a great deal more limited. For example, on the assumption that all of the wage increment is spent on food for the worker, the model argues that rural employers should provide productive wage increases when the energy intake levels of workers is below the efficiency wage (e*). In reality, sharing of the wage increase among household members is likely to result in non-internalized benefits for the employer. The effect on the rural household is likely to be re-allocation of labor time towards home production and human capital formation by members other than the wage laborer, thus increasing their energy needs and making sharing of the wage increment more likely. The results reported by Evenson (1981) for rural Philippines are consistent with this.

Examining available evidence in the context of the efficiency wage hypothesis, and specifically the productivity-energy intake relationship, results in mixed findings. The study with agricultural workers in Guatemala indeed shows that workers consuming higher levels of energy and protein spent more time in both market and home production, and were able to complete standardized tasks in less time, than colleagues with lower intake levels (Viteri 1971). However, these results were obtained retrospectively after a long period of adaptation to higher intake levels by the more productive group. Evidence from short-term energy supplementation studies shows that a positive productivity effect may not be present. A group of 20 rice farmers in India was divided into two sub-samples (Belavady 1966); one group was maintained on 2,400 kcals/day, the other on 3,000 kcals/day, for two periods of 90 and 112 days. No significant differences were found for either period in mean daily work-time, mean daily work output, and work performed per hour. Both groups gained weight, but the increment was greater for the high energy intake group. Wolgemuth et al. (1982) reported that after an average of 53 days of caloric supplementation, the productivity of rural road workers in Kenya increased by 12.5 percent, which is statistically significant only at the .10 probability level.

GUATEMALAN PRODUCTIVITY STUDIES

Two studies were undertaken with sugarcane cutters and coffee pickers in Guatemala. Study data are analyzed cross-sectionally and, in the case of the sugarcane cutters, also longitudinally as this study included an energy supplementation program (Immink et al. 1982; Immink and Viteri 1981a; 1981b).

Sample Description

A group of 158 sugarcane workers who lived in two communities on the plantation were included in the first study. The principal work activities of these workers were sugarcane cutting and loading for a period of approximately 30 weeks (November-June), and canefield maintenance tasks (weeding, fumigation, planting) during the remainder of the year. The sugarcane harvesting season represented a period of unrestricted work availability, during which workers were paid a piece-rate per ton of cane delivered.

These workers can be characterized as mildly to moderately energy deficient, and their body composition described as lean and muscular. Before supplementation their average body weight was 53.3 kg, or 33.4 kg/m height. Mean upper-arm muscle area standardized for height was 28.3 mm²/cm, and mean triceps skinfold was 4.7 mm. They ranged in age from 17 to 73 with a median age of 31, and mean daily energy intake was estimated at 2,971 kcals, or approximately 55 kcals per kg of body weight. Daily protein intake averaged 83 grams, with 19 percent from animal sources. Daily productivity was estimated at 1.22 tons of sugarcane, which is low in comparison with productivity figures reported for sugarcane cutters in Colombia, Jamaica, Tanzania, Sudan, and Zimbabwe.

A second study included 57 coffee pickers from a community organized as a cooperative. These workers ranged in age from 19 to 77 years, also tended to be lean and muscular, and resembled the sugarcane cutters in body composition. They picked coffee beans four months of the year (September-December), a work activity which competed with the need to harvest self-grown maize and/or rice. Workers were paid a piece-rate, and set their own working hours. Mean daily energy intake was estimated to be 43 kcals per kg of body weight.

Energy Supplementation and Productivity

Workers from one community were designated the high energy supplement (HES) group (Table 1), thus assignment to the two treatment groups was non-random. The two supplements consisted of a bottled orange-flavored soft drink distributed 11 times a week. The high energy supplement contained 350 kcals/bottle and, if consistently consumed, provided 550 kcals/day on a weekly basis. The low energy

Table 1

Experimental Design
Energy Supplementation and Productivity of Guatemalan Sugarcane Cutters
1973-77
Supplementation Schedule

Supplementation Groups	N	Delivery Frequency (Week)	Supplement Content (per 350 ml.)			Average Energy Supply/Day (kcals.)
			Energy (kcals.)	Vitamin A (mg.)	Vitamin C (mg.)	
High energy supplement (HES)	95	11	350	3.7	16	550
Low energy supplement (LES)	63	11	15	3.7	16	24

supplement was identical in appearance, contained 15 kcals/bottle, and provided 24 kcals/day. Both supplements contained vitamins A and C and both supplements were well accepted by the workers.

Supplementation was carried out continuously for a period of 28 months (Figure 2). Intensive data collection was initiated 3 months prior to supplementation, although worker productivity records were obtained retrospectively starting 17 months prior to supplementation. Certain data, including productivity records, were obtained during a 10-month period following termination of the supplementation program.

Figure 2

Experimental Design
Energy Supplementation and Productivity of Guatemalan Sugarcane Cutters
1973-1977

DATA COLLECTION

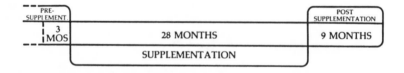

The effectiveness of the program in raising total energy intake levels of the HES workers during the first half of the supplementation period has been reported elsewhere (Immink et al. 1981); therefore, a summary of findings will suffice. Data from the second half of the supplementation period has not yet been analyzed, but is not expected to provide significantly different results.

On the average, the high energy supplement (HES) group raised their total daily energy intake by 10 percent or approximately 300 kcals. The energy intake of the low energy supplement (LES) group remained essentially constant over the supplementation period, but tended to fall towards the end. Workers in both groups remained in energy balance over the whole period, but tended to lose some tricipital adiposity towards the end of each cane harvesting season when work activities intensified. Some substitution of supplement energy for home energy intake took place, with the degree of substitution less among HES workers with low body weights. HES workers appear to have increased their total level of energy expenditure with supplementation.

Time-series of the mean productivity of the two groups during almost 5 harvest seasons are presented in Figure 3. The group means represent 5 week moving averages. No consistent pattern of higher daily productivity by the HES group during supplementation is obvious, but the peaks in HES workers' daily productivity during the 1975/76 harvest season exceed those of the LES group. After termination of the supplementation program, however, the HES workers exhibited extraordinarily high daily productivity levels at the start of the next harvest season. A more detailed statistical analysis of the first half of the supplementation period resulted in the finding that no positive and consistent supplementation effect had been present, even after controlling for several extraneous factors (Immink and Viteri 1981b). It appeared that certain work organization/management practices, instituted whenever effective mill capacity declined, might have affected the productivity of the two groups differently. Since the workers had not been assigned randomly to the two groups, this interaction between selection and history produced a potentially confounding effect.

Figure 3

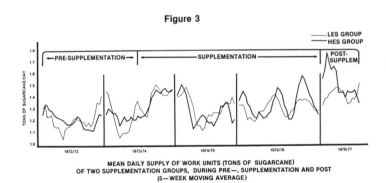

MEAN DAILY SUPPLY OF WORK UNITS (TONS OF SUGARCANE)
OF TWO SUPPLEMENTATION GROUPS, DURING PRE—, SUPPLEMENTATION AND POST
(5—WEEK MOVING AVERAGE)

The data for both the pre- and supplementation periods were submitted to an ARIMA (Auto-Regressive Integrated Moving Average) time series analysis (McCleary and Hay 1980). The results of the analysis demonstrated no abrupt or gradual and sustained supplementation effect on the mean daily output of the HES group; therefore, the findings are not supportive of the efficiency wage hypothesis.

Energy-Protein Intake and Human Capital Formation

The authors found that productivity levels among male Guatemalan sugarcane cutters and coffee pickers are significantly related to indicators of nutritional status and of lean body mass. Some of these results are presented here. Next the analysis was extended in order to look at the implications for human capital formation in these workers.

The following anthropometric measurements are available for assessing the nutritional status of the workers: weight, standing height, mid-upper arm circumference, leg (calf) circumference and tricipital skinfold. Measurements were made in 145 sugarcane cutters who had participated in the longitudinal study. The coffee pickers, members of a coffee cooperative located in the same region of Guatemala, were also included. Workers in both groups were previously described as being lean and muscular. Two additional productivity indicators are also considered for the sugarcane workers: (a) days worked/week during the harvest season, and (b) time required to complete a standardized weeding task during the off harvest season.

A factor analysis was performed on a number of selected anthropometric indicators for each group of workers. The results are presented in Table 2. In order to generate factors which would approximate different aspects of body composition, the following indicators were included: weight adjusted for height, arm muscle circumference, triceps skinfold, and leg (calf) circumference. An Eigenvalue of .5 was specified in order to explain a high percent of the total variance. The matrix was rotated using the varimax method.

The two factors which were generated account for approximately 90 percent of the total variance in each group. Arm muscle circumference, leg (calf) circumference and

Table 2
Factor Analysis of Selected Anthropometric Indicators in Two
Samples of Agricultural Workers in Guatemala
(Varimax Rotation Method)

Anthropometric Indicator	Sugarcane Cutters (n=145)			Coffee Pickers (n=57)		
	Factor Loadings		Communality	Factor Loadings		Communality
	"Factor A"	"Factor B"		"Factor A"	"Factor B"	
Weight/Height	.9146	.3038	.9287	.9116	.3059	.9246
Upper-arm Muscle Circumf.	.9282	.0119	.8618	.9136	.0951	.8436
Tricipital Skinfold	.1556	.9839	.9922	.1809	.9819	.9969
Leg (Calf) Circumference	.8881	1974	.8276	.8856	.1566	.8088
Eigenvalue % Variation	2.74 68.6	0.87 21.7	3.61 90.3	2.76 69.0	0.81 20.3	3.57 89.3

weight/height all entered with a high loading in the first factor ("FACTOR-A"). Triceps skinfold entered with a high loading in the second factor. This paper focuses on the first factor, which is interpreted as an indicator of lean body mass. Using Viteri's data for Guatemalan agricultural workers and military personnel (Viteri 1971) a high correlation was found between this factor and a direct measurement of lean body mass ($r = .82$; $p < .01$), while the correlation with muscle mass was also significant but lower ($r = .49$; $p < .01$).[1]

Correlations between the lean body mass (LBM) factor and several productivity indicators are presented in Table 3. The LBM factor is adjusted for age. The most significant correlation coefficient is obtained for the coffee pickers. Workers with more lean body mass tend to pick more coffee beans a day, cut and load more sugarcane a day, and complete a standardized weeding task in less time. They also tend to have fewer absences from work. These results,

---

[1]An alternative factor, constructed with body surface, arm, and calf circumferences, demonstrated a lower degree of accuracy. FACTOR-A had a maximum absolute error of estimate of 3.5 kg (9.8%) in this sample population.

which are in accord with those published by others (Viteri 1971; Davies 1973), show a high degree of consistency across different agricultural tasks. Further analysis demonstrated that for these workers the relationship is essentially linear, i.e., constant productivity returns to increasing lean body mass values. If workers with more extreme values are included, however, non-linearities may be introduced into these relationships.

Table 3

Productivity of Guatemalan Agricultural Workers Correlated
with an Indicator of Lean Body Mass

Agricultural Task:	Productivity Indicator:	Product-moment Correlation Coefficient:
Coffee Picking (n=57)	Weight of Coffee Beans Picked (kg/day)	.349*
Weeding (n=131)	Task Time (mins/ standard area)	-.175**
Sugarcane Cutting and Loading (n=145)	Weight of Sugarcane delivered (tons/day	.199*
	Days worked/week	.192*

* p < .01
** p < .05

In order to investigate the implications of these findings in terms of human capital formation, the analysis was extended further. The first step was to construct age-earnings profiles associated with different LBM levels within these populations. This approach allows us to estimate the increment, in the stock of human capital of these workers, that may be expected from significant increases in lean body mass.[2]

A simple model demonstrates this:

_____

[2]For references to the human capital approach and the basic human capital model that underlies the analysis here, see Becker (1975) and Ghez and Becker (1975).

$$(1) \qquad I = \frac{d(t) (1 + g)^t}{(1 + i)^t}$$

where I stands for increment in the stock of human capital, d(t) represents the earnings differential of different levels of LBM, g is the time rate of growth in the differential ($g \lesseqgtr 0$), and i is the rate of discount. Estimations for d(t) and g were done statistically, and an 8% discount rate was arbitrarily assumed. Thus, the present value of the lifetime earnings differential at age 17 was calculated, assuming different t's, i.e., different ages during the productive life cycle at which improvement or deterioration in the LBM of workers may take place.

Both groups of workers were divided into two sub-samples, depending on whether their LBM factor scores fell above or below the median factor score (= 0). Regression models were formulated to test whether workers with high LBM values can be expected to be more productive over the life cycle (age 17 to 65) than their colleagues with "low" LBM values. The results of the stepwise regression analysis for the sugarcane cutters were:

(2) P = 29.44* - .0010* (Age squared) + 1.207** (LBMGRP)
     (0.53) (0.0003)   (0.534)

     R = .12   F = 9.13(p<.001)
     *p<.01   **p<.05

where P equals daily cane deliveries and LBMGRP is a dummy variable for high and low LBM values. The term LBMGRP(age squared) was not statistically significant. In terms of our model then: d(t) > 0, and g = 0; sugarcane cutters with relatively high LBM values tend to be consistently more productive at all ages of the productive life cycle than workers with low LBM values. Equation (2) was used to estimate the age-productivity profiles in Figure 4. The shaded area between the two curves represents the estimated productivity differential associated with the two LBM levels. Age squared, rather than age or a polynomial regression, gave the best statistical results, suggesting that the peak of the age-productivity profile tends to come at a very low productive age in these workers. This is consistent with data from the U.S. and elsewhere for workers with low levels of investment in human capital.

Figure 4

ESTIMATED AGE-PRODUCTIVITY PROFILES OF
GUATEMALAN SUGARCANE CUTTERS WITH
TWO DIFFERENT LEVELS OF LEAN BODY MASS (LBM)

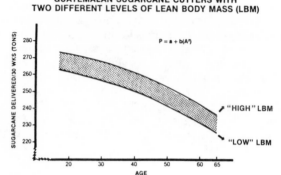

The daily productivity of the coffee pickers were found not to be associated with their age, despite the fact that workers ranged in age from 19 to 77 years. However, there was a significant difference in mean productivity between workers with high and with low LBM factor scores (F = 5.22; p<.03).

In order to estimate the increases in the present value of life-time earnings associated with high LBM values in these populations, the age-productivity profile was converted into life-time earnings using piece-rates paid to the sugar-cane cutters in 1974, and to the coffee pickers in 1977. In these calculations it was assumed that the workers engaged in sugar-cane harvesting and coffee picking year-round, and that no changes in piece-rates will take place during the life cycle. As long as changes over time in piece-rates are not dependent on individual productivity levels, these assumptions have no further consequence. It is the increase in the stock of human capital associated with higher LBM values which is of interest.

Table 4 presents the estimated present value of life-time earnings of sugarcane cutters and coffee pickers with two levels of LBM. For low LBM cutters the present value of life-time earnings was estimated at about $6,400 (at 1974 piece-rates). For cutters who enter the work force with higher LBM values and who maintain them throughout their productive life, the present value of life-time earnings would be a modest 4.3 percent higher. The later the age at which the improvement in LBM takes place, the lower is the percent difference in the life-time earnings because the period over which the productivity benefits are associated with higher LBM values is correspondingly shorter.

Table 4

Present Values (PV)* at Age Seventeen of Life-Time Earnings of Guatemalan Sugarcane Cutters and Coffee Pickers by Two Levels of Lean Body Mass (LBM)

Occupational Group	"Low" LBM Level PV (US$)	LBM Effect at Age:					
		<17		25		35	
		PV (US$)	% Difference with Low	PV (US$)	% Difference with Low	PV (US$)	% Difference with Low
Sugarcane Cutters (1974)	6356	6627	4.3	6489	2.1	6414	1.0
Coffee Pickers (1977)	2130	2595	21.7	2364	11.0	2280	7.1

* Discount rate = 8%

The study results for the coffee pickers are more dramatic, starting with a 22 percent difference for coffee pickers who start with, and maintain throughout the productive life stage, high LBM values.[3] There appears to be a significant association between the lean body mass of these agricultural workers and their productivity and life-time earnings. Within a given range, therefore, more lean body mass represents a form of investment in the stock of human capital of these workers.

The same approach was followed in order to relate an indicator of childhood nutrition to adult productivity. As has previously been shown, adult stature is positively correlated with productivity in sugarcane cutting (Spurr et al. 1977; Morrison and Blake 1974). Genetic as well as environmental factors, including nutrition during the pre- and

---

[3]The significantly lower present values of life-time earnings of coffee pickers compared to the sugarcane cutters are due to the fact that the former were also engaged in the other agricultural activities, predominantly subsistence farming.

post-natal growth period, determine adult height. In poorly nourished populations, however, genetic factors play a lesser role. Parent-child height correlations have been found to be significantly lower among school-age children suffering from energy-protein deficiencies than among well-nourished children (Mueller 1976). Postnatal chronic undernutrition results in both slow height-growth velocity during childhood and a prolonged growth period, leading to a 10 percent reduction in adult stature of poorly nourished populations (Frisancho 1978). Adult stature was also significantly correlated with productivity in the authors' sample of sugarcane cutters. Age-earnings profiles for three different height categories ("short," "medium," and "tall") were estimated. Regression analysis showed that tall workers were significantly more productive than short workers $(d(t)>0)$, with the productivity differential remaining constant over the productive life cycle $(g=0)$.

While tall workers are not more productive than medium workers early in the productive phase, a productivity differential may appear later on. Those workers who suffered most severely from deficient energy-protein intake during childhood and adolescence can expect their productivity in sugarcane cutting to be negatively affected. The increase in life-time earnings, using 1974 data, associated with entering

Table 5

Present Values* of Life Time Earnings up to Age 62 of
a Typical "Short" and "Tall" Sugarcane Cutter

Productivity Indicator Used:	"Tall" Worker (US$)	"Short" Worker (US$)	Difference (%)
A. Sugarcane Delivered (ton)	6,577	6,236	5.5
B. Gross earnings	7,400	6,378	16.0

* Rate of discount = 8%.

the work force as a "tall" rather than "short" cutter is indicated in Table 5. Considering earnings based solely on average daily tonnage of cane cut and loaded, this increase amounts to 5.5 percent. Based upon total gross earnings the increase in life-time earning turns out to be 16 percent. The difference in the estimated life-time earnings differential may be explained in part by the fact that taller workers tended to be absent from work less often. We infer that there may be significant losses in life-time earnings in sugarcane cutting associated with deficient energy-protein intake levels during childhood.

The findings to date from the authors' studies with Guatemalan agricultural workers may be summarized as follows:

1. The sugarcane cutters were moderately energy deficient, as indicated by anthropometric indicators and mean daily energy intake. Energy supplementation resulted in partial substitution of supplement energy for home energy.
2. These workers appeared to have increased their total level of energy expenditure with supplementation; it is most likely that additional energy expenditure took place in non-work activities, as no positive and consistent effect can be demonstrated on worker productivity in sugarcane cutting and loading.
3. The indicator of lean body mass (LBM) explains a part of inter-worker variation in the productivity of sugarcane cutters and weeders, and coffee pickers; low LBM values in these workers are associated with reduced life-time earnings, represent reduced human capital formation, and are thus an economic cost.
4. Low levels of energy intake during the preproductive phase of the life cycle may be an important form of dis-investment in human capital, relative to particular occupations, when it results in decreased adult stature.

SUMMARY

The new home economics approach provides models which explicitly recognize that rural households engage in home production as well as market production. The interdependence of individual production functions of household members is recognized. The approach allows the summary of the total economic effect of low energy intake and of direct and indirect nutrition interventions in one convenient measure: "full income." The methodology to measure full income is in an advanced state of development (Evenson 1981); empirical evidence, however, is grossly lacking.

The interdependence among household members in allocating time inputs among different production activities may provide an explanation of why the results of short-term energy supplementation studies in rural workers do not support the efficiency wage hypothesis. The authors' studies strongly suggest that energy expenditure in off-the-job activities increased with supplementation. Thus, the "full income" of the households of supplemented wage workers may increase even if their productivity in market production remains unchanged. Field studies, in which measurements of worker productivity are made, inherently produce biased results. Such studies a priori exclude adults whose health and nutritional status prevent them from being economically active, thus potentially underestimating the supplementation effect. As Bliss and Stern (1978b) argued, the efficiency curve may be operative only over a certain range of energy intake, above which market wages and the workers' relative preferences for work and leisure determine the supply of work units. This argument can be accommodated easily in the home production model.

The results presented here support the hypothesis that nutritional improvements during childhood represent forms of human capital formation which result in higher life-time earnings in certain occupations. Additionally, such improvements may be associated with upward social and occupational mobility during adulthood, especially if agricultural and rural development is effective. In Latin America, large rural to urban population movements also have that effect. As the economic value of children increases, so does the incentive to invest in them through better child care, nutrition, and health. The old age-social security argument suggests that the economic returns are at least partially internalized by parents. At the same time, the increased need for market goods in human capital formation and the increased value of home production time may serve as inducements to have fewer children (Zeitlin et al. 1982).

Social rates of return may differ from private rates of return thus providing justification for public investment in the nutritional status of children. External benefits may be present in the form of greater involvement in community development activities, better social interactions, improvements in the efficiency of the educational process, etc. Empirically, it is still far from possible to estimate the rates of return from nutritional investments during childhood. In

addition to estimating costs of nutritional inputs, this requires linking those inputs to specific biological and cognitive outcomes and, in turn, linking those to improvements in
human productivity. It is the second linkage which is
difficult to establish because it involves interactions with
cultural, social and economic factors.

This chapter attempts to show that there are significant
gaps in the empirical evidence to indicate:

a) how rural households adapt behaviorally to low levels of
energy intake and what the economic consequences are,
and
b) how rural households re-allocate their resources in
response to either direct nutrition and health interventions, or to improved economic conditions resulting from
long-term agricultural and rural development.

It is clear that additional empirical evidence related to
those questions is required. Longitudinal supplementation
studies are costly and complex, but when measuring the
economic consequences of short-term changes in energy
availability at the household level, it is possible to take
advantage of available information on seasonally occurring
variations in food supplies, disease patterns, and market and
home production opportunities in rural areas. Agricultural
and rural development projects can be used as "intervention
tools" to estimate the economic outcomes at the household
level, and of changes in the cultural, socio-economic, and
physical environments.

Supplemental feeding programs aimed at eliminating or
reducing energy deficiency in rural populations do not
provide the solution to the basic underlying problem - rural
poverty. Such programs, however, may have to be part of
agricultural and rural development efforts. The income
effect may only be felt in the long run, and current energy
intake levels may effectively prevent the optimal participation
by rural households in market, home, leisure and human
capital formation activities.

REFERENCES

1.   Becker GS (1965).   A theory of the allocation of time.
Econ J 75:493-517.

2. Becker GS (1975). "Human Capital. A Theoretical and Empirical Analysis, With Special Reference to Education" (2nd ed.). New York: National Bureau of Economic Research, Inc.
3. Belavady B (1966). Nutrition and efficiency in agricultural labourers. Indian J Med Res 54:971-976.
4. Bliss C and Stern N (1978a). Productivity, wages and nutrition, Part I. The Theory. J Dev Econ 5:331-362.
5. Bliss C and Stern M (1978b). Productivity, wages and nutrition, Part II. Some observations. J Dev Econ 5:363-398.
6. Davies CTM (1973). Relationship of maximum aerobic power output to productivity and absenteeism of east African sugar cane workers. Brit J Industr Med 30:146-154.
7. Evenson RE (1978). Time allocation in rural Philippines. Am J Ag Econ 60:323-330.
8. Evenson RE (1981). Food policy and the new home economics. Food Policy 6:180-193.
9. Frisancho RA (1978). Nutritional influences on human growth and maturation. Yearbook Phys Anthro 21:174-191.
10. Ghez GR and Becker GS (1975). "The Allocation of Time and Goods over the Life Cycle." New York: National Bureau of Economic Research, Inc.
11. Gross DR and Underwood BA (1971). Technological change and calorie costs: sisal agriculture in Northeastern Brazil. Am Anthro 73:725-740.
12. Immink MDC and Viteri FE (1981a). Energy intake and productivity of Guatemalan sugarcane cutters. An empirical test of the efficiency wage hypothesis. Part I. J Dev Econ 9:251-271.
13. Immink MDC and Viteri FE (1981b). Energy intake and productivity of Guatemalan sugarcane cutters. An empirical test of the efficiency wage hypothesis. Part II. J Dev Econ 9:273-287.
14. Immink MDC, Viteri FE and Helms RW (1981). Food substitution with worker feeding programs: energy supplementation in Guatemalan sugarcane workers. Am J Clin Nutr 34:2145-2150.
15. Immink MDC, Viteri FE and Helms RW (1982). Energy intake over the life cycle and human capital formation in Guatemalan sugarcane cutters. Econ Dev Cult Change 30:351-372.

16. Leibenstein H (1957). The theory of underemployment in backward economies. J Pol Econ 65:91-103.
17. Leibenstein H (1958). Underemployment in backward economies: Some additional notes. J Pol Econ 66:256-258.
18. Malina RM (1984). Physical activity and motor development/performance in populations nutritionally at risk. In Pollitt E and Amante P (eds.): "Energy Intake and Activity," New York: Alan R. Liss, Inc. (In Press).
19. McCleary R and Hay RA Jr. (1980). "Applied Time Series Analysis for the Social Sciences." Beverly Hills, CA: Sage Publications, Inc.
20. McGuire JS (1979). "Seasonal Changes in Energy Expenditure and Work Patterns of Rural Guatemalan Women," Ph.D. Dissertation (unpublished). Massachusetts Institute of Technology.
21. Minge-Klevana W (1980). Does labor time decrease with industrialization? A survey of time-allocation studies. Curr Anthro 21:279-298.
22. Mirrlees JA (1976). A pure theory of underdeveloped economies. In Reynolds LG (ed.): "Agriculture in Development Theory," New Haven, CT: Yale University Press.
23. Morrison JF and Blake GTW (1974). Physiological observations on cane cutters. Europ J App Phys 33:247-254.
24. Mueller WH (1976). Parent-child correlations for status and weight among school aged children: A review of 24 studies. Hum Bio 48:379-397.
25. Nag M, White BNF and Peet RC (1978). An anthropological approach to the study of the economic value of children in Java and Nepal. Curr Anthro 19:293-306.
26. Popkin BM (1980). Time allocation of the mother and child nutrition. Ecol Food and Nutri 9:1-14.
27. Sameroff AJ and McDonough SC (1984). The role of motor activity in human cognitive and social development. In Pollitt E and Amante P (eds.): "Energy Intake and Activity," New York: Alan R. Liss, Inc. (In press).
28. Spurr GB (1984). Physical activity, nutritional status and physical work capacity in relation to agricultural activity. In Pollitt E and Amante P (eds.): "Energy Intake and Activity," New York, Alan R. Liss, Inc. (In press).

29. Spurr GB, Barac-Nieto M and Maksud MG (1977). Productivity and maximal oxygen consumption in sugarcane cutters. Am J Clin Nutr 30:316-321.
30. Stiglitz JE (1976). The efficiency wage hypothesis, surplus labour and the distribution of income in L.D.C.'s. Oxford Econ Papers (New Series). 28:185-207.
31. Viteri FE (1971). Considerations on the effect of nutrition on body composition and physical working capacity of young Guatemalan adults. In Scrimshaw NS and Altschul AM (eds.): "Amino Acid Fortification of Protein Foods," Cambridge, Mass: The M.I.T. Press.
32. Viteri FE, Torún B, Immink MDC and Flores R (1981). Marginal malnutrition and working capacity. In Harper AE and Davis GK (eds.): "Nutrition in Health and Disease and International Development," New York: Alan R. Liss, Inc.
33. Wolgemuth JD, Latham MC, Hall A, Chester A and Crompton DWT (1982). Worker productivity and the nutritional status of Kenyan road construction laborers. Am J Clin Nutr 36:68-78.
34. Zeitlin MF, Wray JD, Stanbury JB, Schlossman NP and Meurer MF (1982). "Nutrition and Population Growth: The Delicate Balance," Cambridge, Mass: Oelgeschlager, Gunn and Hain Publishers, Inc.

Energy Intake and Activity, pages 377–394
© *1984 Alan R. Liss, Inc., 150 Fifth Avenue, New York, NY 10011*

POLICY IMPLICATIONS OF RESEARCH ON ENERGY INTAKE AND ACTIVITY LEVELS WITH REFERENCE TO THE DEBATE ON THE ENERGY ADEQUACY OF EXISTING DIETS IN DEVELOPING COUNTRIES

Shlomo Reutlinger

Senior Economist, World Bank

INTRODUCTION

In essence, the central policy question is whether the average energy intake of sub-populations known to have low intakes should be augmented through public intervention. Ideally, the benefits and the costs of such interventions should be determined. As a practical matter, the public policy debate about nutrition has proceeded on another plane. Everyone has accepted too readily the idea of an energy "requirement" level which should be met by all persons (or more correctly, the average person) of the same sex, age, and body size, in all places and at all times. I think this idea was adopted because it was convenient but, while convenience and pragmatism are important, perhaps some improvements might be made if we admit that there are flaws in the reasoning, and then proceed.

Aside from convenience, I believe that the present state of affairs is also the result of insufficient communication between nutritionists, economists, and policy-makers. Nutritionists can and do make estimates of energy "requirements" for achieving very particular results: rates of growth in children, activity levels, etc. They cannot and do not tell us what results "should be" achieved. Nor do economists and policy-makers specify results. They have neither adequate knowledge of the effect of body weight and activity levels on economic performance nor theories about suitable income distribution or acceptable levels of poverty.

In my view, the current flurry of interest among policy-makers and advisors in obtaining solid information about the benefits and costs of augmenting low energy diets has several origins. In recent years economists and statisticians (Dandeker and Rath 1971; Reutlinger and Selowsky 1976; Reutlinger and Alderman 1980; FAO 1977) have attempted to determine the implications of using the same, or similar, energy requirement standards advocated by the FAO/WHO Expert Committee to estimate the percent of the population in developing countries that exists on diets which fall below these standards. Their findings vividly illustrate the potential magnitude of the problems involved with meeting such standards.

These same studies also draw attention to the variation in energy intakes among different socio-economic groups and, therefore, raise questions about the validity of using standards based on country averages for all segments of the population. The financial, administrative and political costs of augmenting the food energy intakes of all people to the level of the FAO/WHO requirement standards are known to be very high. Thus, some basic questions are now being asked, correctly in my view, about the nature of the recommended requirements and whether they could be stated more precisely in reference to particular socio-economic groups. For example: What are the consequences of intakes that are lower than recommended for: children and adults? people exposed to varying degrees of risk for infectious diseases? people accustomed to different activity patterns? and people expected to participate in economic change? Another reason why we see, or should see, increased interest in the relative benefits of augmenting food energy intakes, through monetary assistance to a household, relates to the existing level of intake. If the initial per capita daily energy intake is 1,900 calories rather than 1,500 calories it may require two or three times as large an income transfer, in money or in kind, to induce a household to increase the energy intake by a given amount.

Disenchantment with the energy requirement concept is extended by the growing debate among nutritionists over what is the "correct" level of requirements. It has become increasingly evident that the widely different recommendations suggested by different authorities are not due to differences about the biomedical and scientific interpretations of energy input/output relationships, though that may be a factor. Instead they reflect judgments about lifestyles and the way people should live and function. If this perception is correct, and whether or not they wish to acknowledge it, policy-makers and their advisors must realize quickly that they cannot simply defer to the authoritative judgment of the nutritionist. For an excellent exposition of this point of view, see Beaton (1982).

Finally, as the economic slowdown and rising debt levels have decreased international aid resources and funding as well as government programs, it has become increasingly necessary to reduce food interventions which, in the past, were carried out for political reasons. In addition, policy advisors are frequently asked about the nature and magnitude of the consequences of reducing already established interventions. The case of Sri Lanka is a good example. The nation has had a food rationing program in effect for over 35 years. The rice rationing program has supplied 2-4 lbs. per capita per week, 1-2 lbs. of which was free and the remainder subsidized. The coverage of this program has been nearly universal, primarily because the political cost of universal coverage was far less than the political cost of targeted coverage. It is estimated, however, that the economic cost of this program has amounted to 20% of current expenditures for the last 15 years (Isenman 1980). It is the economic costs of these programs that have recently encouraged Sri Lanka to begin scaling them down and targeting specific population segments.

In principle, for those accustomed to think in terms of economics, this shift in focus from debate over the appropriate "requirement of energy" to the "costs and benefits of different levels of energy" is a welcome, long overdue development. As a practical matter, we all enjoyed the convenience of using a fixed level of "energy requirements" against which to measure international nutritional adequacy and related policy performance. But what is required at this juncture, is a reasonable compromise between the correct approach on theoretical grounds and an approach that is attainable, desirable, and workable. We should stop debate about the correct energy requirement of a population; if we have learned anything from studies of energy input/output relationships and benefit-cost calculations, it is that a unique requirement level does not exist. On the other hand, it would be enormously expensive and utterly impractical to carry out all the studies and calculations needed to

determine optimal energy intakes for each specific population. It will remain necessary, however, to measure energy
intake performance against some "requirement" standards;
not a single standard, but an array of "requirement" levels
each of which reflects levels of adequacy for different
objectives.

In such a context, I am skeptical about the policy
implications of measuring precisely the relationship between
energy intake and activity levels in particular individuals.
This skepticism arises from my understanding of the nature
of policy interventions and the dynamic nature of the environment in which individuals operate (Keys et al. 1950;
Muller-Schwarze et al. 1982; Apfelbaum et al. 1971; Batliwala
1982; and INCAP 1978). Yet it would be quite instructive to
have research designed to identify the entire activity profile
of households at different levels of energy intake, as well as
carefully constructed experiments to identify circumstances
in which energy intake sets undue constraints on activity.

In the remainder of the paper, I will discuss the kinds
of knowledge and judgments needed in order to evaluate
policy options with regard to interventions designed to
satisfy food energy requirements of populations.

THE THEORY OF OPTIMAL ENERGY INTAKE

Whether considering individual household units or
society at large, benefits and costs differ according to levels
of intake. What distinguishes household and societal decisions is the nature and magnitude of the benefits and costs
relevant for those decisions.

Figure 1 illustrates the marginal benefit and cost functions for different levels of energy intake. The optimal
amount of energy intake is obviously at the point at which
the marginal benefit equals the marginal cost. At issue are
the shape of those marginal benefit and cost functions and
how decisions can be made in the presence of a great deal of
ignorance about them.

Let us consider first the individual household and see
why the shapes of the functions are as they are shown.
Unless there is a certain minimum level of energy intake,
there is no life. In this range one cannot speak of the

Figure 1: Marginal Benefit and Cost Functions for Energy Intake of Households

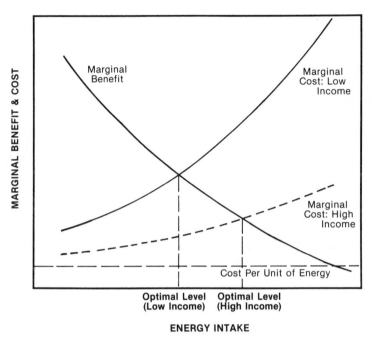

ENERGY INTAKE

benefit of an additional unit of energy--the function does not exist. But, once there is enough energy to survive, additional units of energy are likely to have large benefits: satisfying hunger; preventing disease; performing more work or more household chores, etc. As the energy intake level increases, benefits for the initial accounts will decline and energy will be allocated to other ends with less marginal benefits, such as play, education, and social interaction. There is a good deal of evidence to support this point. In a 1982 study by Muller-Schwarze et al., deer were subjected to an experimentally induced milk shortage. They compensated by reducing play, and increasing foraging activity. It is reasonable to expect that the opposite would have been true had milk intake then increased. In several studies Viteri and collaborators found that increased energy intake resulted in greater energy expenditure both at work and after work, especially among more severely malnourished

individuals (Immink et al., In press). Marginally malnourished workers tended to use the extra energy intake on
after work activities rather than on increasing their work
productivity (Viteri 1975; Viteri et al. 1981; Immink and
Viteri 1981; Immink et al. 1982).

On the cost side, rising marginal costs are the result of
an overall budget constraint. More food means doing with
less clothing, housing, etc. Just as there are diminishing
benefits to increased food energy, the cost of giving up
more and more of the other amenities rises as their consumption levels decrease. In very high income households, the
sacrifice of other consumption items is minuscule as expenditures for energy intake increase, and the marginal cost is
approximately constant at whatever it costs to purchase a
unit of energy.

Society can and does influence the shape of the marginal benefit and cost function: through the prices of every
item in the consumption basket; through the income attained
by the household; through the values of the activities made
possible by the energy intake; and by the provision of
information about the benefits of additional energy utilization. But, in the final analysis, it is the physiological
needs, psychological preferences, and values attached to the
relative welfare of the members of the household which
determine the correct level of energy intake, and its allocation to different uses and to each member of the household.

It is important, for several reasons, to keep in mind
the determinants for decisions about food consumption and
allocation for individual households. First, they illustrate
the difficulty of using public policy to influence selective
uses of energy for purposes which outsiders deem important.
Second, they suggest which policies and interventions might
be most suitable for achieving social objectives. For instance, measures which conserve energy in household chores
might not lead to the allocation of increased energy to work
related activities; the household might choose to decrease
total energy intake and relocate the available energy among
alternative uses. In contrast, providing work related incentives might induce the household to increase energy intake
and to allocate a larger share to work related activities.
Finally, knowledge of how different groups of households
utilize energy is important for selective targeting of interventions designed to achieve specific policy goals.

Although the theoretical framework for public decisions about augmenting energy intake is analogous to the framework for private decisions, the nature and magnitude of relevant benefits and costs may be quite different. Society may count as a benefit only those energy uses which increase overall productivity. When there is a great deal of unemployment, additional work related activity by underachiever households may benefit those households, but may not increase the gross national product. Increased activity by the underachiever households would then be regarded as a benefit only by a government concerned with a more egalitarian income distribution. Such a government may also consider it a benefit if additional energy is used to improve the quality of life. And a government which provides free health services may count it as a benefit if increased energy reduces the demand on these facilities.

On the cost side, rising marginal costs for inducing greater food consumption result from overall constraints set by the government budget, as well as from the escalating amounts of income transfers, in money or in kind, which are necessary to induce households to increase energy intakes as their level of energy intake rises. Again, the case of Sri Lanka is instructive (Isenman 1980). Figure 2 illustrates the levels of optimal energy intake, characterized by respective marginal benefit and cost functions, which occur in different public policy and country scenarios.

THE NATURE OF BENEFITS AND COST OF PUBLIC POLICY INTERVENTION

The Energy Intake of Individuals and Its Allocations to a Specific Use

Unless a government undertakes the feeding of individuals (children or workers) throughout the day, the energy intake of individuals cannot be controlled; therefore, the usual unit of intervention is the household. Moreover, it is likely that any augmentation of individuals' energy intake would have to be far in excess of the requirements for particular "outputs" selected on the basis of narrow policy objectives.

It is easy to document the observation that much of the augmented energy intake in low energy intake households is

Figure 2: Marginal Benefit and Cost of Public Regulation of Household Energy Intake

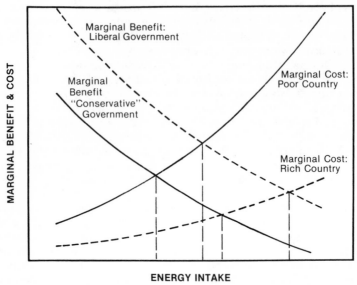

utilized for other than work related activities. Observed differences in energy intakes of households with different incomes are much larger than anything "explainable" on the basis of the differences in energy requirements needed to support the additional income generating activities. How else can one explain the observation in many household surveys that daily energy intakes of adjacent income groups, particularly at the lower end of the income scale, differ by as much as 300 or 400 calories per capita or by 1,500 to 2,000 calories per household? The additional work performed could have required at most 300 to 400 calories. The members of the higher income groups usually have higher body weights and this can account for another 400 to 800 calories. By sheer deduction, the remaining differences in intake must have been utilized in non-work related activities. In this context, it is interesting to note that the transition from very low incomes to higher incomes, particularly in rural areas, may also reduce the energy required for work, particularly as energy use intensive activities such as walking long distances to fetch water and gather firewood are replaced with more convenient arrangements (Batliwala 1982). Thus, the net energy expended on work related activity and "basic life chores" may not increase and may even decline, as income and energy intakes are observed to increase.

In my view, the way energy is utilized in the household has two implications for the relevance of research on the relationship between energy intake and activity. Research limited to the energy requirements of work related activities is of little use. Even if we were interested exclusively in providing for the energy needed in the performance of work tasks, it would not be particularly useful to know how many calories were required for the performance if we did not know the number of calories needed by the household in order to allocate the necessary additional energy to the activity in question. It would be more useful to design studies which show the relationship between household energy intake and, for example, the number of hours in which the income producing members of the household engage in energy intensive activities. Such studies can give meaningful results, however, only when demand for the various activities is the same for all the observed households. We might observe then that 2,000 incremental calories consumed by the household have the effect of allowing the income producing members to spend two additional hours at work. When the marginal energy cost is less than the value of two hours of work, the policy implications are clear. A "pump priming" income transfer, or other intervention to augment the household's energy intake, would be greatly rewarding.

I would like to think that there are many opportunities for "pump priming" interventions, but the little evidence we have so far, particularly from studies conducted at INCAP (Viteri 1975; Viteri et al. 1981; Immink and Viteri 1981; and Immink et al. 1982) suggests that this is not the case. The opportunities for remunerative physical work do not seem to expand as rapidly as the labor force. Moreover, even households with low energy intakes must, and do, give highest priority to the energy needed for sheer survival. Nevertheless, because "pump priming" interventions would be so cost-effective where suitable, we should devote additional research to identifying appropriate opportunities.

The other implication of the observation that augmented energy intakes by households have joint, multiple "products" is that policy-makers must be made aware of the potential benefits of enhanced energy availability for activities other than those related to physical work. Larger body sizes and activity seemingly unrelated to direct work output, such as children and adults exploring and interacting with the environment, may have more development and income distribution benefits, in the long run, than augmented energy expenditure in the performance of physical work. Recognizing and quantifying these non-direct work related energy uses might be particularly important when there is much under- and unemployment and, therefore, little justification on immediate, direct productivity grounds to augment the energy intake of the poorest segments of the population.

While there is probably little disagreement with the contention that non-work related activity could have major long-term consequences, it is questionable whether these can be quantified to the extent necessary for making policy recommendations. On this issue I offer only two brief comments. Even if we cannot predict, for example, the development impact of a more socially active and interacting population, it is important to determine the energy expenditure profiles of households with different energy intakes and the extent to which these affect functional performance, such as educational achievement, adoption of innovation, migration, etc. Since the development impact of enhanced energy intakes is, in many ways, the result of a chain of events evolving over a long period of time, the only hope for unraveling the puzzle is to study separately the links which can be observed at a single point in time. If the research is to bear fruit within the policy context, it is important that we keep in mind the need to study all the links explaining the relationship between energy intake and development and that, within a reasonable time, we join them together.

My other comment is that policy-makers should be warned against basing decisions exclusively on the more easily observable and measurable immediate benefits when, in fact, there are other benefits which are, unfortunately, of an uncertain nature.

The Cost of Public Intervention Programs Designed
to Increase the Energy Intake of Households

While a fairly high level of energy intake may result in
substantial benefits in terms of development, perhaps on the
order of the levels corresponding to moderate activity, we
should not conclude that it is desirable to increase energy
intakes to such high levels through public intervention.
That decision requires knowledge about the marginal cost
function. When considering the cost to the public sector of
augmenting the energy intakes of certain households, it is
useful to be aware that these interventions are affected by:
the opportunity cost of public revenue; the cost of inducing
households to increase their energy intake; and the cost of
administering the intervention.

On at least the first two accounts the marginal cost can
be expected to increase sharply as governments attempt to
satisfy higher energy intake levels for the population. This
is true for several reasons. We will consider first the cost
of inducing households to increase energy intake. The most
straightforward public intervention could take the form of
transfer payments to augment the incomes of low income
households. In this case, a dollar of transfer payments
leads to a dollar of additional income available to the low
income household. Other public intervention programs, such
as subsidized employment schemes or the transfer of subsidized food rations, work in precisely the same way except
that a dollar's worth of the program money may result in
more or less than a dollar of additional income in the recipi-
ent households. In our context, the central determinant of
the induced change in energy intake is the household's
allocation of the dollar received, from the public intervention
program, between more energy intake and other needs.

Figure 3 shows the relative marginal change in income
associated with a one unit increase in energy intake for
households observed at different levels of energy intake in
six separate household surveys. The interpretation is
straightforward. If households allocate only an increasingly
smaller share of additional income to the augmentation of
their energy intake when their per capita intake level rises,
the marginal cost of inducing energy augmentation through
public intervention rises sharply as higher levels of intake
are sought.

Figure 3: Indices of Marginal Cost Per Calorie*

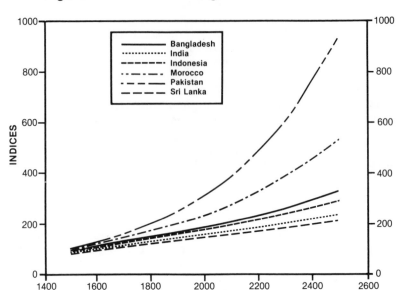

*The semi-log regression equations relating calorie intake to income, and the data sources used in deriving the marginal cost functions in Figure 3 are taken from Knudsen and Scandizzo, 1979. The marginal cost per calorie is the inverse of the marginal propensity to increase energy intake as income rises.

As an illustration, consider a nation in which 5 million people have average daily energy intakes of 1,500 calories, 15 million of 1,600 calories, 20 million of 1,700 calories and the remainder of 1,800 calories and more. Let's further assume that the additional (annual) income required to increase daily energy intake by 100 calories is $10, $15 and $25, respectively, at the level of intake of 1,500, 1,600 and 1,700 calories. If the goal of the public intervention is to assure the entire population a minimum energy intake of 1,600 calories, 5 million people at very low levels of intake would have to get a total cash transfer of 50 million dollars. If the goal were to assure a minimum of 1,700 calories in the population, an additional 15 dollars per capita would have to be provided to the 5 million people with the lowest energy intake as well as to 15 million more people. The additional cost would be 300 million dollars. If a minimum energy intake of 1,800 calories were to be assured, the additional cost would be 1,000 million dollars. Thus the marginal cost of raising minimum energy intakes from 1,700 to 1,800 calories is 20 times the marginal cost of raising minimum intakes from 1,500 to 1,600 calories.

The above calculations are illustrative, but not unrealistic, given what we know about the declining marginal propensities of households, at different levels of energy intake and income, to allocate additional income to energy intake. The marginal cost of public interventions to increase energy intake rises sharply as higher levels of intake are sought, though the marginal cost curve may shift to the right or the left depending on whether a program dollar will deliver more or less than a dollar of income to the target population. If public intervention takes the form of subsidized employment, the cost would be reduced by the extent to which the employment produces positive revenues. Similarly, if instead of money a food is distributed whose cost to the government is less than its worth to the recipients, the marginal cost curve would shift to the left of what it would be if cash were distributed. In the not unlikely case of the government distributing a food which costs more than it is worth to the recipients, the marginal cost curve is shifted to the right.

Clearly, as the size of the program increases, the marginal cost function will be even steeper if we appropriately ascribe rising marginal costs to a dollar used for energy augmentation. In the case of fixed government revenues, a large nutrition program would reduce other high priority public expenditures, whereas a small program could be carried out simply by cutting out some "fat" in other programs. Similarly, taxes can be expected to result in rising marginal costs as they increasingly reduce the incentive to produce and to save.

It is less clear what would happen to political costs and to the marginal cost of administering public intervention programs as increasing levels of energy augmentation are sought. Relevant considerations are economies of scale, the accessibility of different segments of the population to be covered, the type of program, the popular appeal of the interventions, and the portion of the population which is taxed for implementing nutrition interventions.

The Uses of Studies on Activity
Profiles in Groups of Households

In recent years field studies have been conducted to determine the activity profiles of members of households during a typical 24-hour day. The ostensible purpose of these studies usually has been to determine energy requirements more accurately than in the past. These "new" requirements are then substituted for the "old" requirements and it is presumed that the former provide a better estimate of the adequacy of energy levels in existing diets. In my view, studies of activity profiles are potentially useful, but in a different context from the one in which they are currently used.

"Requirements" connote a yardstick by which to measure adequacy. Indeed, if observed activity patterns and observed body weights are judged to be adequate, any discrepancy between energy intakes and the observed requirements (given the observed activity patterns, the relevant energy use coefficients, actual body weights, and the appropriate BMR) are, by definition, only measurement errors in the determinants of the energy requirements and/or intakes. I believe that the proper uses of activity profile studies are to estimate the energy use of the identified activities, and to describe the consequences associated with different levels of energy intake. These are not easily attainable objectives because normally we would encounter an identification problem, i.e., energy intakes could effect the observed intake levels and vice versa. In fact, deliberate experiments may be required whereby "treatments" are assigned at random to the observations in the sample.

I emphasize the importance of performing studies on activity profiles and to analyzing them in the above stated manner because I do not believe that scientists or anyone else should be the final judge of what constitutes adequate energy intakes. To make this determination on the basis of the status quo seems particularly obnoxious. I believe, however, that it is quite appropriate to provide policymakers with some of the information they need (i.e. the particular activity profile, etc. associated with different levels of energy intake) in order to make better informed decisions.

CONCLUDING COMMENTS

I have attempted to draw a brief sketch of how im-proved knowledge about the relationship between energy intake and activity levels fits into the wider concerns of policy-makers and their advisors, as distinct from the pure scientist's interest in the subject. I have explored briefly some theoretical building stones. Public policy intervention presumes an understanding of how groups of households decide to allocate their energy intakes. It has been sug-gested that the final outcome is determined by factors over which the group itself exercises complete sovereignty, i.e. its own preferences for leisure, for work, for present vs. future consumption, for the relative satisfaction they obtain from energy intake/outputs, and other forms of consumption, etc. But the final outcome is also determined by factors in the physical and socio-economic environment over which the group does not exercise control. Public intervention occurs when society is dissatisfied with the levels of energy intake or the levels of energy use observed in some groups of the population, and is prepared to alter them.

Dissatisfaction with privately determined energy input/output levels may arise for several reasons: because present or future national product could be increased by inducing groups to modify their observed energy input/output levels, or because of concern about the welfare of "under-achieving" groups. This distributional concern may be of a non-specific nature, such as dissatisfaction with the level of opportunities or the total level of welfare of groups of households, or with specific aspects of their welfare, such as prevention of disease or excessive mortali-ty, or the ability to work or to be educated.

To predict the relationship between energy intake and energy used in specific activities, it is necessary to know how households behave, not merely their physical input/output coefficients. To determine the most desirable level of energy intake and activity for society, it is necessary to know the shadow prices specific to any given social utility function. To ascertain the social utility function, it is necessary to make normative judgments. This is the realm of philosophy not science.

On the positive side, the disenchantment with using an inflexible requirement concept to judge energy adequacy is a healthy development. Although it is difficult to conceive how even monumental progress in measuring energy input/output relationships could lead to anything like a precise determination of optimal levels of energy intake, such measurements can be helpful in analyzing partial effects on limited objectives. In this context it might be particularly useful to study the entire profile of energy utilization in groups with different levels of energy intake. The studies should take place in circumstances where energy intake levels are not restricted to uses which will be judged privately or socially desirable. In any case, if it is still impossible to state categorically that low levels of energy availability are the binding constraints, we could make the weaker but important statement that increased energy intakes, among other conditions, are necessary for higher levels of functioning.

Finally, while there is a great deal of uncertainty about the marginal benefits of public interventions to augment existing energy intakes, there is a growing body of evidence to support the contention that the marginal cost of public interventions rises sharply with the minimum level of energy intake sought for the population. However, the mere fact that we can measure the costs and know them to be high, and that the benefits are difficult to measure, need not become a justification for laissez-faire. Prescription for social intervention requires knowledge not only of the statistical significance of the evidence, but also Type I and Type II errors and their respective, albeit subjective, social costs. Policy-makers and policy advisors cannot expect to escape making such subjective judgments.

With regard to changing the status quo of energy intake, it is also important to remember that in most cases policy is synonymous with doing something directly about poverty. A supplementary food program, or the availability of foods at subsidized prices, mean that poor households are a little less poor. To what extent they will increase their energy intake, or reduce other deprivations, is primarily their own choice and, for better or for worse, cannot be controlled by governments.

REFERENCES

1. Apfelbaum M, Bostsarron J, and Lacatis D (1971). Effect of caloric restriction and excessive caloric intake on energy expenditure. 24:1405-409.
2. Batliwala S (1982). Rural energy scarcity and nutrition. Econ Pol Wkly 2/27.
3. Beaton G (1982). Some thoughts on the definition of the world nutrition problem. Paper prepared for the Eighth Session of the United Nations Administrative Committee on Coordination--Subcommittee on Nutrition (Bangkok, Thailand).
4. Dandekar VM and Rath N (1971). Poverty in India. Pol Wkly 6:(Nos. 1 and 2) 1/2 and 1/9.
5. Food and Agricultural Organization of the United Nations (1977). "The Fourth World Food Survey, 1977." Rome:FAO.
6. Immink M and Viteri F (1981). Energy intake and productivity of Guatemalan sugarcane cutters, Parts I & II. 9:251-71.
7. Immink M, Viteri F and Helms R (1982). Energy intake over the life cycle and human capital formation in Guatemalan sugarcane cutters. Econ Dev Cult Change 30:351-72.
8. Immink MDC, Viteri FE, Flores R and Torun B (In Press). Microeconomic consequences of energy deficiency in rural populations in developing countries. In Pollit E and Amante P (eds.): "Energy Intake and Activity." New York: Alan R. Liss.
9. Institute of Nutrition of Central America and Panama (1978). The INCAP Longitudinal Study of Malnutrition and Mental Development. Guatemala: INCAP.
10. Isenman P (1980). Basic Needs: The case of Sri Lanka. World Dev 8:237-58.
11. Keys A, Brozek J, Henschel A, Mickelsen O and Taylor HL (1950). "The Biology of Human Starvation." Minneapolis: The University of Minnesota Press.
12. Knudsen O and Scandizzo P (1979). Nutrition and Food Needs in Developing Countries. Staff Working Paper No. 328. Washington, DC: The World Bank.
13. Muller-Schwarze D, Stagge B, and Muller-Schwarze C (1982). Play behavior: Persistence, decrease, and

energetic compensation during food shortage in deer fawns. Science 215:800-12.

14. Reutlinger S and Selowsky M (1976). Malnutrition and Poverty. Occasional Paper, No. 23. Washington, D C: The World Bank.

15. Reutlinger S and Alderman H (1980). The prevalence of calorie-deficient diets in developing countries. World Dev 8:399-411.

16. Viteri F (1975). Nutrition and Work Performance. In "Nutrition and Productivity of Agricultural Laborers," Washington, DC: Pan American Health Organization.

17. Viteri F, Torun B, Immink M, and Flores R (1981). Marginal malnutrition and working capacity. In Harper A E and Davis G K (eds): "Nutrition in Health and Disease and International Development," New York: Alan R Liss.

Energy Intake and Activity, pages 395–403
© 1984 Alan R. Liss, Inc., 150 Fifth Avenue, New York, NY 10011

ADAPTATION TO AND ACCOMMODATION OF LONG TERM
LOW ENERGY INTAKE: A COMMENTARY ON THE
CONFERENCE ON ENERGY INTAKE AND ACTIVITY

George H. Beaton

Department of Nutritional Sciences
Faculty of Medicine, University of Toronto
Toronto, Ontario, Canada

Either our concepts and understanding are wrong or
the data are wrong! That may be the real issue made
apparent by many of the chapters in this publication. When
we try to fit into our physiological and nutritional constructs
some of the more recent observations from populations apparently ingesting chronic low intakes of food, either they do
not fit or they conjure up seemingly impossible situations.
Clearly something is wrong - with the constructs or with the
data - and at present we do not know which. A major
purpose of the conference was to expose some of these
inconsistencies; another was to explore methodologies which
may be applicable to new situations and which could be used
to re-examine and clarify the apparent inconsistencies.
Activity was also an important issue - both as a key component of the energy balance equation and as the almost certain intervening variable in the relationship between intake
and many human functions.

The chapter by Prentice (this volume) is one of several
that could serve as examples of the inconsistency of current
data and existing constructs. In their studies of pregnant
and lactating women in the Gambia, Prentice and colleagues
measured food intake at various stages of pregnancy and
during lactation. They also recorded anthropometric changes
in the women and in the infants after birth. From these
data it is possible to construct hypothetical 12 month intake
estimates (note that in doing this, cross sectional data are
being combined without taking into full account the effect of
seasons). It would appear that these women ingested

approximately 1485 kcal/day during pregnancy and 1615 kcal/day during lactation. Over the twelve month cycle of pregnancy and the first three months of lactation, this amounts to an average of 1520 kcal/day. Use of the 12 month cycle is convenient because, although birth weight differed with season of the year, there was compensatory increase in initial growth rate. As a result, by three months of age there was no seasonal weight difference. The women appear to have accommodated the seasonal changes in food intake and other factors. It was reported also (Prentice 1981, and this volume) that this population showed no clear evidence of a progressive loss of maternal weight with increasing parity. The implication is that a long term stable equilibrium exists between this population and its level of food intake - a "successful" adaptation.

Let us compare this observation with current constructs of the physiology of pregnancy and lactation and implied energy needs. A data base currently being developed on behalf of the UNU Committee on Energy and Protein Require-ments provides regression equations for the prediction of BMR from age, sex, weight, and height. Applying the equation for young adult women to average nonpregnant Gambian women, weight 52.7 kg and height 157.4 cm, the predicted BMR is approximately 1265 kcal/day. Schofield (1983) noted that for a set of Indian data the reported BMR's were about 10% lower than predicted. By comparison, the Gambian mean BMR might be in the order of 1140 kcal/day, or 90% of the expected figure.

Thompson and Hytten (cited in Hytten and Leitch 1971) developed estimates of the additional energy costs of preg-nancy. In keeping with suggestions in that source, tissue gains may be prorated in proportion to mean birth weight of Gambian infants (2900 g rather than 3400 g). The calcula-tion is displayed in Table 1. In these calculations, the energy costs of deposition of tissues were based on the estimates of Keilanowski as presented in the FAO/WHO 1973 report on Energy and Protein Requirements. The changes in tissue metabolism and heart work, etc., associated with increased oxygen consumption, reported are those by Hytten and Leitch (1971). This may represent a source of error in the modeling. It is not clear whether a part of the cost of tissue deposition is already included in the in vitro measures of oxygen consumption by those tissues, nor is it clear whether the "waste heat" generated as a by-product of tissue synthesis decreases the need for heat production (designed inefficiency of conversions) for thermogenesis. Table 1 suggests that the theoretical net increase in BMR is in the order of 10% of the predicted low estimate of nonpregnant BMR; any error of modeling associated with the above argument should fall within this 10% or 115 kcal/d. This possibility can ignored and the net costs taken as 1140 + 160 = 1300 kcal/d, or about 1415 kcal/d, if one assumes the same 10% inefficiency of digestion and absorption of food energy for the BMR component as for the additional costs portrayed in Table 1. If the higher BMR estimate is accepted, the total cost estimate rises to about 1550 kcal/d. All of these estimates are exclusive of any change in maternal adipose tissue. In summary, then, the lowest estimate of energy cost during pregnancy, assuming 100% efficiency of digestion and absorption, would be approximately 1280 kcal/d; assuming a 90% efficiency of food energy absorption and the higher nonpregnant BMR estimate, the average need could be as high as 1565 kcal/d.

Table 1

Estimation of Net Cost of a Pregnancy Resulting in a 2900 g Infant
Exclusive of Adipose Tissue Change

Tissue Deposited	Weight*	Food Energy Equivalent	Cost of Deposition	Total Cost**	Net Cost per Day
	g	kcal/g	kcal/g	kcal	kcal/d
Protein	790	4.0	13.0***	13430	
					70
Fat	480	9.0	4.3***	6385	
Net Increase in Tissue Respiration				24600***	90
		Net Cost/Day Averaged Over Total Pregnancy			160

* Weight of tissues deposited is prorated to a birth weight of 2900 g and excludes any change in maternal adipose tissue

** The net change in BMR would be the sum of these after deducting the allowance for inefficiency of absorption (10%) and the energy equivalent of the tissues deposited (7500 kcal). In this model, the expected net change in BMR would be 32,500 kcal or about 115 kcal/d

*** Theoretical estimates of costs have been increased by 10% to allow for inefficiency of digestion and absorption of dietary energy; actual efficiency is not known.

For lactation, Prentice (1981) and coworkers present actual estimates of milk secretion based upon 12 hour test weighing. These are adjusted to 24 hr secretions by regression equations. Energy equivalents were based upon measured proximate composition. For the first three months of lactation the estimated energy secretions were 450 kcal/d and 440 kcal/d in the dry and wet seasons. These are quite conservative estimates compared with those presented for industrialized countries in support of apparently similar infant growth rates. Prentice and associates assumed 80% efficiency of breast milk secretion yielding an average dietary energy net cost of about 560 kcal/d. If an efficiency of 100% could be assumed for digestion and absorption of dietary energy, this figure might fall to about 500 kcal/d. Assuming the low estimate of BMR and 100% efficiency of absorption, the average energy requirement during the first three months of lactation (exclusive of adipose tissue changes) would be about 1640 kcal/d; assuming a 90% efficiency of absorption and the higher BMR estimate, the average energy requirement could be as high as 1965 kcal/d.

Using these figures, the estimates of average energy requirement across the whole of pregnancy and the first three months of lactation would range from a low of 1370 kcal/d to a high of 1665 kcal/d. These estimates apply regardless of the pattern of adipose tissue deposition and withdrawal, as long as there is no net change in adipose tissue across the whole of the 12 months. The low estimate assumes 100% efficiency of food digestion and absorption and a BMR that is 10% lower than that characteristic of women in industrialized countries. The high estimate assumes 90% efficiency of absorption and a nonpregnant BMR equivalent to that seen in industrialized countries.

If we compare these figures to the reported average food intake of Gambian women during pregnancy and the first three months of lactation, 1520 kcal/d, we find that this is only 150 kcal/d above the low requirement estimate and is some 145 kcal/d below the higher requirement estimate! Neither of the requirement estimates make any provision for physical activity; they are based upon BMR and expected costs of tissue deposition or milk secretion only. Obviously, the women are not physically inactive.

We then have the impossible situation. Either the food intake estimates must be wrong or our current concepts of physiology of energy requirements must be wrong. Either way, the data seem to suggest that activity expenditure of energy must be very low - that to make sense, there must be a major element of behavioral accommodation to establish energy equilibria across this 12 month cycle of pregnancy and lactation. Against this we have the observation that in the face of what appears to be very low energy intake, women in this setting seem to be capable of producing infants of somewhat lower birth weight and of nursing them at a level which supports generally accepted growth rates. Furthermore, in this setting the population of women seem to be able to accommodate seasonal changes without apparent impact on the weight of the three month old infant. This is cited as clear evidence of "adaptation" or "accommodation" to chronic low energy intake. The calculations presented above do not offer any clear basis for assuming that improvements in the efficiency of food absorption or of metabolism are a likely explanation. How then does this operate (Beaton 1983)?

Here I enter the realm of speculation, but I suggest that one element of the energy balance equation may have been ignored too long and may have considerable importance in the context of this publication. If, as has been argued, these women live in agrarian setting and contribute to the agricultural and other "economic" activities of the household, and if these activities are maintained during pregnancy and lactation, then it is at least possible that another class of physical activity is altered as a compensatory accommodation mechanism. This has been given different names, but for the present purpose might be termed "discretionary activity." In point of fact it is the range of activities that are seldom measured in studies of economic productivity - what people do outside of their "working" time. This perspective is portrayed diagrammatically in Figure 1. The point to be made should be obvious. Once we portray the energy balance equation in this manner, we begin to see that physiological perspectives and human functions, including social functions and psychosocial development, merge in an inseparable way. When we talk about "adaptation" or "accommodation" to low energy intake are we addressing the question in physiological terms or are we addressing it in behavioral terms?

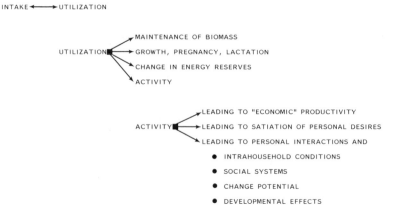

INTAKE ◄───► UTILIZATION

UTILIZATION ■
- MAINTENANCE OF BIOMASS
- GROWTH, PREGNANCY, LACTATION
- CHANGE IN ENERGY RESERVES
- ACTIVITY

ACTIVITY ■
- LEADING TO "ECONOMIC" PRODUCTIVITY
- LEADING TO SATIATION OF PERSONAL DESIRES
- LEADING TO PERSONAL INTERACTIONS AND
  - INTRAHOUSEHOLD CONDITIONS
  - SOCIAL SYSTEMS
  - CHANGE POTENTIAL
  - DEVELOPMENTAL EFFECTS

FIGURE 1

A Perspective of Components of Energy Utilization

In the closing passage of his chapter, Dr. Prentice makes the underlying point. After concluding that "people in developing countries are more efficient than those in developed countries" he suggests that "although it may be possible to survive on much lower intakes than considered possible hitherto, such dietary conditions are almost certainly not compatible with optimum quality of life." In describing the results of supplementation trials in these women, Whitehead, a collaborator in these studies, reported that although there were no clear markers of physiological effects, "in the Gambia the unanimous first reason given by pregnant and lactating mothers for the popularity of the supplement was that it gave them more 'power' for work (Whitehead, 1983, p. 95). Whitehead (personal communication) also reported that when lactating women were given supplements, they sang while they worked. Perhaps we should see in these anecdotal remarks, and in many similar anecdotal reports from other studies, clues to affective behavioral changes.

The final point to be made is relatively simple to state but very difficult to accomplish. With energy, much more than with nutrients, we must recognize that both physiological and socio-psychological aspects of human behavior are

WE KNOW THAT ENERGY EQUILIBRIUM
CAN BE ESTABLISHED AT
DIFFERENT LEVELS OF EXPENDITURE

AS PHYSIOLOGISTS AND BIOLOGISTS, WE CAN ASK
- HOW
- WITH WHAT LEVELS OF PRIORITY FOR THE DIFFERENT COMPONENTS OF EXPENDITURE (WHAT DEMAND FUNCTIONS, WHAT ELAS-TICITIES OF ENERGY EXPENDITURE)
- WITH WHAT DIRECT BIOLOGICAL SEQUELAE

AS SOCIAL SCIENTISTS, WE CAN ASK
- WHAT ACTIVITIES ARE AFFECTED
- WHAT ARE THE EFFECTS OF THESE CHANGES ON PSYCHOSOCIAL PARAMETERS IN THE INDIVIDUAL, THE HOUSEHOLD AND THE COMMUNITY
- WHAT ARE THE POTENTIALS FOR, AND COSTS OF, CHANGING INTAKE

TOGETHER WE CAN ASK
- IS THERE A HUMAN COST ASSOCIATED WITH ESTABLISHING ENERGY EQUILIBRIUM AT A LOW LEVEL (THE APPARENT STATUS QUO SITUATION OF POPULATIONS IN DEVELOPING COUNTRIES)
- WHAT HUMAN FUNCTIONAL BENEFITS, IN WHAT ORDER, MIGHT WE REASONABLY EXPECT AS WE RELEASE EXISTING CONSTRAINTS ON FOOD INTAKE
- WHAT ARE THE EXISTING CONSTRAINTS ON FOOD INTAKE AND HOW MIGHT THEY BE RELIEVED
- WHAT MIGHT IT COST

WILL WE ACCEPT THE CHALLENGE OF THE JOINT APPROACH?

Figure 2
Some Questions to be Addressed

involved. We have known for many years that in physiological terms human populations can accommodate to low intakes of food. The realization is now emerging that this knowledge leads to a series of questions and that the questions are different for biological scientists and for social scientists (Figure 2). Even more important, there is a growing realization that many of the important questions must be phrased and addressed by biological and social scientists working together. The conference from which this book resulted was symptomatic of the recognition of the need to bridge these fields and of the realization that when we discuss energy and activity, the fields become inseparable (or that the separation is artificial). Ultimately the question that must be addressed is "What are the human costs of accommodations to low energy intakes?" That is the all-important policy question. I suggest that it is no longer sufficient to measure it in terms of conventional biological parameters of birth weight, morbidity, and mortality. We must consider also psycho-social effects if, indeed, we truly believe that we should be interested in the potential for human development rather than mere survival. I suggest that such an approach will require an increased degree of interaction of biological science and social science approaches. That is the challenge that characterizes this publication.

REFERENCES

1. Beaton GH (1983). W.O. Atwater Memorial Lecture. Energy in human nutrition: Perspectives and problems. Nutr Revs 41(11):325-340.
2. Prentice AM (1984). Adaptations to long-term low energy intake. In Pollitt E and Amante P (eds.): "Energy Intake and Activity," New York: Alan R Liss, Inc. (In press)
3. Prentice AM, Whitehead RG, Roberts SB, and Paul AA (1981). Long term energy balance in child-bearing Gambian women. Am J Clin Nutr 34:2790-2799.
4. Schofield, WN (1983). The computation of Equations to Estimate Basal Metabolic Rate from Age, Sex, Height and Weight. Unpublished Report.
5. Hytten RE and Leitch I (1971). "The Physiology of Human Pregnancy, Second Edition," London: Blackwell Scientific Publications.

6. FAO/WHO Joint Ad Hoc Expert Committee on Energy and Protein Requirements (1973). WHO Tech Rept Ser No. 52.
7. Whitehead RG (ed.) (1983). Maternal Diet, Breast Feeding Capacity and Lactational Infertility. UNU Food and Nutrition Bulletin, Supplement 6.
8. Whitehead RG. Personal communication.

Index

Absorption of dietary energy, increased efficiency of, as energy sparing mechanism, 22–23

Accelerometers, physical activity measurement in free-living children with, 176

Active tissue mass, energy conservation and, 17–18

Activity diary, energy expenditure measurement and, 106, 124, 135–136

Activity meters, energy expenditure measurement and, 124

Activity recall, energy expenditure measurement and, 124

Actometer, physical activity measurement in children with, 175, 194–196

Adaptation to low energy intake
basal metabolic rate and, 101
cultural and genetic components of, 304
evolution vs. adaptation and, 23–24
limits of homeostasis and, 73
policy-making implications of, 395–402
potential energy sparing mechanisms of, 15–24
in pregnant and lactating women, 3–25, 33–53
quality of life and, 24–25
stature and, 17
See also Autoregulation of energy balance; Energy sparing mechanisms

Adaptive thermogenesis, defined, 116

Adiposity, nutritional status and, 224

Aerobic power. *See* Maximum oxygen output and uptake

Affective-cognitive development, in motorically-impaired children, 347–349

Agricultural activities
energy costs of, 139–152, 207–208, 215–218
physical activity measurement in, 133–136
See also Agricultural productivity

Agricultural productivity, physical activity, nutritional status, and physical work capacity related to, 207–251
See also Productivity

Anabolism, sleep in malnourished infants and, 325–326

Anthropometric measurements
changes in pregnancy and lactation, 44–50
energy balance measurement and, 106
in Guatemalan productivity study, 364–365
in marginally malnourished school-age girls, 267–269
motor development and, 295

Appetite, regulation of energy balance and, 60

Ascorbic acid, physical work capacity and, 223–224

ATP synthesis, non-shivering thermogenesis and, 19

Autoregulation of energy balance, 57–74
historic background, 57–59
homeostatic nature of, 62–71

E